4TH EDITION

medically important fungi
A GUIDE TO IDENTIFICATION

4TH EDITION

medically important fungi

A GUIDE TO IDENTIFICATION

Davise H. Larone

MT(ASCP), Ph.D., F(AAM)
Diplomate, American Board of Medical Microbiology

Associate Professor
Department of Pathology and
Department of Microbiology and Immunology
Weill Medical College of Cornell University

Director of Clinical Microbiology
Cornell Medical Center, New York-Presbyterian Hospital
New York, New York

Illustrated by the Author

ASM
PRESS

Washington, D.C.

Copyright © 1976, 1987, 1995, 2002
ASM Press
American Society for Microbiology
1752 N Street, N.W.
Washington, DC 20036-2904

Library of Congress Cataloging-in-Publication Data

Larone, Davise Honig, 1939–
    Medically important fungi / Davise H. Larone; illustrated by the author.— 4th ed.
        p.; cm.
    Includes bibliographical references and index.
    ISBN 1-55581-172-8
    1. Pathogenic fungi—Identification. 2. Fungi—Cultures and culture media.
    3. Medical mycology. I. Title.
        [DNLM: 1. Fungi—pathogenicity—Laboratory Manuals. 2. Fungi—cytology—
    Laboratory Manuals. 3. Mycology—Laboratory Manuals. QW 25
    L331m 2002]
    QR245 .L37 2002
    616′.015—dc21

                                                                          2002018279

Current printing (last digit)
10 9 8 7 6 5 4 3 2 1

Address editorial correspondence to: ASM Press, 1752 N St., N.W., Washington, DC
20036-2904, U.S.A.

Send orders to: ASM Press, P.O. Box 605, Herndon, VA 20172, U.S.A.
Phone: 800-546-2416; 703-661-1593
Fax: 703-661-1501
Email: books@asmusa.org
Online: www.asmpress.org

Dedicated with love
to
Ronit
Gary
Jessie
Beth
and, with loving memory,
to John D. Lawrence

Contents

PART I Direct Microscopic Examination of Clinical Specimens

PART II Identification of Fungi in Culture

PART III Laboratory Technique

Preface to the Fourth Edition

The constant increase of fungal infections in humans, the seemingly neverending occurrence of fungi that were not previously encountered as opportunistic pathogens, and my unremitting desire to continuously improve and expand the contents of this book constituted the impetus for this 4th edition. Also, as medical technology programs become more scarce, and clinical laboratory personnel receive less formal training in mycology, it is all the more important to have an up-to-date bench-side guide and teaching aid for the identification of clinically encountered fungi.

This edition varies from the previous one in several distinct ways.

- By popular demand, the book is now hardcover with a sewn binding. This was by far the most common change requested whenever I asked readers for suggestions for future editions. Although it will probably diminish sales (i.e., replacement issues for those that fell apart will no longer be purchased!), it is hoped that this binding will withstand the heavy usage to which it is routinely subjected in the laboratory and that it will serve the users well.

- The section on direct microscopic examination of specimens has been greatly expanded in an effort to more completely instruct and assist in the reading and interpretation of tissue sections as well as direct smears. Histological terminology, tissue reactions to fungal infections, and stains employed are covered in a relatively elementary manner designed for microbiologists or students of pathology. A guide based on drawings and brief descriptions of the fungi leads the user to pages of detailed descriptions of each mycosis; for each disease this segment provides delineation of the etiologic agent(s), the typical sites of infection, the usual tissue reactions, and the microscopic morphology of the organism as seen on direct examination of specimens, along with a line drawing and a photomicrograph. Subsequently, a presumptive, or in some cases a quite definitive, identification may be reached.

- Seven organisms have been added to the section of Part II that provides detailed descriptions of fungi on culture. Ten additional tables have also been included to display more clearly the differential characteristics of organisms that are similar to one another. Major among the new tables are those (i) providing the characteristics that assist in differentiating *Candida dubliniensis* from *Candida albicans* and discussing the caveats that must be considered with each of the tests involved (Table 5); (ii) covering the fungi in which arthroconidia predominate (Table 21); (iii) delineating the differences between the organisms that are suggestive of, but unique from, *Phialophora* and *Acremonium* (Table 13); and (iv) defining the differences between *Chrysosporium* and *Sporotrichum,* two genera that have in the past been confused with one another and commonly misidentified (Table 25).
- All guides, descriptions of organisms, and laboratory techniques have been updated, and some have been expanded, as have the suggestions of sources for further information. Many of the standard texts suggested in previous editions remain, but the reader will notice the repeated citation of two recently published books that can be extremely helpful, i.e., *Atlas of Clinical Fungi,* 2nd edition, by de Hoog et al., and *Laboratory Handbook of Dermatophytes* by Kane et al. I highly recommend them as additions to any clinical mycology laboratory's library of reference books to be used in concert with this Guide.
- A section of color plates has been added to exhibit the colony morphology of selected fungi and to demonstrate microscopic images and test reactions that require color for meaningful visualization and interpretation.

As this edition goes to press, I am already considering the next. My intent has always been to provide relevant, reliable, and practical information in an easy-to-understand manner and, in so doing, to make mycology a rewarding and enjoyable experience for those involved in it. The ultimate goal would then be achieved, i.e., heightened assurance of rapid and accurate results for the clinicians and their patients. These objectives can best be reached and maintained by my receiving forthright feedback from the users. All comments, suggestions, or requests aimed at fulfilling the needs of the readership and making this Guide the best and most useful that it can possibly be will be most greatly and sincerely appreciated.

New York City
January 2002

Preface to the First Edition

More than ever, clinical laboratory personnel with limited experience in mycology must culture and identify fungi isolated from clinical specimens. Even after attending a course in the subject, technologists often need guidance in identifying the great variety of organisms encountered in the lab. With the advent of proficiency testing by local and national organizations, technologists have a need and opportunity to practice and increase their skills in the medical mycology laboratory.

Most classic texts, though rich in information, are arranged according to the clinical description of the infection; the textual discussion of any particular fungus can be located only from the index or table of contents. Since the technologist doesn't know the name of an unidentified fungus and usually has little or no knowledge of the clinical picture, these texts are at best difficult to use effectively. The unfortunate result is the all-too-common practice of flipping through an entire mycology textbook in search of a picture that resembles the organism under examination. Such a practice may make the more accomplished mycologist's hair stand on end, but it is a fact to be acknowledged.

This guide is not meant to compete with these large texts, but to complement them. The material here is so arranged that the technologist can systematically reach a possible identification knowing only the macro- and microscopic morphology of an isolated organism. Reference can then be made to one of the classic texts for confirmation and detailed information.

Many possible variants of organisms are found under several categories of morphology and pigment. The outstanding characteristics are listed on the page(s) apportioned to each organism, and references are suggested for further information and confirmation (see How To Use the Guide).

Medically Important Fungi avoids the jargon so commonly and confusingly used in most mycology books. Drawings are used wherever possible to illustrate organisms described in the text. To ensure clarity, a glossary of terms is included, as well as a section on laboratory techniques for observing proper morphology. Another section includes use of the various media, stains, and tests mentioned in the book.

The actinomycetes, although now known to be bacteria rather than fungi, are included because they are frequently handled in the mycology section of the clinical laboratory.

It is believed that this guide will enable students and medical technologists to culture and identify fungi with greater ease and competency and in so doing to develop an appreciation of the truly beautiful microscopic forms encountered.

I wish to acknowledge with gratitude the encouragement and advice received from my co-workers at Lenox Hill Hospital, and Dr. Norman Goodman, Mr. Gerald Krefetz, Mr. Bill Rosenzweig, Ms. Eve Rothenberg, Dr. Guenther Stotzky, Mr. Martin Weisburd, Dr. Irene Weitzman, and Dr. Marion E. Wilson.

New York
December 1975

Acknowledgments

A publication of this sort can never be accomplished without the assistance of a number of people. For their generous new contributions of isolates, photomicrographs, or wise counsel to this edition, I would like to thank Jim Harris, Evelyn Koestenblatt, Bill Merz, Ron Neafie, Ann Nelson, Jean Pollack, Tomas Roges, Stanley Rosenthal, Ira Salkin, Wiley Schell, Lynne Sigler, Jim Snyder, and Alice Weissfeld. My gratitude is also everlastingly extended to the many colleagues who assisted during the preparation of previous editions; most of their contributions are now substantive and integral parts of the ongoing Guide.

Joan Barenfanger and Sara Peters are invaluable contributors to the enhanced section on direct microscopic examination (Part I). It was their knowledge of histology and anatomic pathology, in concert with their enthusiastic assistance through tutoring, writing, reviewing, and supplying slides and photomicrographs, that enabled me to fulfill the vision I had of it. Doug Flieder deserves special recognition for so willingly coming to my rescue by providing additional pathology slides and photomicrographs that I needed for completion of the section. Thanks also goes to the pathology residents Sun Mi Chung, Timothy Hilbert, and Erika Resetkova for reviewing that portion of the manuscript and making some very worthwhile suggestions.

The cultures for color photographs and many of the slides for photomicrographs were prepared in the Clinical Microbiology Laboratory of Weill Cornell Medical Center by Nadine Butler, Benjamin See, and Riva Zinchuk. I owe a debt of gratitude to them as well as to Betty Panik, manager of our laboratory, and to the other members of my staff who were extremely patient and supportive during the writing of this edition.

The improvement in the black and white photomicrographs and the high quality of the newly added color photographs are due to the talent and dedication of Alan Arellano, Pat Kuharic, and Aaron Cormier of the Medical Art, Photogaphy, and Digital Imaging Department of Weill Medical College of Cornell University. Their talent, cooperativeness, and commitment to perfection are unparalleled and deserving of the highest esteem.

Last, but definitely not least, my gratitude goes to the marvelous staff and associates of the ASM Press with whom I worked during the creation of this edition: Jeff Holtmeier, Director; Ellie Tupper, Senior Production Editor; Elizabeth McGillicuddy, copyeditor; and Susan Schmidler, book designer. They have been extraordinarily wise, helpful, creative, diligent, flexible, and dedicated partners in this publication.

How To Use the Guide

Before beginning to use the guide, the reader should understand several points.

Fungi often appear different in living hosts than they do in cultures. Part I (pp. 9–63) is designed as a guide for preliminary identification of fungi seen on direct microscopic examination of clinical specimens.

In Part II (pp. 65–289), the descriptions of the macroscopic and microscopic morphologies of the cultured fungi pertain to those on Sabouraud dextrose agar unless otherwise specified.

Many moulds begin as white mycelial growths, and coloration occurs at the time of conidiation or sporulation. Hence, organisms are listed under their most likely color(s) at maturity, when the typical microscopic reproductive formations are more readily observed.

This book is a *guide to identification*. The standard texts should be used for additional information concerning clinical disease, history, ecology, immunology, and therapy.

Instructions for general procedures prior to identification, i.e., collection of specimens, direct microscopic preparations, primary isolation, slide cultures, special tests, and the like, are given in Part III (pp. 291–349). Staining methods are described on pp. 313–323; the preparation and use of media are explained on pp. 325–349.

Once the organism has been properly collected, cultured, isolated, and observed microscopically, use of the guide is quite simple.

1. Note the morphology of the unknown fungus.
   a. Is it a filamentous bacterium, yeastlike, thermally dimorphic, or a thermally monomorphic mould?
   b. Record color of surface and reverse (underside) of colony.

1

2. Using the initial "Guide to Identification of Fungi in Culture" on pp. 67–96, refer to a page that shows drawings of the microscopic morphologies of organisms having the appropriate macroscopic appearance. Here one may see either the exact organism under examination or several possibilities.

3. Proceed to the page written in parentheses next to the likely organism(s) and find more detailed information, including pathogenicity, rate of growth, colony morphology, an enlarged drawing of the microscopic appearance, a photomicrograph, and references for additional information. Where applicable, there will be indications of tables and color plates* and discussions of tests or characteristics that may help to differentiate extremely similar organisms.

4. Ordinarily, the identification will be quite certain. If, however, any doubt remains, the organism should be sent to a reference laboratory for confirmation of identification as discussed in the following section.

* The color plates are found on pp. 351–378.

Use of Reference Laboratories

Rare or atypical fungi can be difficult to identify even for a very experienced microbiologist or medical technologist. After a possible identification of an isolated organism is reached, confirmation is often necessary.

When the identification of an isolated fungus is dubious or when the fungus appears to be one that the laboratory worker has never before encountered, a reliable reference laboratory should be asked to confirm the identification. Because of the toxicity of antifungal medications, it is especially important to confirm the identification of organisms suspected of causing systemic mycoses. Ordinarily, the state health department acts as a reference laboratory; otherwise, a reputable commercial laboratory of proven competency should be chosen to provide the service.

Cultures sent to reference laboratories should be pure, young, and actively growing on agar slants. Petri plates should not be used. For details on the labeling, mailing, and delivering of potentially pathogenic isolates, one should consult the reference laboratory for specific requirements and comply with the shipping codes.

At the time of writing, the U.S. Department of Transportation and the International Air Transport Association (IATA) are revising their requirements for packaging and shipment of etiologic agents and infectious substances. It is expected that the rules will be somewhat changed; the following guidelines include notations on some of the possibilities.

1. The tube containing the slanted culture must be labeled with the organism identification (in general terms if the identification

is unknown) and must be securely closed and watertight (waterproof tape seal may be required). The culture tube is considered the primary container.

2. Place enough packing and absorbent material at the top, bottom, and sides of the culture tube to prevent breakage and to absorb the entire volume of the culture in case of leakage (this material may be more specifically defined). If more than one tube is being transported, each one must be wrapped individually to ensure that contact between them, and consequent breakage, is prevented.

3. Insert the wrapped culture tube(s) into a secondary durable, watertight container (it must be made of material that is certified for ability to withstand an increased amount of pressure if it is to be shipped by air). Although several culture tubes may be placed in a single secondary container, the total contents cannot exceed 50 ml (if the volume exceeds 50 ml, shock-absorbent material must be placed between the secondary container and the outer shipping container).

4. Place the secondary container(s) in an outer shipping container constructed of cardboard, metal, or other material of equivalent strength (an itemized list of the contents must be enclosed between the secondary and outer containers).

5. Affix the address label to the outer shipping container (the return address should contain the sender's telephone number); include an official "Etiologic Agent" label, which is available from the Centers for Disease Control and Prevention (CDC) and label manufacturers.

6. If the organism being transported is suspected of being *Coccidioides immitis* or *Histoplasma capsulatum,* it must be shipped in a manner that provides for sending notification of receipt back to the sender. If receipt is not confirmed within 5 days following the anticipated delivery date, the sender must notify the CDC.

As of 1 June 2001, new IATA rules concerning the Shipper's Declaration of Dangerous Goods went into effect. Federal Express is requiring compliance. The rule requires that the Shipper's Declaration of Dangerous Goods be *either typewritten or computer generated.* The form must have the red-and-white "candy stripe" border. At least one manufacturer of packaging materials provides online software to generate the form (http://www.saftpak.com/fx12.htm); others may also supply this service.

For updates on the regulations, consult the following websites.

1. Centers for Disease Control and Prevention
   http://www.cdc.gov/od/ohs/biosfty/shipdir.htm
   http://www.cdc.gov/od/ohs/biosfty/shipregs.htm

2. U.S. Department of Transportation
   http://hazmat.dot.gov (follow the path: Rules and Regulations → Hazardous Materials Regulations → 49 CFR Regulations → Part 173 → Subpart E → 173.196)

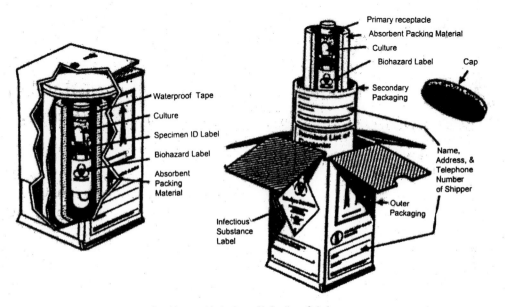

Waterproof Tape

Culture

Specimen ID Label

Biohazard Label

Absorbent Packing Material

Primary receptacle

Absorbent Packing Material

Culture

Biohazard Label

Cap

Secondary Packaging

Name, Address, & Telephone Number of Shipper

Infectious Substance Label

Outer Packaging

Packing and Labeling of Infectious Substances

Safety Precautions

Since many fungi produce conidia or spores that easily become airborne, precautions are essential to prevent contamination of the laboratory environment and infection of personnel.

- A suitable biological safety cabinet (class 1 or 2) should be used when dealing with moulds. Yeast cultures can be handled on the bench in the same manner that bacterial cultures are routinely handled.

- Care must be taken not to spatter infectious material by careless flaming of wire needles or loops. Benchtop microbiology incinerators are recommended to avoid this hazard. Sterile disposable implements may provide the best solution by eliminating the need to flame.

- Tubed slants of media are safer to handle than plates. If plates are used, shrink seals should be employed. Petri plates should NEVER be used if *Coccidioides immitis* is suspected or if a culture is to be mailed or otherwise transported to another laboratory.

- A wet preparation should be made of all moulds before setting up a slide culture; do NOT set up slide cultures of isolates that may be *Histoplasma, Blastomyces, Coccidioides,* or *Paracoccidioides* spp. or *Cladophialophora bantiana.*

- Supernatants should be decanted into containers of disinfectant.

- All contaminated materials must be autoclaved before being discarded.

- Personnel must wash their hands thoroughly with a disinfectant soap after handling mycology cultures.

- The work area must be cleaned with disinfectant at least daily.

- Laboratory coats must be worn at all times in the work area.
- Mouth pipetting must NOT be done.
- There can be no smoking, drinking, eating, gum chewing, application of cosmetics, or insertion of contact lenses in the laboratory.
- A fungal culture must NEVER be sniffed to determine whether it has an odor.

PART I Direct Microscopic Examination of Clinical Specimens

Written with the assistance of:
Joan Barenfanger, M.D., Ph.D., Department of Pathology, Memorial Medical Center, Springfield, Ill.
and
Sara B. Peters, Ph.D., M.D., Department of Pathology, New York Weill Cornell Medical Center, New York, N.Y.

Introduction

Specimens submitted to the mycology laboratory from skin, tissue, or normally sterile body fluids, as well as any specimen from a patient strongly suspected of having a fungal infection, should be examined microscopically for the presence of fungal elements. This examination is important for several reasons.

- It may provide the physician with a rapid diagnosis and information regarding the possible need for treatment.
- It is helpful in determining the significance of an organism that may later be definitively identified on culture. If the cultured organism is one that is only sometimes pathogenic and it is seen on direct microscopic examination in appreciable numbers, it is more likely to be involved in a disease process and not merely present as a contaminant. Also, in cases of suspected candidiasis, pseudohyphae invading tissue indicate infection as opposed to colonization.
- Observation of unique fungal elements may indicate the need for special media, additional specimens from other sites, and/or serological tests.
- All too often, tissue sections are submitted to the anatomic pathology laboratory in fixative, rendering the specimens unsuitable for culture. In these situations, the direct microscopic examination of the tissue plays the principal role in diagnosis.
- Some organisms do not grow in vitro, rendering direct microscopic examination the only method of detection and identification.

It is not uncommon for microbiologists to be requested to examine tissue sections from the anatomic pathology laboratory when fungal infection is suspected or apparent. To attain an acceptable level of comfort and expertise in this responsibility, it is imperative to have at least a cursory knowledge of tissue reactions to mycoses. To familiarize the microbiologist with the histologic responses to fungal infection, the following pages present definitions of pertinent terms, descriptions of the various tissue reactions, and a discussion and table of the stains employed.

The Guide to Interpretation of Direct Microscopic Examination is intended for use as a quick guide in reading direct smears as well as tissue sections. It is intended to allow rapid comparative viewing of the possible interpretations of the structures in the specimen and to direct the reader to the appropriate pages for more detailed descriptions of the direct microscopic appearance of each of the mycoses.

The detailed description of each mycosis includes (i) the etiologic agent(s), (ii) the likely anatomic site(s) of infection, (iii) the tissue reactions most commonly produced, (iv) the microscopic morphology of the implicated organism, and (v) a line drawing and photomicrograph of the organism on direct microscopic examination. In some cases, the direct microscopic examination yields a relatively certain identification of the organism (yet presumptive, to be confirmed by culture); in many other instances, culture is the only means of identification. **Every effort should be made to train physicians to submit specimens for culture whenever an infectious process is in the differential diagnosis.** The most beneficial specimens are obviously obtained prior to initiation of antimicrobial therapy.

Characteristics of various stains are summarized in Table 1, p. 22. Methods for direct microscopic examination of specimens are outlined in Part III, pp. 293–312. Staining methods are described in Part III, pp. 313–324.

For further information and excellent photomicrographs of fungi in tissue, see
  Chandler and Watts, 1987
  Connor et al., 1997

Histological Terminology

Abscess   Localized collection of suppurative inflammatory cells (poly-morphonuclear neutrophils). In some instances, neutrophils and necrotic tissue are surrounded by a zone of granulation tissue. In time, the abscess may become walled off by connective tissue that limits further spread. (Color Plate 1.)

Acanthosis   Increase in the thickness of the epidermis.

Calcification   Deposition of calcium in tissue; with H&E, calcium stains as an amorphous purple deposit. (Color Plates 14 and 15.)

Caseous necrosis   Histologically, amorphous, granular debris of frag-mented, coagulated cells (Color Plates 12 and 13); on gross examination, it is white to yellowish or grayish and has a "cottage cheese" consistency.

Collagen   Structural fibrous protein that provides support; collagen first appears as pink fibrils (with H&E) in early wound healing; later coalesces into dense organized bands in mature scars. (Color Plate 7.)

Connective tissue   Tissue that binds together and supports various struc-tures of the body. It is made up of fibroblasts, collagen, elastin, blood ves-sels, etc.

Cyst   Cavity or sac lined by epithelial cells; it usually contains liquid or semisolid material.

Dermis   Broad, dense connective tissue layer of the skin located under the epidermis. (Color Plate 19.)

Eosinophil   A white blood cell containing a bilobulated nucleus and eosinophilic cytoplasmic granules. It is an acute inflammatory cell. (Color Plate 4.)

Eosinophilic   Easily stained with eosin dyes; eosinophilic structures stain deep pink with H&E stain.

13

Epidermis   The outer, thinner layer of the skin; it consists of layers of stratified squamous epithelium. (Color Plate 19.)

Epithelioid cell   A cell having characteristics resembling those of an epithelial cell; usually derived from a macrophage. A relatively large polygonal or elongated cell with a pale nucleus, pale pink granular cytoplasm (H&E stain), and indistinct cell boundaries. The ratio of the size of the nucleus to total cell size is approximately 1:4. (Color Plate 5.)

Fibroblast   An elongated, flattened, spindle-shaped cell with cytoplasmic projections at each end; common in connective tissue that is growing; gives rise to collagen fibers. (Color Plate 7.)

Fibrosis   Mature, organized bands of collagen; scar tissue. It appears as pink, smooth collagen bundles. (Color Plates 8 and 15.)

Giant cell   Multinucleated cell created by fusion of macrophages. (Color Plates 9, 10, and 13.)

GMS   Gomori methenamine silver (stain).

Granulation tissue   Early reparative tissue composed of capillaries, fibroblasts, young collagen, and leukocytes (mostly mononuclear). As healing continues, granulation tissue becomes organized to form fibrous tissue (fibrosis). Note: this term should not be confused with "granuloma." (Color Plate 6.)

Granuloma   Distinct circumscribed pattern of chronic inflammation in which the predominant cell is the macrophage with epithelioid appearance, with or without the formation of giant cells. A granuloma generally has a pink center (H&E) with epithelioid cells or necrosis surrounded by a rim of mononuclear leukocytes (predominantly lymphocytes, possibly giant cells, and occasionally plasma cells); older granulomas may have an outer rim of fibroblasts, connective tissue, and fibrosis. (Color Plates 10, 11, 12, and 13.)

H&E   Hematoxylin and eosin (stain).

Histiocyte   A large mononuclear phagocyte; an activated macrophage. (Color Plate 4.)

Hyperkeratosis   Increase in the thickness of the stratum corneum.

Hyperplasia   Abnormal increase in the number of cells in the tissue.

Infarct   An area of tissue that has undergone necrosis as a result of obstruction of blood supply. (Color Plate 18.)

Lymphocyte   A leukocyte that is relatively small and has scant cytoplasm, yielding a higher ratio of the size of the nucleus to total cell size (approximately 1:1.2) than that of a monocyte. It is characteristic of chronic inflammation. (Color Plates 2 and 4.)

Macrophage   Term applied to a monocyte when it is seen in tissue; a large, mononuclear, phagocytic cell.

Monocyte   White cell (leukocyte) found in the blood. A large round to oval cell with a large curved or horseshoe-shaped nucleus and a moderate amount of cytoplasm. The ratio of the size of the nucleus to total cell size is approximately 1:3.

Necrosis Spectrum of morphologic changes that follow cell death; results from progressive degenerative action of enzymes on the lethally injured cell. Histologically, there is increased eosinophilia (pink with H&E) of the cell; the cytoplasm may appear vacuolated and moth-eaten, while the nucleus shows shrinkage and fragmentation. The overall resulting image is one of amorphous cellular debris. (Color Plates 12, 13, 15, 16, and 17.)

Neutrophil White blood cell (WBC) with a multilobulated nucleus that appears as 2 to 4 small round to ovoid nuclei connected by thin filaments of nuclear material; a polymorphonuclear leukocyte, commonly called a "poly." It is a granulocytic WBC that is neither eosinophilic nor basophilic. This cell is characteristic of acute inflammation. (Color Plates 1 and 2.)

Parakeratosis Persistence of nuclei in the cells of the stratum corneum of the skin, which is normally devoid of nucleated cells.

PAS Periodic acid-Schiff (stain).

Plasma cell A type of lymphocyte that is specialized for production of antibodies. It has an eccentric nucleus near one edge of the cytoplasm. The nucleus has a speckled chromatin pattern that has been likened to a clock face. The Golgi complex, next to the nucleus, produces a clear, pale-stained area. The ratio of the size of the nucleus to total cell size is approximately 1:2. (Color Plate 4.)

Pseudoepitheliomatous hyperplasia Extensive increase in the thickness of the epidermis that is benign but may resemble squamous cell carcinoma microscopically.

Splendore-Hoeppli phenomenon The development of eosinophilic material around certain infectious agents in tissue. (Color Plate 20.)

Stratum corneum The outermost layer of the epidermis; it consists of flat, denucleated cells that are composed of keratin. (Color Plate 19.)

Suppurative inflammation An acute reaction characterized by a large number of polymorphonuclear leukocytes and necrotic cells and a large amount of edema fluid. (Color Plates 1 and 2.)

Tissue Reactions
to Fungal Infection

After damage of any kind, including infection, the body responds in a fairly predictable manner consisting of three major steps: (i) inflammatory cells (white blood cells) migrate to the damaged area in order to remove dead tissue and the etiologic agent; (ii) damaged areas are initially repaired by the production of granulation tissue, which is composed of macrophages, fibroblasts, collagen, and capillaries; and (iii) the granulation tissue is then replaced by fibrous tissue, commonly known as scar tissue.

While no tissue reactions during this process of inflammation and repair are absolutely diagnostic of a specific organism, they can be highly suggestive of the general category of fungal infection and in some instances can narrow the spectrum of possible fungal agents. Generally, the most common tissue findings suggestive of fungal infection are necrotizing granulomatous reactions, but several genera are associated with more suppurative reactions, i.e., with polymorphonuclear leukocytes predominating.

Usually, the infectious agent is present where the inflammation is the most pronounced. If a tissue has many inflammatory cells, it is likely that the etiologic agent can be observed; if the tissue is healed with little inflammatory component remaining, the organisms are less likely to be detected.

It should be kept in mind that patients who are immuno-compromised, due to immunosuppressive drugs or an immune deficiency disease, often do not produce a pronounced cellular response to fungal infections.

The following are the major tissue reactions observed with fungal infections.

Acute Suppurative Inflammation and Microabscess

Suppurative inflammation is an acute reaction and is characterized by the predominance of polymorphonuclear neutrophilic leukocytes. The suppurative area may be walled off by repair tissue, forming an abscess cavity. (Color Plate 1.)

Chronic Inflammation

Areas of acute inflammation that do not heal in a relatively short time will be replaced by a predominance of mononuclear cells (lymphocytes, plasma cells, and histiocytes). This reaction is nonspecific; it is seen in a variety of fungal infections, as well as in inflammatory reactions caused by other agents. (Color Plates 3 and 4.)

Granulomatous Inflammation (Granuloma)

The term **granulomatous** refers to a type of chronic inflammation characterized by aggregates of large mononuclear cells (macrophages or histiocytes) that often fuse to form multinucleated **giant cells**. In fungal diseases (as well as in tuberculosis), the nuclei are arranged along the inner periphery of the giant cell (known as a Langhans giant cell) (Color Plate 9); in foreign body or tumor giant cells, the nuclei are irregularly placed throughout the cytoplasm.

The **tuberculoid granuloma** is commonly associated with mycobacterial infections but is also seen with many fungal diseases. It is a relatively well circumscribed accumulation of epithelioid macrophages surrounded by a border of lymphocytes; varying numbers of giant cells and caseous necrosis occur. (Color Plates 10 and 11.)

A **necrotic granuloma** is composed of a central area of dead tissue or necrotic debris surrounded by inflammatory cells (mainly epithelioid macrophages) that are in turn surrounded by a layer of fibrous tissue. (Color Plates 12 and 13.)

Pyogranulomatous inflammation is a combination of suppurative and granulomatous reactions. Neutrophils typical of acute suppurative inflammation are present, as well as the mononuclear cells typical of chronic granulomatous reactions.

Necrosis

Following cell death, there are a spectrum of morphologic changes due to progressive degenerative enzymatic action on the dead cell; the sum of these changes is known as necrosis. Histologically, the cytoplasm of the cell shows increased eosinophilia (pink with H&E stain) and may appear vacuolated and moth-eaten; nuclear changes include nuclear shrinkage (pyknosis), increased blueness (basophilia) with H&E stain, breaking up of the nuclear chromatin (karyolysis), and fragmentation of the shrunken nucleus (karyorrhexis). (Color Plate 16.)

Caseous necrosis is a form of necrosis that upon gross examination has a cottage cheese-like consistency. It is devoid of viable cells and microscopically appears as homogeneously staining, amorphous, finely granular material within which giant cells may be seen; caseous necrosis often accompanies granulomatous inflammation. (Color Plates 12 and 13.)

Angioinvasion, Infarction, and Necrosis

The zygomycetes, *Aspergillus* spp., and a few other fungi, such as *Pseudallescheria boydii* and *Fusarium* spp., have a tendency to invade blood vessels, blocking the lumen of the vessel, stopping the flow of blood, and causing death of the tissue deprived of blood supply. This process is known as infarction. Histologically, angioinvasion appears as infected thrombotic material blocking the lumen of arteries or veins with the surrounding tissue being hemorrhagic and necrotic; polymorphonuclear neutrophils and monocytic cells, as well as a large amount of degenerated cellular debris, are usually present. (Color Plates 17 and 18.)

Splendore-Hoeppli Phenomenon

The Splendore-Hoeppli reaction is indicative of a localized immunologic host response to antigens of a variety of infectious agents, including some fungi and bacteria; it is characterized by Splendore-Hoeppli material coating or bordering the microorganisms. Histologically, it appears as radiating homogeneous, refractile, eosinophilic (pink with H&E) clublike material surrounding a central eosinophilic focus. (Color Plate 20.) Fungi associated with the phenomenon are *Coccidioides immitis, Sporothrix schenckii,* and those causing mycetoma and some forms of dermatophytosis. The actinomycetes and the nonfilamentous bacteria causing botryomycosis also generate the phenomenon.

Fungus Ball

A fungus ball results when filamentous fungi (most commonly, but not exclusively, *Aspergillus*) colonize a previously formed cavity that has access to oxygen. There is minimal to no invasion of the tissues unless the host is immunocompromised. Hyphae and sometimes conidial heads, complete with phialides and conidia, develop. Fungal masses are seen lying free within the cavity; the hyphae are not usually attached to the cavity wall. Surrounding inflammation may be minimal, or there may be fibrosis with chronic inflammation made up of lymphocytes and other mononuclear inflammatory cells.

Stains

Although fungi may be seen in tissue with the routinely used hematoxylin and eosin (H&E) stain, there are special stains that enhance their detection. The most commonly used stains are summarized in Table 1, p. 22. The Gomori methenamine silver (GMS) stain is generally the preferred method for tissue sections and also for smeared material that requires a permanent stain; it is routinely performed in the histology laboratory. If there is debris in the tissue background that, when stained with GMS, mimics fungi (e.g., yeastlike black pigment in the lung or hypha-like elastic fibers in skin or lymph node), an alternative stain, such as periodic acid-Schiff (PAS) or Gridley fungus stain, can be useful.

On wet preparations of specimens or on smeared and dried material, the fluorescent Calcofluor White (CFW) stain (p. 316), with or without potassium hydroxide (KOH), is far superior to the traditional KOH alone. CFW is also useful in detecting sparse amounts of fungi in deparaffinized tissue sections.

Some stains are used as supplements to aid in more specific identification of an organism after detection with a preliminary fungal stain. For example, GMS readily detects yeast in tissue, but the mucicarmine stain can subsequently be performed on the tissue to determine whether the yeast has a polysaccharide capsule, typical of *Cryptococcus neoformans*. Similarly, GMS will detect the yeast cells of *Blastomyces* but it will not reliably demonstrate the doubly refractile wall, which can be better seen with a PAS or H&E stain.

The Fontana-Masson (FM) stain is used for detecting melanin, or its precursors, in cell walls. It can be helpful in the rare case of a capsule-deficient strain of *C. neoformans*, as the melanin in the cell wall will stain dark brown. FM is known to intensely stain dematiaceous fungi in tissue sections; in a recent study (Kimura and McGinnis, 1998), a varying, and always lesser, degree of staining was exhibited by other fungi, notably some zygomycetes, *Aspergillus*, and *Trichosporon*. *Candida*, *Fusarium*, and *Pseudallescheria* were consistently negative. These findings accentuate the need to carefully evaluate the morphology and depth of color of positive FM-stained hyphae that appear hyaline with H&E stain.

See Part III, pp. 313–324, for further information on the stains most commonly performed in the clinical mycology laboratory.

TABLE 1 Stains for direct microscopic observation of fungi and filamentous bacteria in tissue

Stain (abbreviation)	Characteristics
Brown and Brenn (B&B)	Gram stain for bacteria; demonstrates the bacterial filaments of the actinomycetes, e.g., *Nocardia*, *Actinomadura*, etc.
Calcofluor White (CFW)	Stains the chitin in fungal cell walls; extremely useful for smeared preparations; fluorescence microscope required.
Fontana-Masson (FM)	Stains select fungi brown to black. It was originally thought to stain only dematiaceous fungi and *Cryptococcus neoformans* (organisms known to contain melanin or melanin precursors), but it has now been shown to stain variably, but less intensely, *Aspergillus fumigatus*, *Aspergillus flavus*, *Trichosporon* sp., and some zygomycetes.[a]
Giemsa	Most organisms (fungi and also bacteria) stain blue-purple. It enables visualization of *Histoplasma capsulatum* and *Penicillium marneffei* in bone marrow and blood smears.
Gomori methenamine silver (GMS)	Fungi including *Pneumocystis carinii* are gray to black; background is green. It also stains *Nocardia* and other actinomycetes. Its drawback is that it often stains fungi too densely to observe structural details.
Gridley fungus (GF)	Fungi stain purplish red; filaments of the actinomycetes are NOT stained.
Hematoxylin & eosin (H&E)	Stains some fungal elements violet to bluish purple in mild to moderate contrast to the lighter background tissue. Has advantage of allowing observation of natural pigment of fungi. It is the best stain to demonstrate host tissue reaction.
Modified acid-fast	Filaments of *Nocardia* stain at least partially acid fast (pink); *Actinomyces* and other actinomycetes are negative.
Mucicarmine	Stains the capsule of *Cryptococcus* pinkish red and may also stain the cell walls of *Blastomyces dermatitidis* and *Rhinosporidium seeberi*.
Periodic acid-Schiff (PAS)	Stains fungi pinkish red. Demonstrates the double-contoured refractile walls of *Blastomyces dermatitidis* that may not be visible with GMS stain. It is the fungal stain of choice of many dermatopathologists.

[a]Kimura and McGinnis, 1998.

Guide to Interpretation of Direct Microscopic Examination

Abbreviations: GMS, Gomori methenamine silver stain; H&E, hematoxylin and eosin stain; GF, Gridley fungus stain; PAS, periodic acid-Schiff stain.

For further information and excellent photomicrographs, see Chandler and Watts (1987) and Connor et al. (1997).

Observation	Brief description	Interpretation
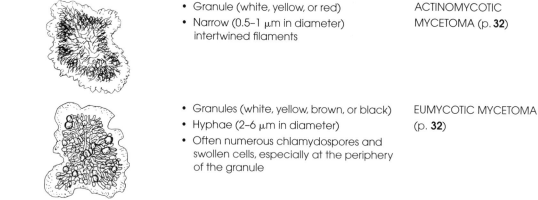	• "Sulfur granules" (30–3,000 μm or more in diameter) • Delicate (<1-μm diameter) branched filaments • Gram positive and non-acid fast • Stain with GMS and Giemsa stains but not with H&E, GF, and PAS	ACTINOMYCOSIS (p. **31**)
	• Granule (white, yellow, or red) • Narrow (0.5–1 μm in diameter) intertwined filaments	ACTINOMYCOTIC MYCETOMA (p. **32**)
	• Granules (white, yellow, brown, or black) • Hyphae (2–6 μm in diameter) • Often numerous chlamydospores and swollen cells, especially at the periphery of the granule	EUMYCOTIC MYCETOMA (p. **32**)
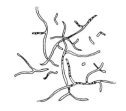	• Delicate narrow (0.5–1.0 μm in diameter) filaments • Tendency to branch at right angles • Frequently appear beaded or granular • Partially acid fast	NOCARDIOSIS (p. **34**)
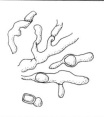	• Hyphae broad (3–25 μm in diameter; average, 12 μm) • Almost nonseptate, with nonparallel sides • Branching is nondichotomous; irregular; sometimes at right angles	ZYGOMYCOSIS (p. **35**)

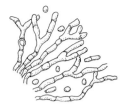

- Septate hyphae (3–12 μm in diameter)
- Dichotomous branching at 45° angles
- Tendency to grow in radial pattern
- Hyphae nearly parallel to one another

ASPERGILLOSIS (p. **36**)

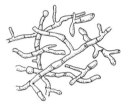

- Septate hyphae (2–8 μm in diameter)
- Hyphae irregular and haphazardly arranged
- Branching at 45 and 90° angles
- Phialides and conidia may form in closed lesions

HYALOHYPHOMYCOSES (p. **38**)

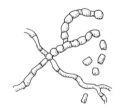

- Colorless, branched, septate hyphae
- Hyphae often break up into chains of arthroconidia
- Other conidia do not form in tissue

DERMATOPHYTOSIS (tinea, ringworm) (p. **40**)

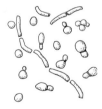

- Septate hyphal elements (2.5–4.0 μm in diameter)
- Hypha elements short, slightly curved, form short chains
- Oval to round thick-walled yeastlike cells (3–8 μm in diameter)
- Produce buds through small phialidic collarettes
- "Spaghetti and meatball" appearance

TINEA VERSICOLOR (p. **41**)

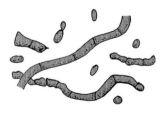

- Darkly pigmented septate hyphae (1.5–3.0 μm in diameter)
- Sometimes elongated budding cells (1.5–5.0 μm in diameter)
- Occasionally chlamydoconidia

TINEA NIGRA (p. **42**)

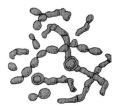

- Brown-pigmented septate hyphae (2–6 μm in diameter)
- Dark budding yeastlike forms may also occur

PHAEOHYPHOMYCOSIS (p. **43**)

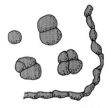

- Sclerotic bodies (5–12 μm in diameter):
    Brown pigmented
    Thick walled
    Have horizontal and vertical septations
- Occasionally, brown septate hyphae (3–8 μm in diameter)

CHROMOBLASTOMYCOSIS (p. **44**)

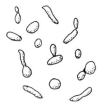

- Yeastlike cells:
    Various sizes and shapes
    Round to oval (2–6 μm in diameter)
    Bud on narrow base
    Some characteristically elongated "cigar bodies" (2 × 3 to 3 × 10 μm)

SPOROTRICHOSIS (p. **45**)

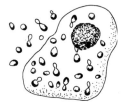

- Yeastlike cells:
    Small (2–4 μm in diameter); usually ovoid
    Budding on a narrow base at the smaller end
    Characteristically within macrophages or monocytes
    Commonly remain clustered when extracellular

HISTOPLASMOSIS CAPSULATI (p. **46**)

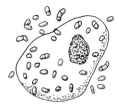

- Yeastlike cells:
    Round or oval (approximately 3 μm in diameter)
    Characteristically within macrophages or monocytes
    May elongate somewhat when extracellular
    Have central septum; do not bud

PENICILLIOSIS MARNEFFEI (p. **48**)

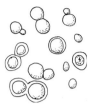

- Yeastlike cells:
  - Round to oval (3–30 μm in diameter; usually 8–15 μm)
  - May appear thick walled
  - Budding on a broad base

BLASTOMYCOSIS (p. **50**)

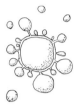

- Yeastlike cells:
  - Round to oval; large (3–30 μm in diameter)
  - Multiple budding
  - Buds are attached to the parent cell by narrow connections

PARACOCCIDIOIDO-MYCOSIS (p. **51**)

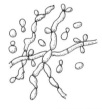

- Round to oval budding yeast cells (3–6 μm in diameter)
- Branching septate hyphae and pseudohyphae
- Chains of budding cells

CANDIDIASIS (CANDIDOSIS) (p. **52**)

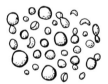

- Yeastlike cells:
  - Mostly round; some oval (2–20 μm in diameter)
  - Encapsulated
  - Thin dark walls
  - Budding on a narrow base

CRYPTOCOCCOSIS (p. **54**)

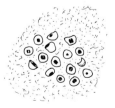

- Round, ovoid, or collapsed crescent forms (3–5 μm in diameter)
- Nonbudding
- Appear in small clusters on a thick foamy background
- Comma- or parenthesis-shaped focal thickenings in wall

PNEUMOCYSTOSIS (p. **56**)

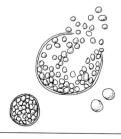

- Round or oval sporangia (range, 2–25 μm in diameter)
- Round or polyhedral endospores in sporangia
- No budding

PROTOTHECOSIS (p. **57**)

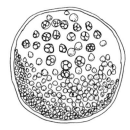

- Spherules (10–100 μm or more in diameter)
- Mature spherule relatively thin walled (1–2 μm thick)
- Round endospores (2–5 μm in diameter) in mature spherules
- No budding

COCCIDIOIDOMYCOSIS (p. **58**)

- Large round sporangia (100–350 μm in diameter when mature)
- Sporangia thick walled (approximately 5 μm)
- Endospores vary in size (1–10 μm in diameter)
- Endospores are arranged in zonal pattern in mature sporangia
- Inner surface of sporangial wall and walls of endospores stain with mucicarmine
- No budding

RHINOSPORIDIOSIS (p. **59**)

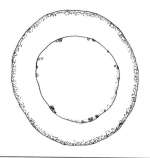

- Large round adiaconidia (200–400 μm in diameter)
- Adiaconidia very thick walled (20–70 μm)
- Interior of adiaconidium usually appears empty
- No budding

ADIASPIROMYCOSIS (p. **61**)

Detailed Descriptions

Actinomycosis

ETIOLOGIC AGENTS: *Actinomyces israelii* (in humans), *Actinomyces bovis* (in animals), and other *Actinomyces* spp.; occasionally *Arachnia, Rothia*, and *Eubacterium* spp.

SITES OF INFECTION: Neck and face area, lung, thoracic cavity, abdomen, pelvis, multiple systemic sites.

TISSUE REACTION: Typically suppuration with abscesses containing granules composed of the bacterial filaments. The innermost portion of the wall of the abscess sometimes contains foamy macrophages. Palisading epithelioid macrophages and giant cells often surround the abscess and may be encapsulated by fibrosing granulation tissue. Splendore-Hoeppli material usually radiates around the abscesses. Sinus tracts connecting the abscesses or opening to the body surface are common.

MORPHOLOGY OF ORGANISM: Granules from an abscess or draining sinus tract are 30–3,000 μm or more in diameter and are commonly called "sulfur granules" (due to their yellow color, which resembles elemental sulfur, but they do not contain sulfur). When crushed, the granules appear microscopically as opaque masses with peripheral, gelatinous, club-shaped bodies. The granules are composed of numerous delicate (less than 1 μm in diameter) bacterial filaments that branch (often at right angles) and may exhibit beading (but not as commonly as does *Nocardia*). In some instances, only small groups of branching filaments form instead of the characteristic granules. (Color Plate 21.) The organisms are gram positive and nonacid fast; they stain well with GMS and Giemsa stains but not with H&E, PAS, and Gridley fungus. Other anaerobic bacteria may also be present.

Branching filaments of *Nocardia* are morphologically similar, but most (although not all) *Nocardia* are partially acid fast. Culture (aerobic and anaerobic) is required for definitive identification of the etiologic agent.

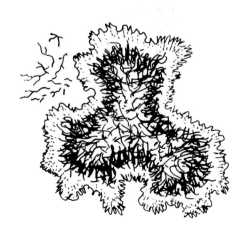

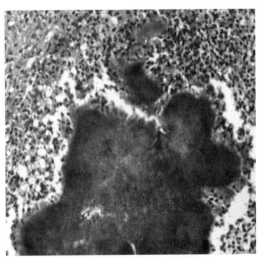

Courtesy of Joan Barenfanger.

Mycetoma (Actinomycotic or Eumycotic)

ETIOLOGIC AGENTS:
Actinomycotic: *Nocardia* spp., *Actinomadura* spp., *Streptomyces* spp.
Eumycotic: *Pseudallescheria boydii, Madurella* spp., *Exophiala jeanselmei, Acremonium* spp., *Fusarium* spp., *Curvularia* spp., and occasionally other moulds.

SITES OF INFECTION: Subcutaneous tissue and skin; long-standing infections may involve muscle, fascia, and bone. The infection is most commonly on lower leg or foot, rarely disseminated.

TISSUE REACTION: Similar reactions are seen with all mycetomas, i.e., both actinomycotic and eumycotic. Multiple draining sinus tracts with neutrophilic abscesses containing granules (composed of the etiologic agent) and necrotic debris are characteristic. The abscesses and sinus tracts are surrounded by chronic inflammation consisting of palisading epithelioid macrophages, multinucleated giant cells, lymphocytes, and plasma cells. Between the abscesses is granulation tissue that is usually vascular and contains many inflammatory cells. Splendore-Hoeppli material very often surrounds the granules. Fibrosis may occur in long-standing infections.

MORPHOLOGY OF ORGANISM: The etiologic agent typically organizes into aggregates in infected tissue to form granules ranging in size from 25 μm to 5 mm.

* Actinomycotic Mycetoma: Granules (white, yellow, or red) are composed of narrow (1 μm or less in diameter) intertwined filaments that are radially oriented and most numerous at the edge of the granule. *Nocardia* spp. are usually at least partially acid fast, while *Actinomadura* and *Streptomyces* spp. are not acid fast. All are gram positive and stain well with GMS and Giemsa, but not with H&E, PAS, or Gridley fungus.
* Eumycotic Mycetoma: Granules (white, yellow, brown, or black) contain septate, variously shaped, somewhat distorted hyphae (2–6 μm in diameter) that are often accompanied by numerous chlamydoconidia and swollen cells; the fungal forms are most commonly visible at the periphery of the granule. (Color Plate 22.)

Mycetoma (Actinomycotic or Eumycotic) *(continued)*

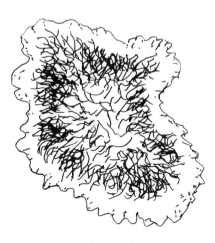

Actinomycotic

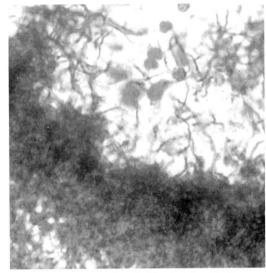

Edge of actinomycotic granule.

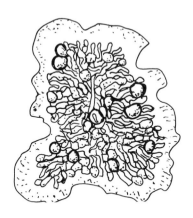

Eumycotic

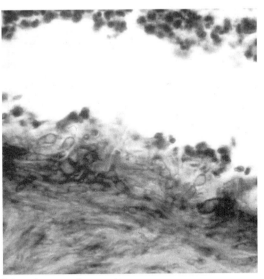

Edge of eumycotic granule.

Nocardiosis

ETIOLOGIC AGENTS: *Nocardia asteroides* (most common), *Nocardia brasiliensis*, *Nocardia otitidiscaviarum* (formerly *Nocardia caviae*), and rarely other *Nocardia* spp.

SITES OF INFECTION: Lung, central nervous system, skin and subcutaneous tissue, multiple systemic sites.

TISSUE REACTION: Generally, the reaction is suppurative, sometimes necrotizing. Poorly defined, variably encapsulated abscesses may form. Occasionally, granulomatous tissue is seen in chronic infections. The Splendore-Hoeppli phenomenon is rare in *Nocardia* infections.

MORPHOLOGY OF ORGANISM: Delicate, narrow (0.5–1.0 μm in diameter) filaments that tend to branch at right angles; coccobacillary elements may also form. Organisms characteristically appear beaded and may be so numerous and highly branched that they have been described as resembling "Chinese letters." They are partially acid fast when stained with the modified Kinyoun stain (p. 315) or other acid fast stain using a weak acid solution for decolorization. (Color Plate 23.) The organisms are gram positive and stain well with GMS, especially when the staining time in the silver nitrate solution is increased; they do not reliably stain with H&E, PAS, or Gridley fungus.

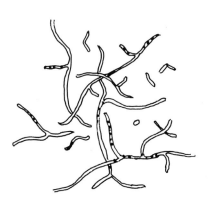

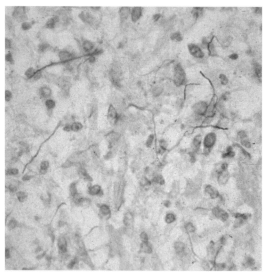

Courtesy of Ron C. Neafie.

Zygomycosis (Mucormycosis)

ETIOLOGIC AGENTS: *Rhizopus* spp., *Mucor* spp., *Rhizomucor* sp., *Absidia corymbifera, Apophysomyces elegans, Saksenaea vasiformis, Cunninghamella bertholletiae* (*Basidiobolus* and *Conidiobolus* spp. cause subcutaneous zygomycosis, known as entomophthoromycosis).

SITES OF INFECTION: Lung, nasal sinus, brain, eye, skin, mucous membranes, multiple systemic sites.

TISSUE REACTION: Suppurative necrosis and occasionally granulomatous reactions occur. Zygomycetes (of the order Mucorales [p. 163]) have a predilection for invasion of blood vessels, causing thrombosis and infarction. These agents must be differentiated from *Aspergillus* and other hyphomycetes that also commonly invade blood vessels.

MORPHOLOGY OF ORGANISM: The key features are (i) broad hyphae (5–25 μm in diameter; average, 12 μm) with nonparallel walls; (ii) hyphae almost nonseptate—the thin walls and lack of regular septation decreases the internal support of these broad hyphae and allows them to become characteristically twisted, collapsed, and folded in a ribbonlike fashion; (iii) branching that is irregularly spaced, nondichotomous, and at various angles (often at right angles) to the parent hypha. (Color Plate 24.) Thick-walled chlamydospores (15–30 μm in diameter) may form.

The special fungus stains (GMS, PAS, and Gridley fungus) generally do not color the zygomycetes as deeply as they do other fungi.

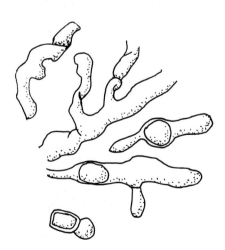

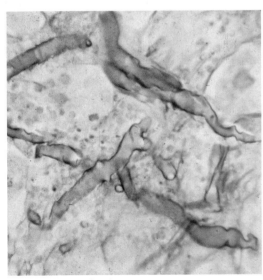

Courtesy of Morris Gordon.

Aspergillosis

ETIOLOGIC AGENTS: *Aspergillus fumigatus, Aspergillus flavus, Aspergillus niger,* and other *Aspergillus* spp.

SITES OF INFECTION: Lung, paranasal sinus, ear, eye, skin, mucous membranes, and multiple systemic sites.

TISSUE REACTION: Invasive aspergillosis is characterized by acute inflammation (neutrophils) and necrotic debris. In severely neutropenic patients, the acute inflammatory response is greatly reduced. Occasionally, a granulomatous response occurs. *Aspergillus* has a predilection for invading blood vessels (angioinvasion; see p. 19), causing blockage of blood vessels (thrombosis), tissue death and necrosis (infarction), and presence of red blood cells outside of the blood vessels (hemorrhage). Fungi causing other hyaline hyphomycoses cause similar tissue reactions.

Allergic or hypersensitivity aspergillosis can occur in several forms, but most will result in tissue reactions that involve hypersecretion of mucus with neutrophils and eosinophils. Charcot-Leyden crystals are sometimes seen; they are formed from breakdown products of eosinophils and are intensely pink, long, narrow, widening at the center, and tapered to a point at each end. Granulomatous inflammation develops in some instances. Mucus plugs are sometimes expectorated and have concentric layers of eosinophils, epithelial cells, necrotic cellular debris, and possibly Charcot-Leyden crystals.

When fungus balls (aspergillomas; see p. 19) form, the wall of the cavity is often eroded and composed of inflammatory granulation tissue; calcium oxalate crystals may be seen in the ball (especially if composed of *A. niger*).

MORPHOLOGY OF ORGANISM: The key features include (i) septate hyphae, mostly 3–6 μm in diameter; (ii) dichotomous branching (i.e., each branch is approximately equal in width to the originating parent hypha) at 45° angles; and (iii) tendency to grow from hematogenous lesions in tissues in a radial fashion, like the spokes of a wheel, with the hyphae appearing nearly parallel to one another. (Color Plates 25, 26, and 27.) In chronic lesions, short, distorted hyphae may be as wide as 12 μm. Conidial heads (vesicle, phialides, and conidia) may occasionally form in areas exposed to air, e.g., in pulmonary cavities, nasal-sinus aspergillomas, and ear or skin infections.

Many other fungi appear similar to the aspergilli in tissue or other clinical specimens; however, there are subtle differences. Zygomycetes have hyphae that are almost nonseptate, are commonly broader (up to 25 μm in diameter), show random branching, often appear collapsed and twisted, are irregular and nonparallel, and usually stain lighter with GMS than do the aspergilli. *Candida* spp., in addition to hyphae, form pseudohyphae (typically showing distinct constrictions at the septa) and budding yeast cells; but when the hyphae of *Aspergillus* are cut on cross section, they may be mistaken for nonbudding yeast cells. Hyphae of other opportunistic hyaline moulds may be indistinguishable from *Aspergillus* in tissue (see "Miscellaneous Hyalohyphomycoses," p. 38).

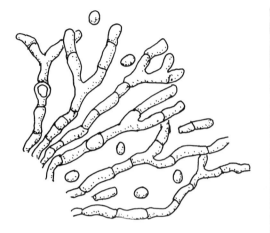

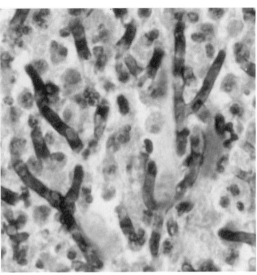

Miscellaneous Hyalohyphomycoses (Other than Aspergillosis)

ETIOLOGIC AGENTS: Any mould that forms colorless, septate hyphae in host tissue, e.g., *Fusarium, Paecilomyces, Acremonium, Scedosporium* (and *Pseudallescheria*).

SITES OF INFECTION: Almost any body site; much more likely to be recovered in blood culture than is *Aspergillus*.

TISSUE REACTION: The most common tissue responses are acute inflammation and necrosis with occasional granulomatous inflammation. Invasion of blood vessels with subsequent thrombosis and infarction also occurs.

MORPHOLOGY OF ORGANISMS: The hyphae are usually irregular and haphazardly arranged, with considerable variation in diameter (2–8 μm); they typically exhibit both 45 and 90° branching. These traits suggest an etiologic agent other than *Aspergillus* (p. 268), but it is usually not possible to reliably differentiate any of these agents from *Aspergillus* in tissue unless there is production of conidia. All hyphomycetes differ from the zygomycetes in forming hyphae that are narrower, are regularly septate, and are less prone to ribbonlike folding. These miscellaneous hyphomycetes differ from both the aspergilli and the zygomycetes in having the capacity to produce conidia and phialides within a **closed** lesion. Phialides usually appear as tapering structures (some are slightly flask shaped or bottle necked) along the sides or at the ends of the hyphae; a broad, darkly staining band can be seen on the sides of the neck of the phialide after production of multiple conidia. The conidia commonly have a rounded apex and a flat basal scar when detached; those of *Pseudallescheria/Scedosporium* may be brown. Occasionally hyphae that are somewhat constricted at the septa, along with the presence of phialoconidia, can resemble the pseudohyphae and budding yeasts seen in candidiasis. Culture is almost always required for definitive identification of the etiologic agent.

For further information, see
  Liu et al., 1998

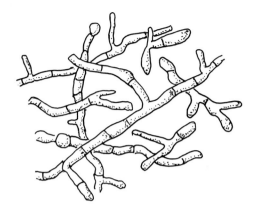

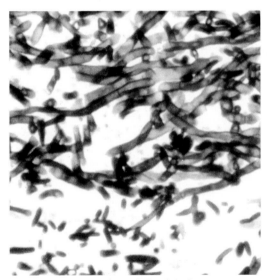

Hyphal elements. Courtesy of Wiley Schell.

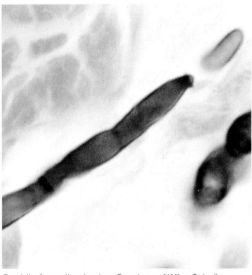

Conidia formation in vivo. Courtesy of Wiley Schell.

Dermatophytosis (Tinea, Ringworm)

ETIOLOGIC AGENTS: *Microsporum* spp., *Trichophyton* spp., *Epidermophyton floccosum*.

SITES OF INFECTION: Skin, hair, nails.

TISSUE REACTION: Skin specimens usually show hyperkeratosis and various degrees of acanthosis, parakeratosis, and increased space between the cells (spongiosis). When present, the inflammatory response is usually mild and predominantly mononuclear. If the deep nonkeratinized layers of the skin are involved, a suppurative or granulomatous reaction may occur; Splendore-Hoeppli material may also be present. The etiologic agent is most commonly found in the stratum corneum (the outermost layer of the epidermis, consisting of keratinized, nonnucleated cells).

MORPHOLOGY OF ORGANISM: All of the dermatophytes appear in the host as colorless, branched, septate hyphae that characteristically break up into chains of arthroconidia. Other conidia do not form in tissue. When hair is involved, the pattern of infection depends on the species of dermatophyte, i.e., arthroconidia may form on the outside of the hair (ectothrix type of invasion) or inside the hair (endothrix type); hyphae can be found within the hair in either case; there is also a favic pattern of invasion in which hyphae, arthroconidia, and empty spaces form inside the hair.

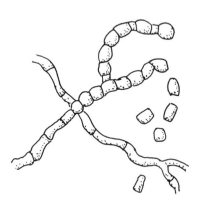

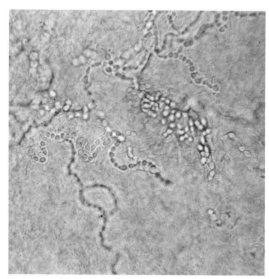

Courtesy of Tomas Roges.

Tinea versicolor

ETIOLOGIC AGENT: *Malassezia furfur.*

SITES OF INFECTION: The stratum corneum (the outermost layer of the skin); the organisms can therefore be readily seen in skin scrapings.

Note: The etiologic agent can also cause fungemia and occasionally systemic infection (most frequently involving the lung) in patients receiving prolonged infusion of lipids through contaminated central venous catheters.

TISSUE REACTION: Mild to moderate hyperkeratosis and acanthosis is usually seen. There may be a minimal mononuclear response in the dermis. The causative organism is usually seen in the stratum corneum.

MORPHOLOGY OF ORGANISM: Short, slightly curved, septate hyphal elements (2.5–4.0 μm in diameter) typically form in short chains. These are accompanied by clusters of oval to round thick-walled cells (2.5–8 μm in diameter) that appear yeast-like but are actually phialidic; they are characteristically round at one end and have a flat collarette at the opposite end through which "buds" are produced. (Color Plate 28.) The organisms are routinely observed in skin scrapings with a KOH preparation and/or with Calcofluor White; in biopsy specimens, they can be seen with H&E but are best demonstrated by special stains for fungus, preferably PAS (to better see the defining lines of the organism). The etiologic agent, *M. furfur*, will grow only on media that have been overlaid or supplemented with olive oil or another long-chain fatty acid.

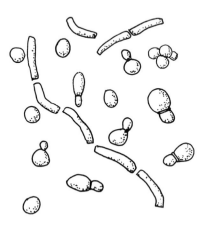
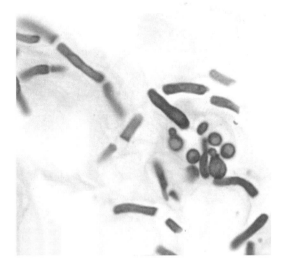

Tinea nigra

ETIOLOGIC AGENT: *Phaeoannellomyces werneckii.*

SITES OF INFECTION: Palms of hands, soles of feet; rarely on other skin surfaces. Only the stratum corneum (outermost layer of the skin) is involved.

TISSUE REACTION: Mild to moderate hyperplasia and/or hyperkeratosis is seen in the epidermis. A minimal mononuclear cell infiltrate may occur in the dermis. The fungi are easily detected in the stratum corneum.

MORPHOLOGY OF ORGANISM: Darkly pigmented, branched, septate, narrow hyphae (1.5–3.0 μm wide) usually accompanied by elongated budding cells (1.5–5.0 μm in diameter). The organism stains well with the special fungus stains, but the natural pigmentation can be best seen with H&E.

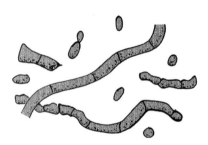

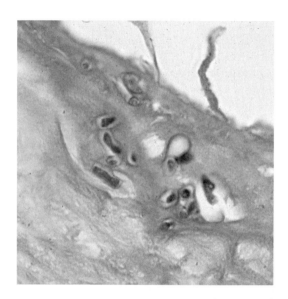

Phaeohyphomycosis

ETIOLOGIC AGENTS: *Exophiala jeanselmei, Phaeoacremonium parasiticum, Phialophora richardsiae, Wangiella dermatitidis, Bipolaris* sp., *Alternaria* sp., *Cladophialophora bantiana* (in the brain), and a large variety of other dematiaceous fungi.

SITES OF INFECTION: Most commonly in skin and subcutaneous tissue; also occurs in the brain and occasionally in a variety of other body sites. Severe disseminated infection has also been reported.

TISSUE REACTION: The more common etiologic agents elicit encapsulated cystic granulomas in the dermis and subcutaneous tissue; the epidermis is seldom affected. The center of the granuloma contains a suppurative exudate that often liquifies; it is surrounded by a wide zone of granulation tissue. Multiple abscesses may occur in early infection. The less common etiologic agents produce a dispersed granulomatous inflammation. In cerebral infections, the characteristic inflammatory response is suppurative and granulomatous with abscess formation.

MORPHOLOGY OF ORGANISM: Brown-pigmented hyphae (2–6 μm wide) occur singly or in small aggregates. They often have closely spaced, constricted septations producing a moniliform ("string of beads") appearance. Large, bizarre, thick-walled vesicular swellings (≥25 μm in diameter) resembling chlamydoconidia may be seen along, or at the ends of, the hyphae. Yeastlike cells producing buds singly or in chains are also commonly present. The pigment is usually visible in unstained or H&E-stained specimens, but the Fontana-Masson stain can be used to further demonstrate the melanin in the cell wall. (Color Plate 29.) The organism also stains well with the special stains for fungus.

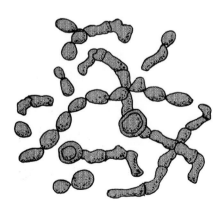
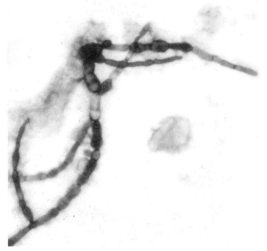

Courtesy of Joan Barenfanger.

Chromoblastomycosis

ETIOLOGIC AGENTS: *Fonsecaea pedrosoi, Fonsecaea compacta, Phialophora verrucosa, Cladophialophora carrionii, Exophiala jeanselmei, Exophiala spinifera,* and *Rhinocladiella aquaspersa.*

SITES OF INFECTION: Skin and subcutaneous tissue.

TISSUE REACTION: In skin, a characteristic pseudoepitheliomatous hyperplasia with hyperkeratosis and parakeratosis occurs. Inflammation is generally granulomatous; it is often accompanied by a suppurative reaction, possibly from a secondary infection, causing satellite microabscesses.

MORPHOLOGY OF ORGANISM: Brown-pigmented, round to polyhedral, thick-walled sclerotic bodies (5–12 μm in diameter) having horizontal and/or vertical septations are diagnostic. These structures are also referred to as Medlar bodies or "copper pennies." (Color Plate 30.) Brown, branched, distorted, septate hyphae (3–5 μm in diameter) may also be present. The fungi typically migrate to the surface of the skin and are seen as black dots in the keratin scales; sclerotic bodies and sometimes short hyphae are seen microscopically.

The structure and pigment of the organism is usually well demonstrated with H&E stain.

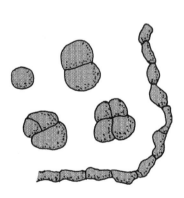

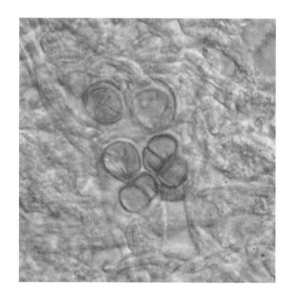

Sporotrichosis

ETIOLOGIC AGENT: *Sporothrix schenckii.*

SITES OF INFECTION: Skin, subcutaneous tissue, and contiguous lymphatics; rare dissemination to bones, joints, lungs, and other internal organs.

TISSUE REACTION: *S. schenckii* usually provokes a mixed suppurative and granulomatous inflammatory reaction that is often accompanied by fibrosis and microabscess formation; this mixed inflammatory reaction is seen in the dermis and subcutaneous tissue as well as in disseminated disease. Splendore-Hoeppli material typically forms around the yeastlike cells. Lesions of cutaneous infections usually exhibit hyperkeratosis, parakeratosis, and pseudoepitheliomatous hyperplasia.

MORPHOLOGY OF ORGANISM: Yeastlike cells are of various sizes and shapes; they may be round to oval (usually 2–6 μm in diameter) and often have elongated "pipe stem" buds. Budding is on a narrow base. Characteristic elongated "cigar bodies" are most commonly seen in disseminated lesions. In cutaneous lesions, the organisms are usually very sparse, and special stains for fungus (e.g., GMS or PAS) are required. Fluorescent-antibody staining is extremely helpful in observing the organism, but it is not readily available in most laboratories.

    S. schenckii and *Histoplasma capsulatum* var. *capsulatum* may both appear as small, round or oval cells, but the neutrophilic inflammatory reaction seen in the mixed suppurative and granulomatous reaction of sporotrichosis is not characteristic of histoplasmosis. *Candida glabrata*, which also appears as small, oval yeast cells, produces a suppurative tissue reaction but does not usually generate granulomas; this fact might assist in differentiating it from *Sporothrix*.

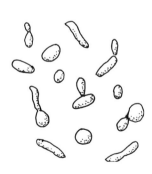

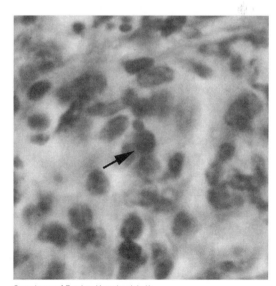

Courtesy of Evelyn Koestenblatt.

Histoplasmosis capsulati

ETIOLOGIC AGENT: *Histoplasma capsulatum* var. *capsulatum.*

SITES OF INFECTION: Lung, blood, bone marrow, multiple systemic sites.

TISSUE REACTION: The initial reaction is histiocytic. In acute pulmonary infections, macrophages and giant cells that are packed with yeast cells fill the alveolar spaces. Parenchymal necrosis develops, along with epithelioid and giant-cell granulomas, and often eventual cavitation. Healing is typified by the granulomas becoming fibrocaseous nodules that commonly calcify. (Color Plates 14 and 15.) Although *Candida glabrata* is similar in size and shape to *H. capsulatum*, the infections differ histologically in that *Candida* almost always produces a suppurative tissue reaction; *Sporothrix schenckii*, which is also a small yeast, differs in commonly producing a mixed suppurative and granulomatous reaction.

MORPHOLOGY OF ORGANISM: Small yeast cells (2–4 μm in length) are usually ovoid with budding on a narrow base at the smaller end. The yeasts reproduce within monocytes or macrophages and, when released, often remain in clusters. In Giemsa- or Wright-stained preparations, a pale blue ring (the fungus cell wall) surrounds the darker blue cytoplasm that retracts from the wall, often giving the false impression of a capsule; the chromatin stains dark violet and appears as a crescent-shaped mass within the cell. A halo or pseudocapsule also appears with H&E, but the organism stains well and evenly with GMS or PAS.

Differentiation of *Histoplasma* from other small yeasts and a few parasites can be difficult, but a few factors may be helpful.

- The yeastlike cells of *Penicillium marneffei* do not bud; they have a prominent transverse septum and reproduce by fission.
- The yeast cells of *Candida glabrata* are more variable in size, stain better with H&E, and do not demonstrate a pseudocapsule. Also, *Candida* spp. generate a suppurative tissue reaction, not a granulomatous one.
- *Sporothrix schenckii* causes a mixed suppurative and granulomatous reaction rather than the purely granulomatous reaction seen in histoplasmosis. In sporotrichosis, the yeast cells are often fewer, and they may be more elongated and variably shaped than those of *Histoplasma.*
- *Cryptococcus* yeast cells have a dark wall (accentuated with Fontana-Masson stain), are rounder, and consistently appear in a large variety of sizes. Their capsular material stains with mucicarmine.
- The endospores of *Coccidioides* are about the same size as the yeast cells of *Histoplasma*, but the endospores are rounder, do not bud, and are typically accompanied by spherules.
- Some protozoans can mimic *Histoplasma* but are different in that they stain entirely with H&E, do not form a pseudocapsule, do not reliably stain with special histologic fungal stains, and do not bud. Additionally, amastigotes of *Leishmania* sp. and *Trypanosoma cruzi* have paranuclear bar-shaped kinetoplasts that can be seen with H&E under oil immersion.

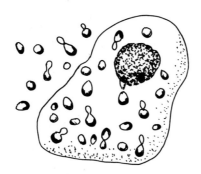

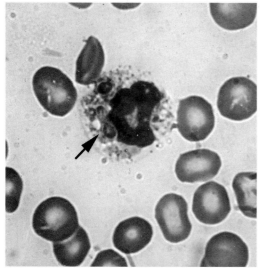

Bone marrow; intracellular.

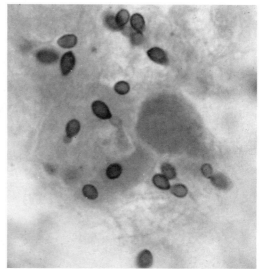

Lung; extracellular. Courtesy of Joan Barenfanger.

Penicilliosis marneffei

ETIOLOGIC AGENT: *Penicillium marneffei.*

SITES OF INFECTION: Blood, bone marrow, skin, lung, liver, lymph nodes, and multiple systemic sites.

TISSUE REACTION: Histiocytes predominate in early lesions. As the lesion progresses, central necrosis develops, with infiltration of neutrophils and formation of abscesses. Granulomas slowly evolve in the lung and may lead to fibrosis and cavitation. Calcification does not usually occur (in contrast to histoplasmosis). In the severely immunocompromised patient, the inflammatory response may be minimal or absent.

MORPHOLOGY OF ORGANISM: Oval yeastlike cells are 2.5–5 μm in length and multiply within histiocytes in tissue (or within monocytes in blood or bone marrow). Budding does not occur; a prominent central septum forms, and reproduction is by fission (arthroconidium-like). Outside of histiocytes, yeast cells are up to 8 μm in length, may have several septa, and are sometimes curved. The organisms stain well with GMS or PAS; they give a false impression of having a capsule when stained with H&E, so they can very closely mimic *Histoplasma capsulatum* var. *capsulatum*, especially when intracellular (but the yeast cells of *Histoplasma* reproduce by budding).

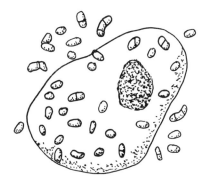

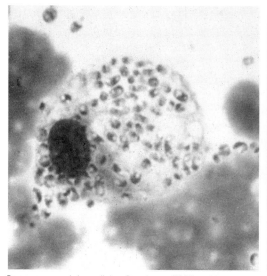

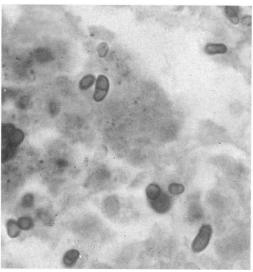

Bone marrow; intracellular. Courtesy of William Merz.

Bone marrow; extracellular. Courtesy of Ron C. Neafie.

Blastomycosis

ETIOLOGIC AGENT: *Blastomyces dermatitidis.*

SITES OF INFECTION: Lung, skin, bones, multiple systemic sites.

TISSUE REACTION: *Blastomyces* evokes a suppurative and/or granulomatous response. In young lesions, neutrophils predominate (eosinophils may also be present). In older lesions, the suppurative reaction decreases and granulomas, which may contain central abscesses and/or caseation, predominate. Long-standing infections commonly show fibrosis and sometimes cavitation. In skin, hyperplasia occurs.

MORPHOLOGY OF ORGANISM: Yeastlike cells (3–30 μm in diameter; most commonly 8–15 μm) are round to oval, with sharply defined refractile cell walls that are commonly referred to as "double contoured." The thick wall is seen with H&E and PAS, and it is sometimes lightly colored with mucicarmine stain, but it is not always conspicuous with GMS stain. Shrinkage of cytoplasmic contents and retraction from the rigid cell walls during fixation and processing creates clear spaces, or "halos," in the fungal cells. Each yeast cell produces only one bud, which is distinctively attached to the parent cell on a very **broad base** (average, 4–5 μm); the bud characteristically grows to the same size as the parent cell before detaching. (Color Plates 31 and 32.) Budding in vivo may be relatively infrequent.

Small spherules of *Coccidioides* may be easily mistaken for yeast cells of *Blastomyces*, especially if two spherules abut one another and give the impression of broad-based budding. Both organisms have thick refractile walls, but close examination should reveal typical single spherules with endospores.

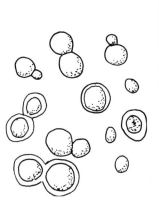

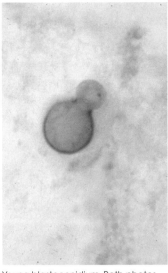

Young blastoconidium. Both photos courtesy of Joan Barenfanger.

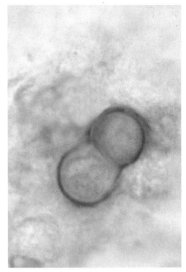

Mature blastoconidium.

Paracoccidioidomycosis

ETIOLOGIC AGENT: *Paracoccidioides brasiliensis.*

SITES OF INFECTION: Lung, skin, mucous membranes, multiple systemic sites.

TISSUE REACTION: A mixed suppurative and granulomatous inflammatory response is elicited by *P. brasiliensis* in pulmonary infections. Neutrophilic abscesses may predominate in one area of tissue while another area contains mainly granulomas. In rapidly progressing lesions, necrosis is frequently observed. In long-standing disease, fibrosis is common and calcification may occasionally occur. In mucocutaneous infections, ulceration and pseudoepitheliomatous hyperplasia may be seen.

MORPHOLOGY OF ORGANISM: Yeastlike cells are round to oval and can become quite large (3–30 μm or more in diameter). The outstanding characteristic is the presence of multiple buds that are attached to the parent cell by narrow connections. Buds may be small and all approximately the same size or fairly large and of unequal sizes and shapes. A large parent cell surrounded by small buds creates the classic "ship's wheel" appearance; parent cells with fewer, but larger, buds are common, and single budding may also be seen.

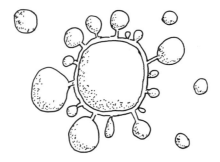

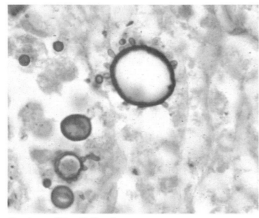

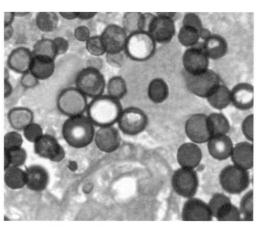

Courtesy of Ron C. Neafie.

Courtesy of Douglas Flieder.

Candidiasis (Candidosis)

ETIOLOGIC AGENTS: *Candida albicans, Candida tropicalis, Candida glabrata, Candida parapsilosis*, other *Candida* spp.

SITES OF INFECTION: Blood, mucous membranes, skin, nails, multiple systemic sites (appearance in the urine can be an early indication of candidemia).

TISSUE REACTION: In systemic infections, *Candida* spp. most commonly elicit an acute suppurative inflammation, sometimes forming abscesses composed of polymorphonuclear as well as mononuclear cells. Coagulative necrosis replaces the suppurative reaction in neutropenic patients. Granulomas only rarely occur (generally with chronic systemic candidiasis); other yeastlike fungi are more likely than *Candida* to form granulomatous lesions. *Candida* spp. are also known to invade blood vessels and produce infarcts (see p. 19).

MORPHOLOGY OF ORGANISM: All species of *Candida* form round to oval budding yeast cells (blastoconidia, 3–6 μm in diameter) singly, in chains, or in small loose clusters. Most species, when invading tissue, form both pseudohyphae and true hyphae. Pseudohyphae are actually chains of blastoconidia that have elongated and have not separated from one another. They can be recognized by the distinct constrictions at the septa; also, pseudohyphal branching will only occur at the site of a septation. True hyphae have no, or only slight, constrictions at the septa, and there is often no septation at the initiation of a branch. Blastoconidia develop along the sides of both types of hyphae.

C. glabrata is unique in that it is slightly smaller (2–5 μm in diameter) than the other species of *Candida*, and it does not produce any hyphal forms. The small yeast cells often aggregate in clusters and may closely resemble *Histoplasma capsulatum*, but no halo or pseudocapsular effect is seen when the cells are stained with H&E.

Culture is required to identify any *Candida* to species level.

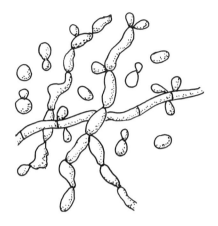

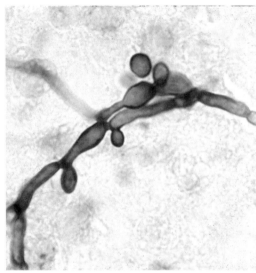

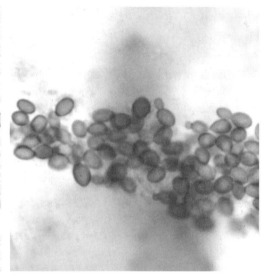

Candida albicans.

Candida glabrata. Both photos courtesy of Joan Barenfanger.

Cryptococcosis

ETIOLOGIC AGENT: *Cryptococcus neoformans.*

SITES OF INFECTION: Lung, meninges and cerebrospinal fluid, blood, skin, mucous membranes, multiple systemic sites.

TISSUE REACTION: In immunocompetent patients, *C. neoformans* evokes a mixed suppurative and granulomatous reaction or a purely granulomatous reaction with various degrees of necrosis. Chronic pulmonary infection results in the formation of residual granulomas (cryptococcomas). Healing is by fibrosis, generally without calcification.

In immunocompromised patients, the reaction may be minimal or absent. In this case, the yeasts proliferate abundantly, creating mucoid "cystic" lesions packed with round, encapsulated cryptococci that resemble "soap bubbles"; these are seen most frequently in the brain. The number of organisms present in the tissue is inversely proportional to the number of inflammatory cells.

Candidiasis differs from cryptococcosis by most commonly producing a purely suppurative reaction.

MORPHOLOGY OF ORGANISM: The yeast cells (i) are 2–20 μm in diameter (usually 4–10 μm); (ii) vary in size within the microscopic field; (iii) may be oval, but are more typically round with thin dark walls; (iv) bud on a narrow base; and (v) characteristically produce thick capsules, but cells relatively deficient in capsular material sometimes occur.

Capsules should be suspected when the yeast cells do not appear to touch one another (due to the surrounding mucopolysaccharide capsular material). In smeared specimens, capsules are demonstrated with India ink. (Color Plate 33.) Tissues stained with mucicarmine show the capsule as bright carmine red, often with a spiny or scalloped appearance. (Color Plate 34.) The mucicarmine stain may also color the cell walls of *Rhinosporidium seeberi* and *Blastomyces dermatitidis*. The cryptococcal yeast cell (but not the capsule) is stained by GMS. Because the cell walls of *C. neoformans* contain melanin-like substances, they become brown to black with the Fontana-Masson stain. Drying, fixing, and staining may cause the yeast cells to collapse or become crescent shaped.

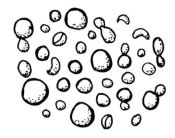

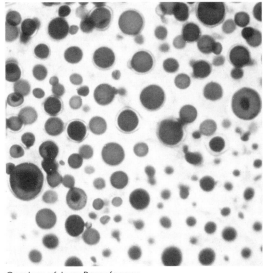

Courtesy of Joan Barenfanger.

Pneumocystosis

ETIOLOGIC AGENT: *Pneumocystis carinii*.*

SITE OF INFECTION: Lung.

TISSUE REACTION: The prominent characteristic in the lung is a foamy exudate in the alveolar spaces; this foam can be observed in lung biopsies as well as in specimens of bronchoalveolar lavage and, in many cases, induced sputum; this reaction is almost diagnostic of infection with *P. carinii*. The organisms are seen in the foamy exudate. Granulomatous reaction has been reported on rare occasions.

MORPHOLOGY OF ORGANISM: The most commonly used stains for *Pneumocystis* (GMS, CFW, and toluidine blue O) stain the cyst form, not the trophozoite. The cysts (4–7 mm in diameter) are nonbudding and are round, ovoid, or collapsed crescent forms; they characteristically have focal thickenings in the wall that appear as single or double "commas" or a set of "parentheses." The organisms occur in small clusters on a thick foamy background. (Color Plate 35.) Immuno-specific stain is commercially available. *P. carinii* does not grow on routine culture.

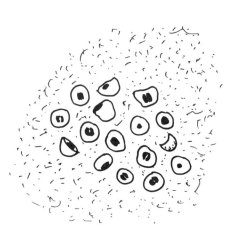
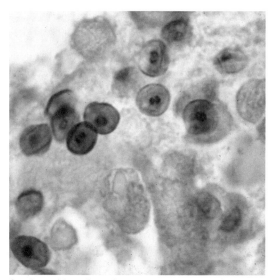

Courtesy of Joan Barenfanger.

---

*The taxonomic position of *P. carinii* is controversial; phylogenically it appears to belong in the periphery of the kingdom Fungi.

Protothecosis

ETIOLOGIC AGENTS: *Prototheca wickerhamii* (the species more commonly encountered in human infections) and *Prototheca zopfii*. They are actually achlorophyllous algae.

SITES OF INFECTION: Skin and subcutaneous tissue, bursa of the elbow, very rarely systemic sites.

TISSUE REACTION: Skin biopsies show varying degrees of nonspecific changes, including hyperkeratosis, parakeratosis, and acanthosis. The inflammatory response may be minor or absent, or it may consist of mononuclear and/or granulomatous infiltrates, with or without necrosis. Bursitis of the elbow typically exhibits necrotizing granulomas.

MORPHOLOGY OF ORGANISM: Round or oval sporangia of *P. wickerhamii* vary from 3–15 μm in diameter, while those of *P. zopfii* are 7–30 μm in diameter. Each sporangium of *P. wickerhamii* contains 2–20 endospores; only 4–8 are usually visible in one plane, and they appear round, polyhedral, or wedge shaped in a radial arrangement. The spores are densely basophilic, staining deep purplish blue with H&E. The organisms are best seen with the special stains for fungi. Hyaline, nonviable ghostlike forms may also be present.

    P. zopfii can be similar to *P. wickerhamii*, but it frequently forms oval, non-endosporulating cells, each having vacuolated cytoplasm and a single, discrete, basophilic nucleus.

    The size of the mother cells and differences in the number and morphology of endospores help differentiate *Prototheca* from *Coccidioides*.

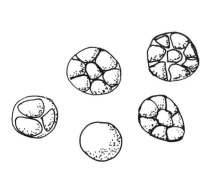

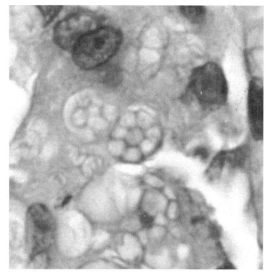

Courtesy of Evelyn Koestenblatt.

Coccidioidomycosis

ETIOLOGIC AGENT: *Coccidioides immitis.*

SITES OF INFECTION: Lung, skin, bone, meninges; dissemination to multiple systemic sites.

TISSUE REACTION: A granulomatous reaction develops in the presence of spherules, and a predominantly suppurative reaction occurs in response to released endospores; both of the forms and reactions commonly occur simultaneously. Splendore-Hoeppli material sometimes surrounds spherules and aggregates of endospores.

MORPHOLOGY OF ORGANISM: Round spherules can be as small as 5 μm in diameter when immature (nonendosporulating) and grow to 30–100 μm or more in diameter upon maturity (endosporulating). Immature spherules stain well with PAS and GMS, but mature spherules are GMS variable and PAS negative due to the high phospholipid content of the mature cell wall (1–2 μm in width). Endospores are round (2–5 μm in diameter) and uninucleate and have walls and cytoplasmic inclusions that are GMS and PAS positive. (Color Plate 36.) The spherules and endospores stain with H&E and are readily visible in sufficient numbers. Fragmented or empty ruptured spherules are common. Septate hyphae and barrel-shaped arthroconidia are sometimes observed in cavitary and necrotic lesions.

When only endospores are seen, they may initially be confused with yeasts, but endospores do not bud. When two immature spherules abut one another, they can give the impression of broad-based budding cells of *Blastomyces dermatitidis.*

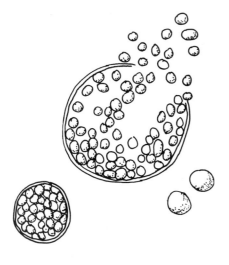

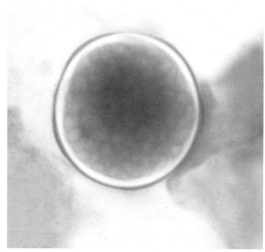

Courtesy of Joan Barenfanger.

Rhinosporidiosis

ETIOLOGIC AGENT: *Rhinosporidium seeberi* (does not grow on synthetic media).

SITES OF INFECTION: Mucocutaneous tissue, primarily involving the nasal cavity, nasopharynx, and oral cavity; secondary skin infections and rarely limited systemic dissemination have been reported.

TISSUE REACTION: In the submucosa or dermis, a chronic inflammatory response (mostly lymphocytes, plasma cells, and various numbers of epithelioid cells and neutrophils) with granulation tissue is typically seen. If the sporangia rupture and endospores are released, a granulomatous reaction is likely, but in some instances a suppurative response may occur.

MORPHOLOGY OF ORGANISM: Mature sporangia are thick walled (~5 μm wide), round, large (100–350 μm in diameter; most commonly 100–200 μm), and contain numerous sporangiospores (endospores) that range from 1–10 μm in diameter. A zonal pattern of sporangiospore development is uniquely characteristic of this pathogen: small, young spores are seen peripherally along the inner wall or form a crescent-like mass at one pole of the sporangium; medium-size, enlarging spores are between the periphery and the center; and the larger, mature spores are centrally located. Mature sporangiospores appear lobulated due to globular eosinophilic inclusions and, when released into the tissue, can be suggestive of *Prototheca* (p. 139). The walls of the sporangiospores and the mature sporangia are GMS and PAS positive. Mucicarmine also will stain the walls of the spores and the inner surface of the sporangial wall. (Color Plate 37.) Special fungal stains are seldom necessary, as the organism is readily seen with H&E.

Trophocytes (immature sporangia) are 10–100 μm in diameter with refractile eosinophilic walls approximately 2–3 μm thick. Trophocytes contain granular or flocculent cytoplasm and a round pale nucleus with a prominent nucleolus or karyosome. They are readily seen with H&E but do not stain well with GMS.

The etiologic agent, *R. seeberi*, cannot be cultured; diagnosis depends on direct examination of infected tissue.

(continued on following page)

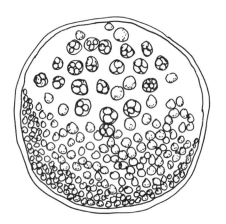

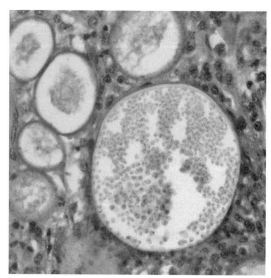

Courtesy of Douglas Flieder.

Adiaspiromycosis

ETIOLOGIC AGENT: *Emmonsia crescens.*

SITE OF INFECTION: Lung.

TISSUE REACTION: The typical inflammatory response is granulomatous and fibrotic. A granuloma forms around each adiaconidium (formerly adiaspore), which in turn is surrounded by dense fibrous connective tissue. Giant cells are often in contact with the outer spore wall. Polymorphonuclear leukocytes, especially eosinophils, may also be seen in the presence of small, immature adiaconidia. Necrosis or caseation is almost never seen. In some individuals, there is little, or no, host response (regardless of the level of immunocompetence).

MORPHOLOGY OF ORGANISM: Mature adiaconidia are round, large (200–400 µm in diameter), and thick walled (20–70 µm in width). The narrow outer layer of the adiaconidial wall is eosinophilic; a thin middle layer of the wall has irregular perforations that may appear as unstained spots; the inner layer of the wall is broad, hyaline, and composed predominantly of chitin. The walls can be readily seen with H&E and stain extremely well with GMS, PAS, and Gridley fungus stains. The interior of the conidium usually appears empty, but small (1–3 µm in diameter), refractile, eosinophilic hyaline globules may be seen along the inner surface of the wall. There is no evidence of replication, i.e., no budding or endosporulation.

If starch granules of lentils and other legumes are aspirated into the lungs, a pneumonitis may develop that can somewhat resemble adiaspiromycosis, but the starch granules of the legumes will have thinner walls and contain loculated material that can be seen with PAS and other stains.

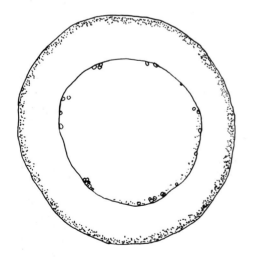

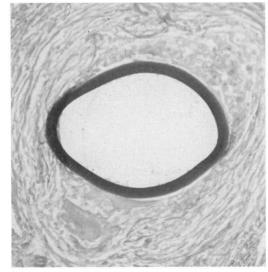

Courtesy of Ron C. Neafie.

Special References

For further information and additional photomicrographs, see:

Chandler, F. W., and J. C. Watts. 1987. *Pathologic Diagnosis of Fungal Infections*. American Society of Clinical Pathology Press, Chicago, Ill.

Connor, D. H., F. W. Chandler, D. Schwartz, H. Manz, and E. Lack. 1997. *Pathology of Infectious Diseases*. Appleton & Lange, Stamford, Conn.

Kimura, M., and M. R. McGinnis. 1998. Fontana-Masson-stained tissue from culture-proven mycoses. *Arch. Pathol. Lab. Med.* **122:**1107–1111.

Koneman, E. W., and G. D. Roberts. 1991. Mycotic disease, p. 1099–1130. *In* J. B. Henry (ed.), *Clinical Diagnosis and Management by Laboratory Methods*, 18th ed. The W. B. Saunders Co., Philadelphia, Pa.

Kwon-Chung, K. J., and J. E. Bennett. 1992. *Medical Mycology*. Lea & Febiger, Philadelphia, Pa.

Liu, K., D. N. Howell, J. R. Perfect, and W. A. Schell. 1998. Morphologic criteria for the preliminary identification of *Fusarium*, *Paecilomyces*, and *Acremonium* species by histopathology. *Am. J. Clin. Pathol.* **109:**45–54.

Salfelder, K. 1990. *Atlas of Fungal Pathology*. Kluwer Academic Publishers, Dordrecht, The Netherlands.

Identification of
PART II Fungi in Culture

Guide to Identification of Fungi in Culture

FILAMENTOUS BACTERIA

Very thin (1 μm or less in diameter) branching filaments*
Aerobic Actinomycetes

Nocardia (p. **104**)

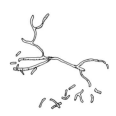

Streptomyces (p. **106**)

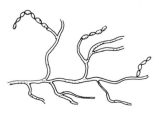

Actinomadura (p. **107**)

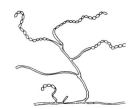

Nocardiopsis (p. **108**)

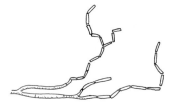

---

*Growth characteristics and biochemical tests must be utilized for identifications; these are summarized in Table 2 (p. 103).

MONOMORPHIC YEASTS AND YEASTLIKE ORGANISMS

Yeastlike at 25–30°C and also at 35–37°C if growth occurs
All rapid growers except *Ustilago* spp.
All WHITE, CREAM, or TAN except *Rhodotorula* and *Sporobolomyces* spp.

Microscopic morphology on Cornmeal-Tween 80 agar (Dalmau plate)*

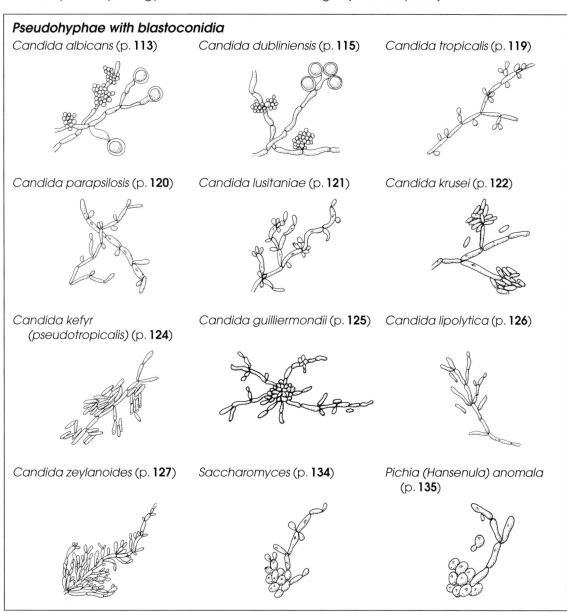

Pseudohyphae with blastoconidia

Candida albicans (p. **113**)   *Candida dubliniensis* (p. **115**)   *Candida tropicalis* (p. **119**)

Candida parapsilosis (p. **120**)   *Candida lusitaniae* (p. **121**)   *Candida krusei* (p. **122**)

Candida kefyr (pseudotropicalis) (p. **124**)   *Candida guilliermondii* (p. **125**)   *Candida lipolytica* (p. **126**)

Candida zeylanoides (p. **127**)   *Saccharomyces* (p. **134**)   *Pichia (Hansenula) anomala* (p. **135**)

*Morphology alone cannot be relied upon for identification. Use procedure on p. 305 and Tables 3 through 9 (pp. 114, 116, 118, 123, 130, and 131) for identification of genus and species.

MONOMORPHIC YEASTS AND YEASTLIKE ORGANISMS

Yeastlike at 25–30°C and also at 35–37°C if growth occurs *(continued)*
All rapid growers except *Ustilago* spp.
All WHITE, CREAM, or TAN except *Rhodotorula* and *Sporobolomyces* spp.

Microscopic morphology on Cornmeal-Tween 80 agar (Dalmau plate)*

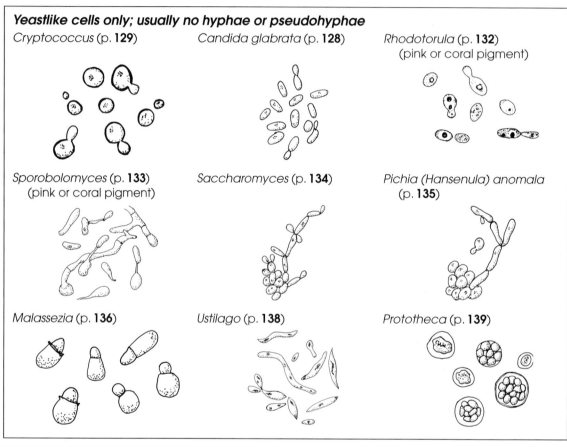

Yeastlike cells only; usually no hyphae or pseudohyphae

Cryptococcus (p. **129**)

Candida glabrata (p. **128**)

Rhodotorula (p. **132**)
(pink or coral pigment)

Sporobolomyces (p. **133**)
(pink or coral pigment)

Saccharomyces (p. **134**)

Pichia (Hansenula) anomala
(p. **135**)

Malassezia (p. **136**)

Ustilago (p. **138**)

Prototheca (p. **139**)

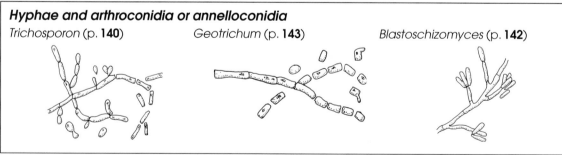

Hyphae and arthroconidia or annelloconidia

Trichosporon (p. **140**)

Geotrichum (p. **143**)

Blastoschizomyces (p. **142**)

*Morphology alone cannot be relied upon for identification. Use procedure on p. 305 and Tables 3 through 9 (pp. 114, 116, 118, 123, 130, and 131) for identification of genus and species.

THERMALLY DIMORPHIC FUNGI

Filamentous when cultured at 25–30°C; yeastlike when cultured at 35–37°C*

Sporothrix schenckii (p. 148)	*Histoplasma capsulatum* (p. 150)	*Blastomyces dermatitidis* (p. 152)	*Paracoccidioides brasiliensis* (p. 154)	*Penicillium marneffei* (p. 156)

25°C mould phase on Sabouraud dextrose agar

MACROSCOPICALLY:

Wrinkled, leathery, some short aerial mycelium when old	Loose, cottony	Smooth, then prickly, then cottony	Heaped; short mycelium	Flat, velvety
White, then tan or black	White or brownish	White, then brownish	White, then brownish	Tan, then reddish yellow and bluish green; red diffusing pigment

MICROSCOPICALLY:

Fine, branched, septate hyphae, "flowerette" conidial form	Branched, septate hyphae; microconidia; knobby macroconidia in 3–4 weeks	Branched, septate hyphae, single small conidia	Septate hyphae, chlamydoconidia, few microconidia	Septate hyphae, metulae, phialides, chains of conidia

37°C yeast phase on brain heart infusion agar

MACROSCOPICALLY: All cream or tan

MICROSCOPICALLY:

Round, oval, or "cigar"-shaped	Small budding cells	Large, double-contoured cells budding on a broad base	Large, multiple budding cells, "ship's wheel"	Oval cells with central septum; no budding

*See p. 309 for method of converting filamentous forms to yeast phase.

THERMALLY MONOMORPHIC MOULDS

Filamentous when cultured at 25–30°C and also at 35–37°C if growth occurs
SURFACE: WHITE, CREAM, OR LIGHT GRAY*
REVERSE: NONPIGMENTED

Having microconidia or macroconidia

Streptomyces** (p. **106**)

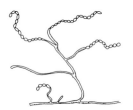

Microsporum vanbreuseghemii (p. **239**)

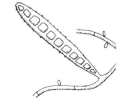

Trichophyton ajelloi (p. **252**)

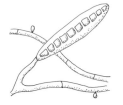

Trichophyton mentagrophytes (p. **241**)

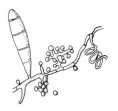

Trichophyton rubrum (p. **243**)

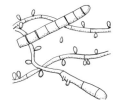

Tricophyton tonsurans (p. **244**)

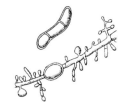

Trichophyton terrestre (p. **245**)

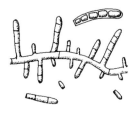

Fusarium (p. **280**)

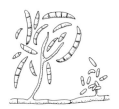

Acremonium (p. **279**)

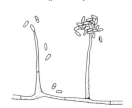

Phialemonium (p. **191**)

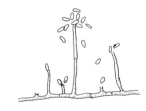

Verticillium (p. **278**)

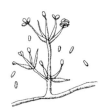

Beauveria (p. **277**)

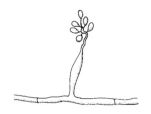

---

*Also see p. 71, as several thermally dimorphic fungi may fit this description at 25–30°C.

**Streptomyces is a filamentous bacterium.

THERMALLY MONOMORPHIC MOULDS

SURFACE: WHITE, CREAM, OR LIGHT GRAY*
REVERSE: NONPIGMENTED *(continued)*

Having microconidia or macroconidia (*continued*)

*Emmonsia*** (p. **265**)

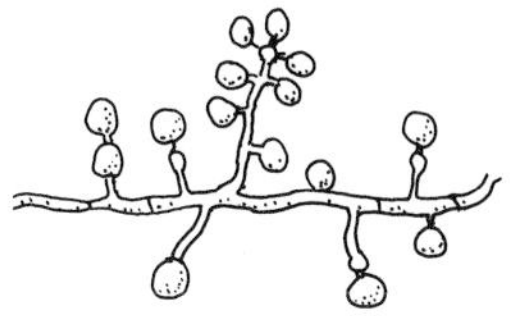

Pseudallescheria boydii (p. **197**) (*Scedosporium apiospermum*)

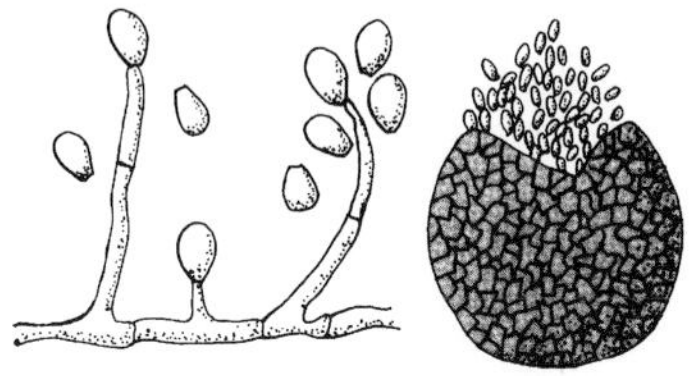

Chrysosporium (p. **284**)

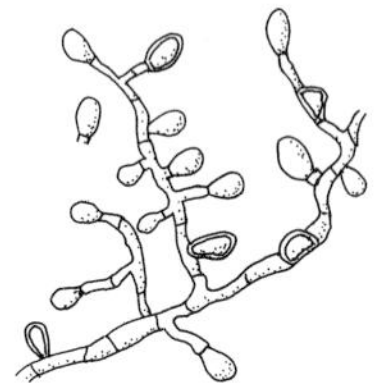

Sporotrichum (p. **287**)

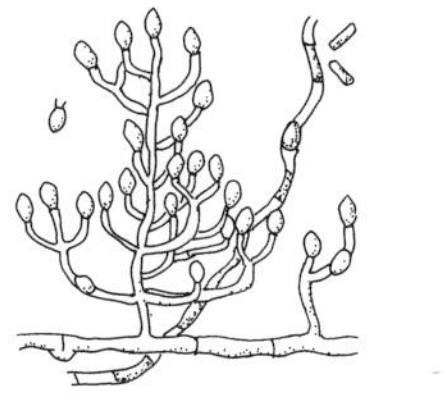

Sepedonium (p. **288**)

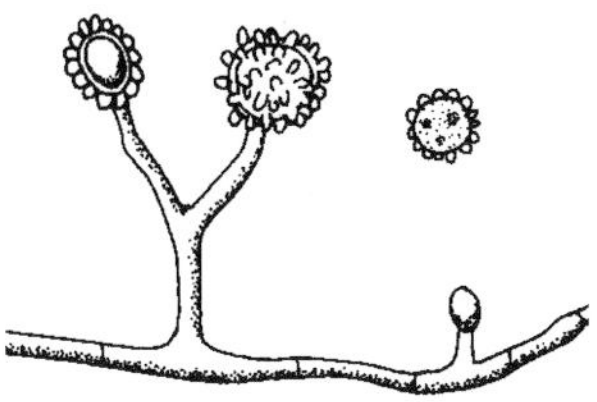

Graphium (p. **215**)

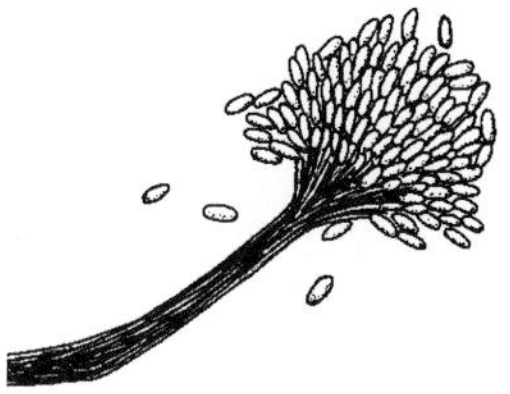

Stachybotrys (p. **214**)

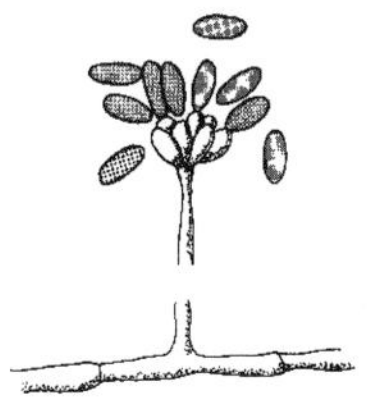

*Also see p. 71, as several thermally dimorphic fungi may fit this description at 25–30°C.
**Large adiaconidia form at ≥37°C.

THERMALLY MONOMORPHIC MOULDS

SURFACE: WHITE, CREAM, OR LIGHT GRAY*
REVERSE: NONPIGMENTED *(continued)*

Having sporangia or sporangiola

Rhizopus (p. **166**)

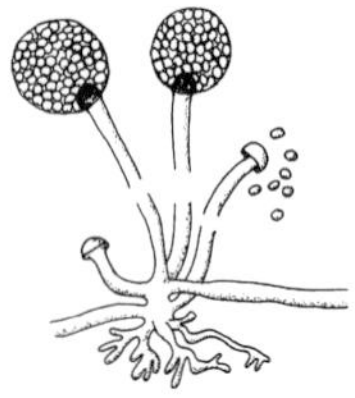

Mucor (p. **167**)

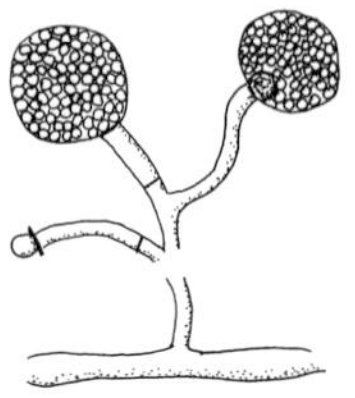

Rhizomucor (p. **168**)

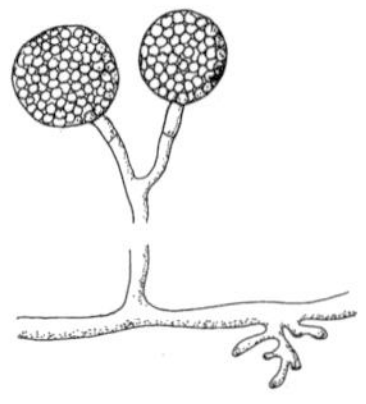

Absidia (p. **169**)

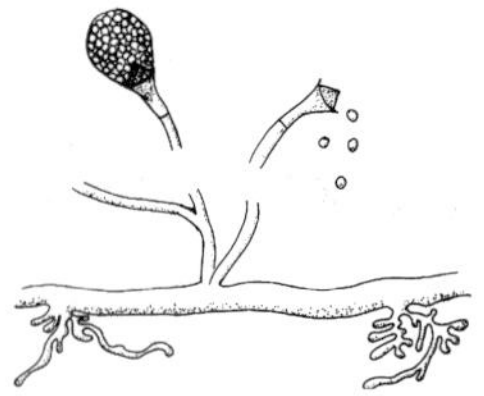

Apophysomyces (p. **170**)

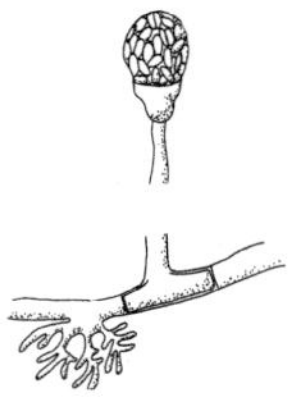

Saksenaea (p. **172**)

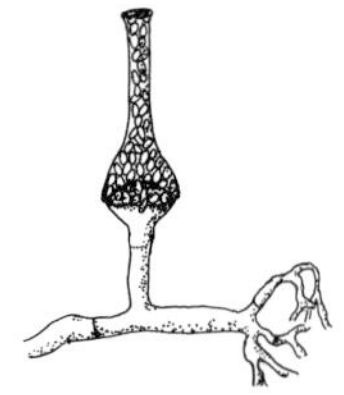

Cunninghamella (p. **174**)

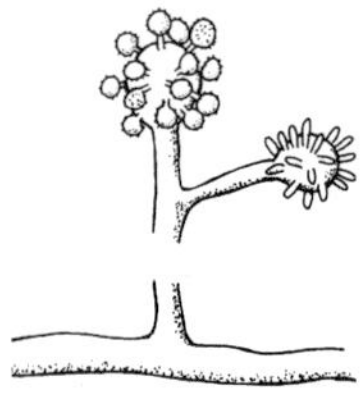

Basidiobolus (p. **176**)

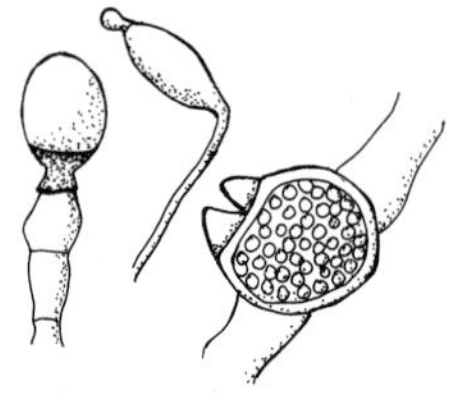

Conidiobolus (p. **177**)

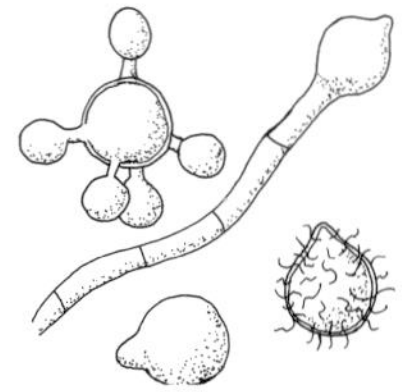

---

*Also see p. 71, as several thermally dimorphic fungi may fit this description at 25–30°C.

THERMALLY MONOMORPHIC MOULDS

SURFACE: WHITE, CREAM, OR LIGHT GRAY*
REVERSE: NONPIGMENTED *(continued)*

Having arthroconidia

Coccidioides (p. **259**)   Malbranchea (p. **261**)   Geomyces (p. **262**)

Arthrographis (p. **263**)   Geotrichum (p. **143**)   Scytalidium (p. **211**)

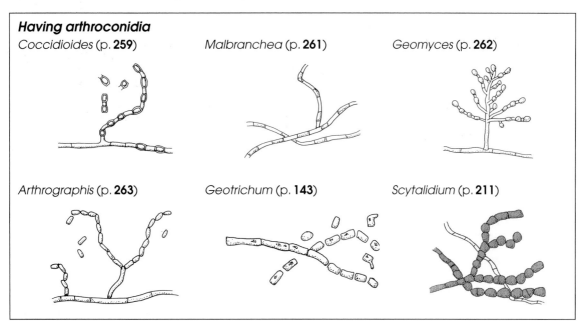

Having only hyphae with chlamydoconidia

Microsporum ferrugineum
   (p. **240**)   Trichophyton schoenleinii
   (p. **249**)   Trichophyton verrucosum
   (p. **250**)

Trichophyton violaceum (p. **251**)

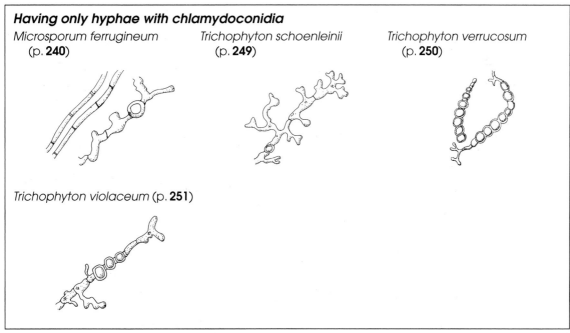

*Also see p. 71, as several thermally dimorphic fungi may fit this description at 25–30°C.

THERMALLY MONOMORPHIC MOULDS

SURFACE: WHITE, CREAM, BEIGE, OR LIGHT GRAY
REVERSE: YELLOW, ORANGE, OR REDDISH

Microsporum audouinii (p. **232**)

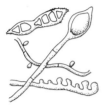

Microsporum canis var. *canis* (p. **233**)

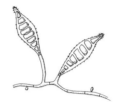

Microsporum canis var. *distortum* (p. **234**)

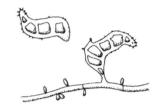

Microsporum gypseum (p. **236**)

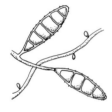

Microsporum nanum (p. **238**)

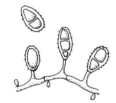

Microsporum vanbreuseghemii (p. **239**)

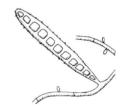

Trichophyton mentagrophytes (p. **241**)

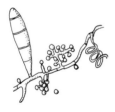

Trichophyton rubrum (p. **243**)

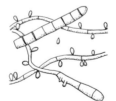

Trichophyton tonsurans (p. **244**)

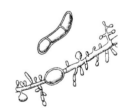

THERMALLY MONOMORPHIC MOULDS

SURFACE: WHITE, CREAM, BEIGE, OR LIGHT GRAY
REVERSE: YELLOW, ORANGE, OR REDDISH *(continued)*

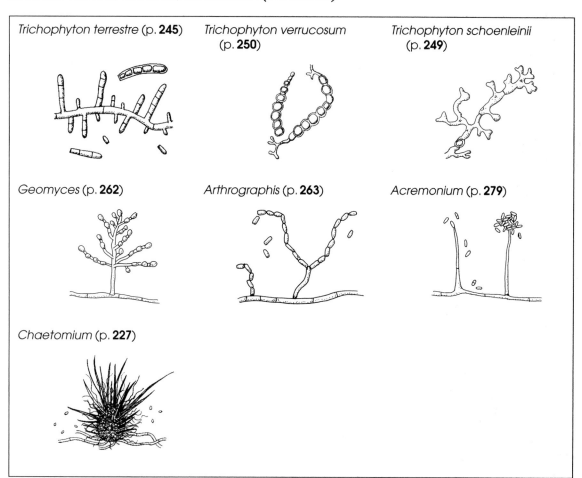

Trichophyton terrestre (p. **245**)

Trichophyton verrucosum (p. **250**)

Trichophyton schoenleinii (p. **249**)

Geomyces (p. **262**)

Arthrographis (p. **263**)

Acremonium (p. **279**)

Chaetomium (p. **227**)

THERMALLY MONOMORPHIC MOULDS

SURFACE: WHITE, CREAM, BEIGE, OR LIGHT GRAY
REVERSE: DEEP RED TO PURPLE

Microsporum gypseum (p. **236**)   *Microsporum cookei* (p. **235**)   *Microsporum gallinae* (p. **237**)

Trichophyton ajelloi (p. **252**)   *Trichophyton rubrum* (p. **243**)   *Trichophyton megninii* (p. **246**)

Trichophyton mentagrophytes (p. **241**)   *Penicillium marneffei** (p. **156**)

P. marneffei is thermally dimorphic.

THERMALLY MONOMORPHIC MOULDS

SURFACE: WHITE, CREAM, BEIGE, OR LIGHT GRAY
REVERSE: BROWNISH

Madurella mycetomatis
    (p. **204**)

Microsporum audouinii (p. **232**)

Microsporum ferrugineum
    (p. **240**)

Trichophyton schoenleinii
    (p. **249**)

Microsporum canis (p. **233**)

Microsporum gypseum (p.**236**)

Microsporum nanum (p. **238**)

Trichophyton mentagrophytes
    (p. **241**)

Trichophyton rubrum (p. **243**)

THERMALLY MONOMORPHIC MOULDS

SURFACE: WHITE, CREAM, BEIGE, OR LIGHT GRAY
REVERSE: BROWNISH *(continued)*

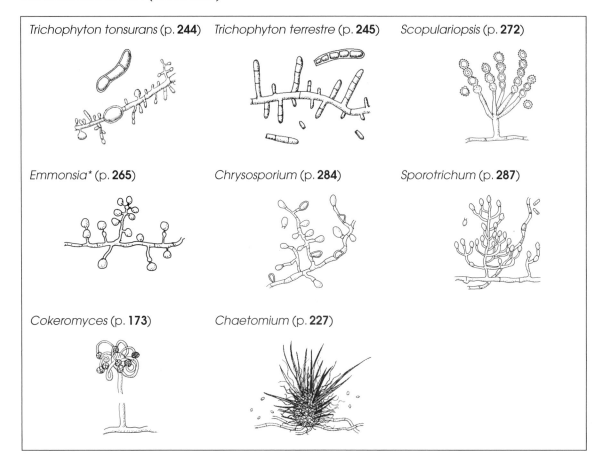

Trichophyton tonsurans (p. **244**)   Trichophyton terrestre (p. **245**)   Scopulariopsis (p. **272**)

Emmonsia* (p. **265**)   Chrysosporium (p. **284**)   Sporotrichum (p. **287**)

Cokeromyces (p. **173**)   Chaetomium (p. **227**)

*Large adiaconidia form at ≥37°C.

THERMALLY MONOMORPHIC MOULDS

SURFACE: WHITE, CREAM, BEIGE, OR LIGHT GRAY
REVERSE: BLACKISH

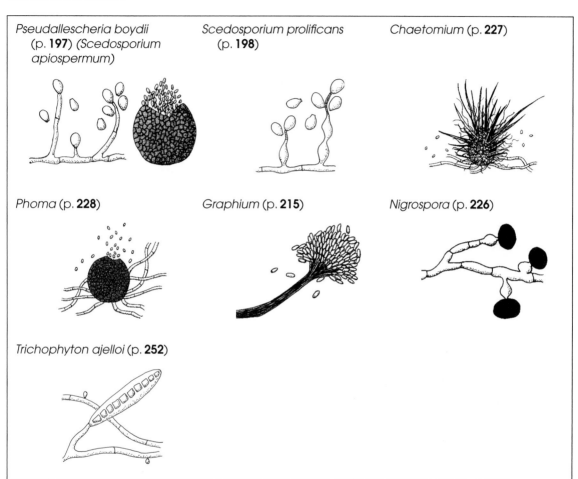

Pseudallescheria boydii (p. **197**) (Scedosporium apiospermum)

Scedosporium prolificans (p. **198**)

Chaetomium (p. **227**)

Phoma (p. **228**)

Graphium (p. **215**)

Nigrospora (p. **226**)

Trichophyton ajelloi (p. **252**)

THERMALLY MONOMORPHIC MOULDS

SURFACE: TAN TO BROWN*

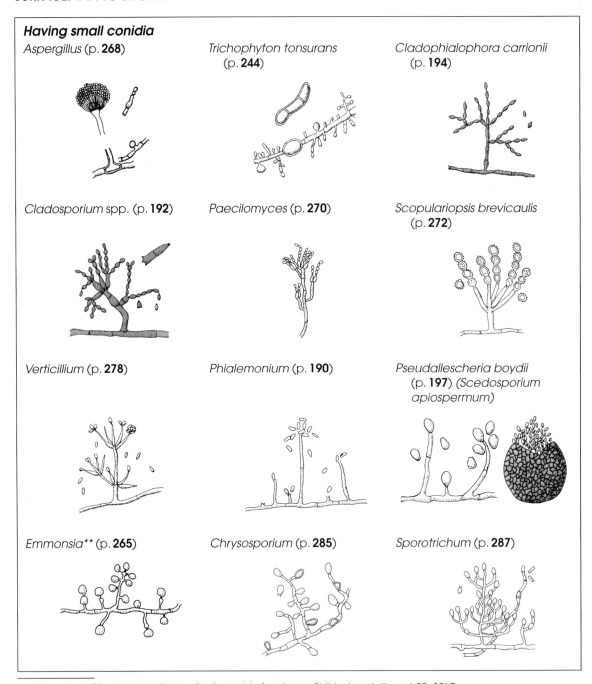

Having small conidia

Aspergillus (p. **268**)

Trichophyton tonsurans (p. **244**)

Cladophialophora carrionii (p. **194**)

Cladosporium spp. (p. **192**)

Paecilomyces (p. **270**)

Scopulariopsis brevicaulis (p. **272**)

Verticillium (p. **278**)

Phialemonium (p. **190**)

Pseudallescheria boydii (p. **197**) (Scedosporium apiospermum)

Emmonsia** (p. **265**)

Chrysosporium (p. **285**)

Sporotrichum (p. **287**)

*Also see p. 71, as several thermally dimorphic fungi may fit this description at 25–30°C.
**Large adiaconidia form at ≥37°C.

THERMALLY MONOMORPHIC MOULDS

SURFACE: TAN TO BROWN* *(continued)*

Having small conidia *(continued)*

Dactylaria (p. **199**)　　　Phialophora richardsiae (p. **188**)　Botrytis (p. **213**)

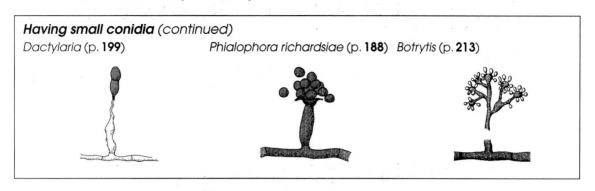

Having large conidia or sporangia

Rhizopus (p. **166**)　　　Mucor (p. **167**)　　　　Rhizomucor (p. **168**)

Apophysomyces (p. **170**)　　Cokeromyces (p. **173**)　　Basidiobolus (p. **176**)

Conidiobolus (p. **177**)　　Alternaria (p. **221**)　　Stemphylium (p. **223**)

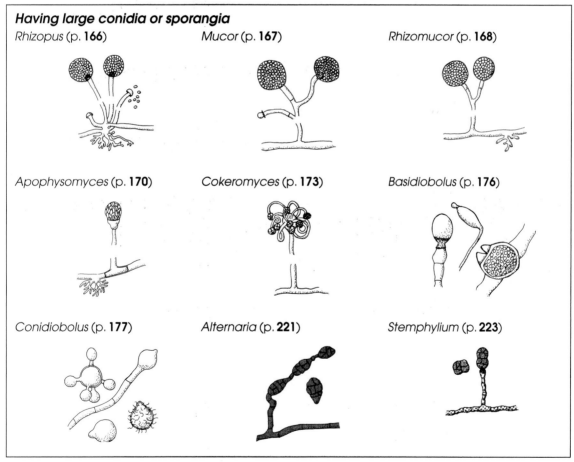

*Also see p. 71, as several thermally dimorphic fungi may fit this description at 25–30°C.

THERMALLY MONOMORPHIC MOULDS

SURFACE: TAN TO BROWN* *(continued)*

Having large conidia or sporangia (continued)

Ulocladium (p. **222**)

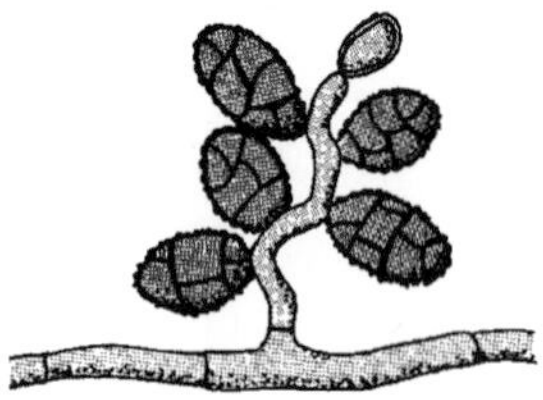

Epicoccum (p. **225**)

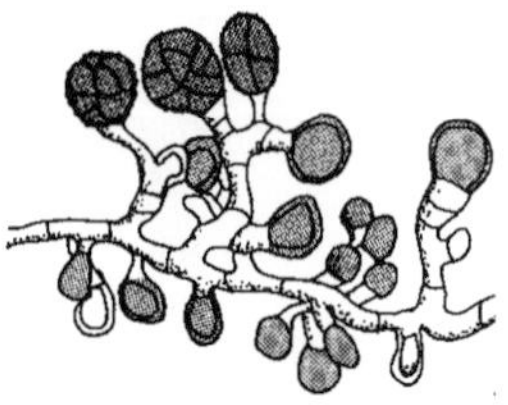

Curvularia (p. **216**)

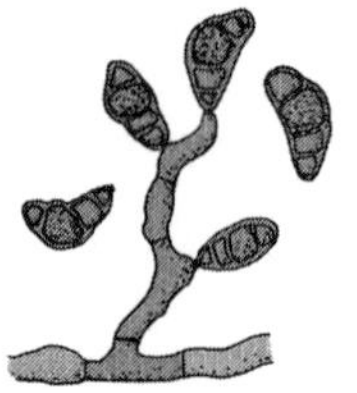

Bipolaris (p. **217**)

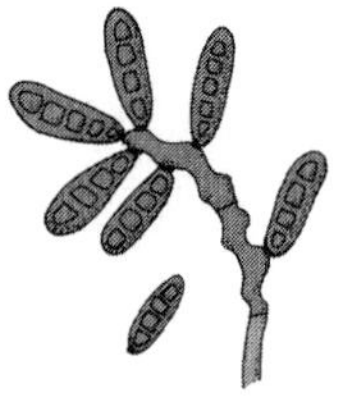

Microsporum gypseum (p. **236**)

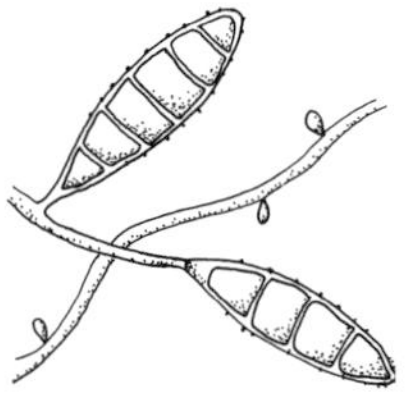

Microsporum cookei (p. **235**)

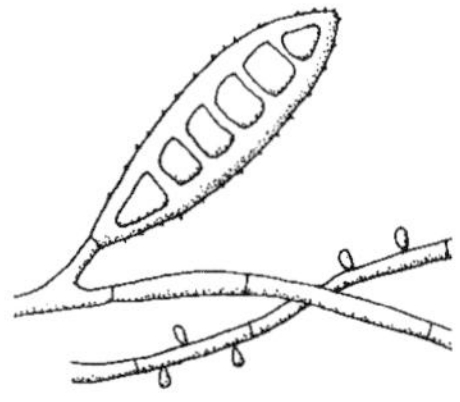

Microsporum nanum (p. **238**)

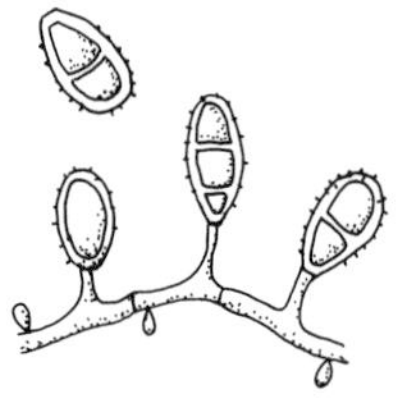

Microsporum vanbreuseghemii (p. **239**)

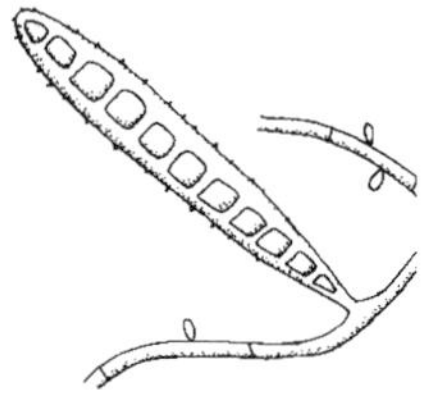

Trichophyton ajelloi (p. **252**)

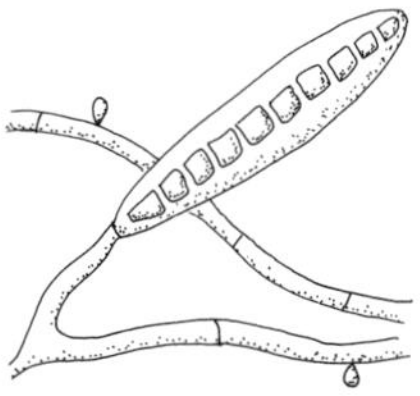

Epidermophyton floccosum (p. **253**)

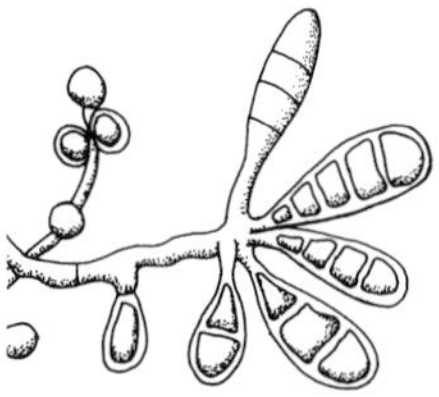

Fusarium (p. **280**)

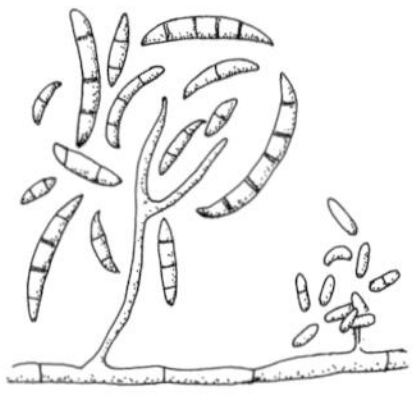

Botrytis (p. **213**)

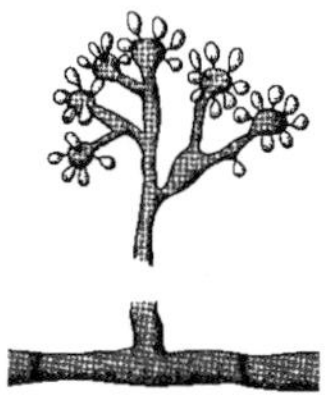

*Also see p. 71, as several thermally dimorphic fungi may fit this description at 25–30°C.

THERMALLY MONOMORPHIC MOULDS

SURFACE: TAN TO BROWN* *(continued)*

Having arthroconidia

Coccidioides (p. **259**)

Malbranchea (p. **261**)

Aureobasidium pullulans
(p. **208**)

Hormonema dematioides
(p. **210**)

Scytalidium (p. **211**)

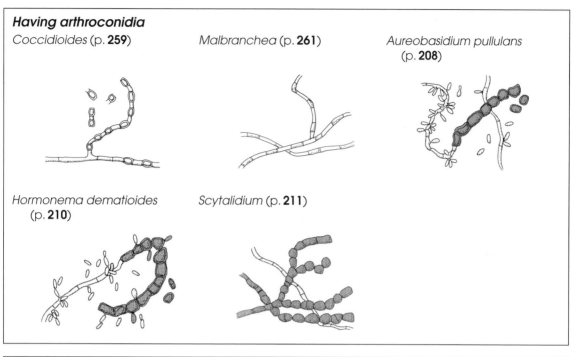

Having miscellaneous microscopic morphology

Ustilago (p. **138**)

Madurella mycetomatis
(p. **204**)

Madurella grisea (p. **205**)

Phoma (p. **228**)

Chaetomium (p. **227**)

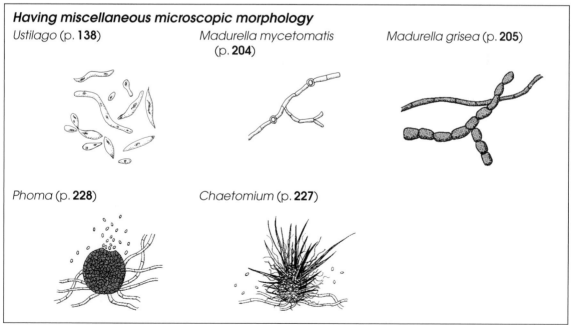

*Also see p. 71, as several thermally dimorphic fungi may fit this description at 25–30°C.

THERMALLY MONOMORPHIC MOULDS

SURFACE: YELLOW TO ORANGE

*Nocardia** (p. **104**)

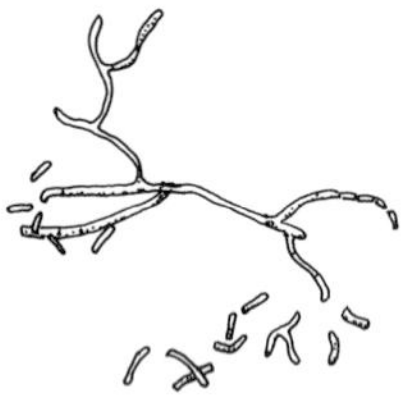

*Streptomyces** (p. **106**)

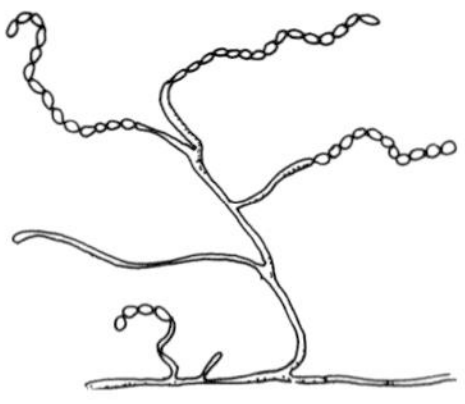

*Actinomadura** (p. **107**)

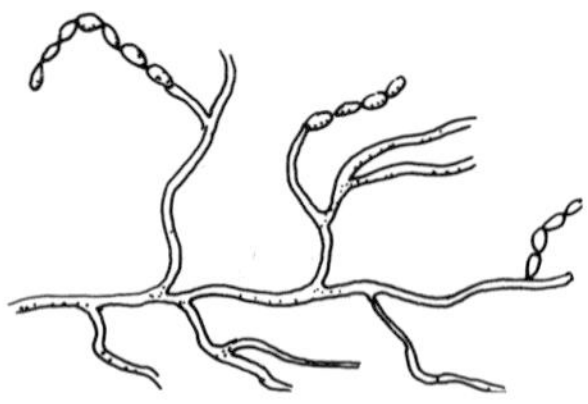

*Nocardiopsis** (p. **108**)

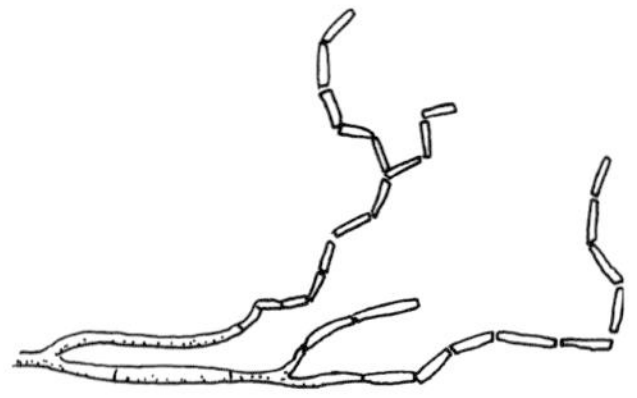

Trichophyton tonsurans (p. **244**)

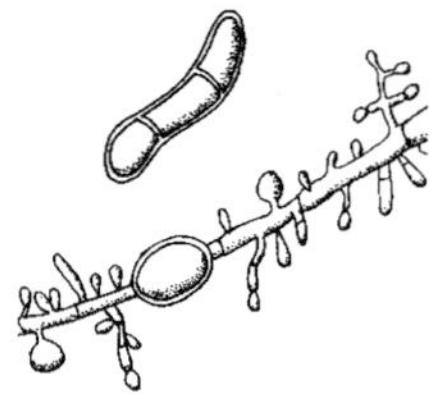

Trichophyton terrestre (p. **245**)

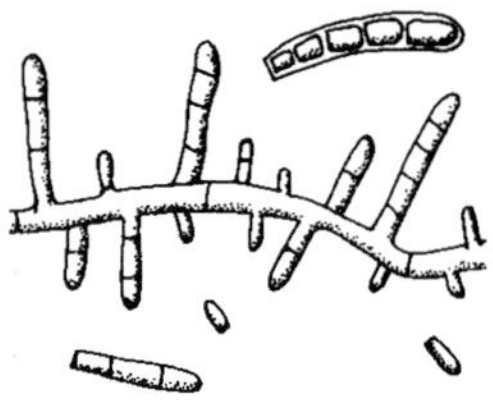

Microsporum ferrugineum (p. **240**)

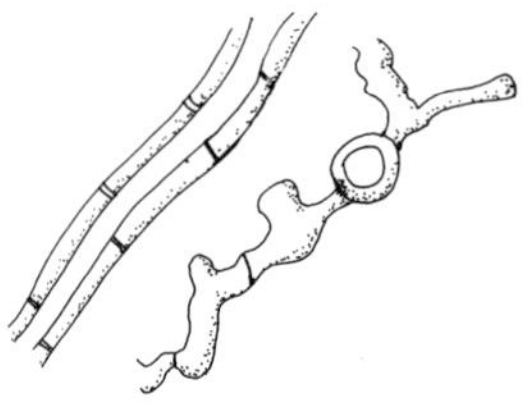

Trichophyton soudanense (p. **247**)

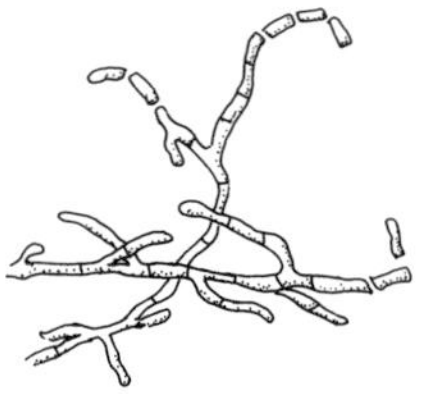

Trichophyton verrucosum (p. **250**)

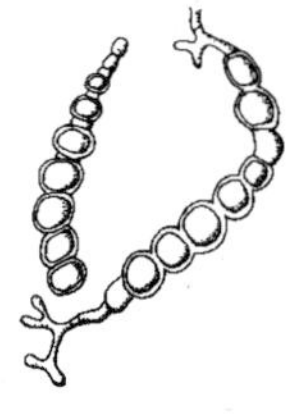

*These organisms are actinomycetes.

SURFACE: YELLOW TO ORANGE (continued)

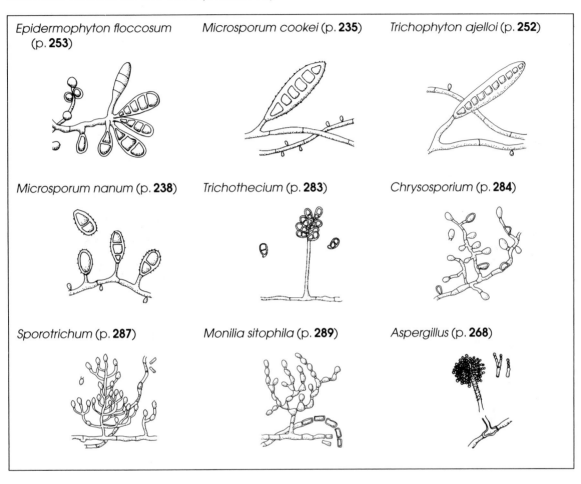

Epidermophyton floccosum (p. 253)

Microsporum cookei (p. 235)

Trichophyton ajelloi (p. 252)

Microsporum nanum (p. 238)

Trichothecium (p. 283)

Chrysosporium (p. 284)

Sporotrichum (p. 287)

Monilia sitophila (p. 289)

Aspergillus (p. 268)

SURFACE: YELLOW TO ORANGE *(continued)*

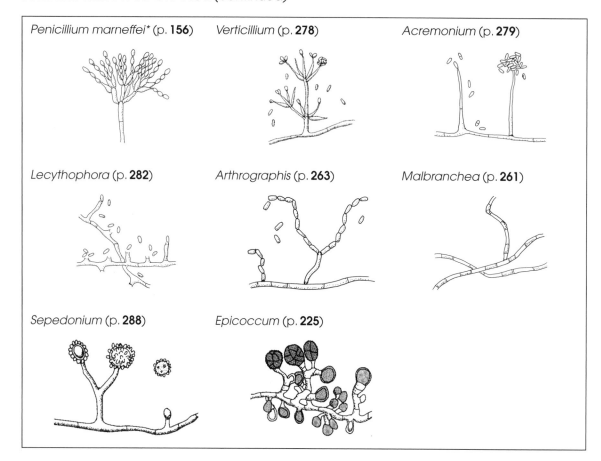

Penicillium marneffei (p. **156**) *Verticillium* (p. **278**) *Acremonium* (p. **279**)

Lecythophora (p. **282**) *Arthrographis* (p. **263**) *Malbranchea* (p. **261**)

Sepedonium (p. **288**) *Epicoccum* (p. **225**)

---

*P. marneffei is thermally dimorphic.

THERMALLY MONOMORPHIC MOULDS

SURFACE: PINK TO VIOLET

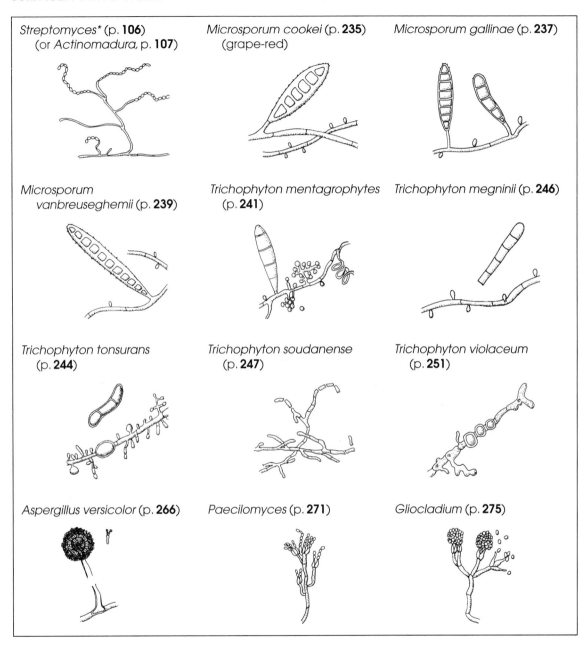

Streptomyces* (p. **106**)
  (or Actinomadura, p. **107**)

Microsporum cookei (p. **235**)
  (grape-red)

Microsporum gallinae (p. **237**)

Microsporum
  vanbreuseghemii (p. **239**)

Trichophyton mentagrophytes
  (p. **241**)

Trichophyton megninii (p. **246**)

Trichophyton tonsurans
  (p. **244**)

Trichophyton soudanense
  (p. **247**)

Trichophyton violaceum
  (p. **251**)

Aspergillus versicolor (p. **266**)

Paecilomyces (p. **271**)

Gliocladium (p. **275**)

---

*Streptomyces and Actinomadura are filamentous bacteria.

SURFACE: PINK TO VIOLET *(continued)*

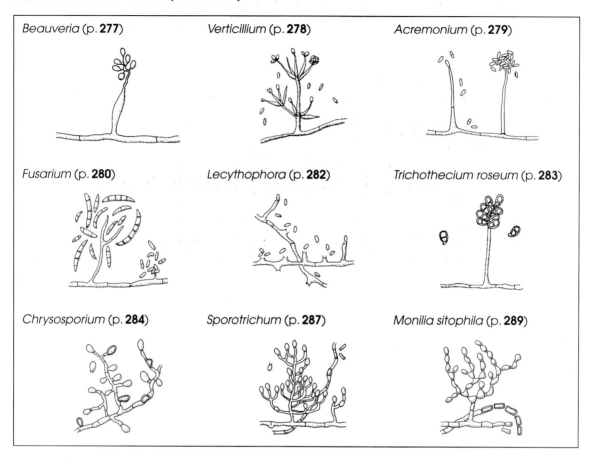

Beauveria (p. **277**)

Verticillium (p. **278**)

Acremonium (p. **279**)

Fusarium (p. **280**)

Lecythophora (p. **282**)

Trichothecium roseum (p. **283**)

Chrysosporium (p. **284**)

Sporotrichum (p. **287**)

Monilia sitophila (p. **289**)

THERMALLY MONOMORPHIC MOULDS

SURFACE: GREEN
REVERSE: LIGHT

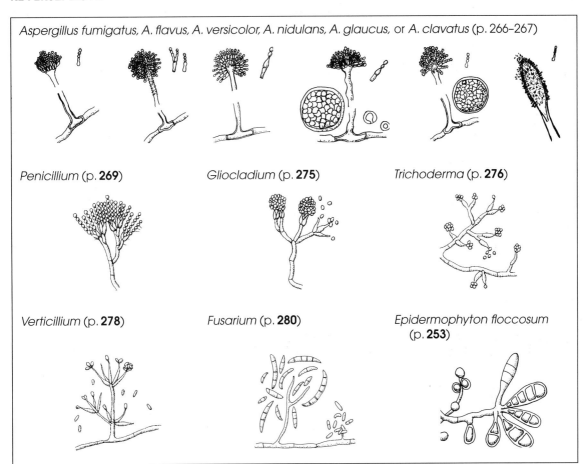

Aspergillus fumigatus, A. flavus, A. versicolor, A. nidulans, A. glaucus, or *A. clavatus* (p. 266–267)

Penicillium (p. **269**) *Gliocladium* (p. **275**) *Trichoderma* (p. **276**)

Verticillium (p. **278**) *Fusarium* (p. **280**) *Epidermophyton floccosum* (p. **253**)

SURFACE: DARK GRAY OR BLACK
REVERSE: LIGHT

Syncephalastrum (p. **175**)

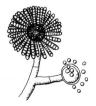

Aspergillus niger (p. **266**)

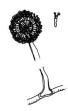

THERMALLY MONOMORPHIC MOULDS

SURFACE: GREENISH, DARK GRAY, OR BLACK
REVERSE: DARK

*Having small conidia**

Fonsecaea pedrosoi (p. **183**)

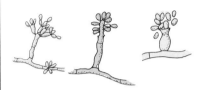

Fonsecaea compacta (p. **185**)

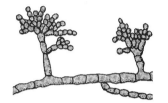

Phialophora verrucosa (p. **187**)

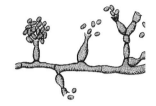

Phialophora richardsiae (p. **188**)

Cladosporium sp. (p. **192**)

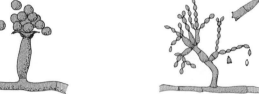

Cladophialophora carrionii (p. **194**)

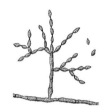

Cladophialophora bantiana (p. **195**)

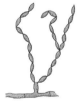

Phaeoacremonium parasiticum (p. **189**)

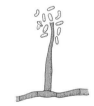

Exophiala jeanselmei (p. **201**)

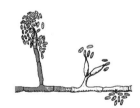

Wangiella dermatitidis (p. **202**)

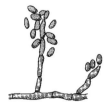

Phaeoannellomyces werneckii (p. **203**)

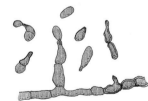

Pseudallescheria boydii (Scedosporium apiospermum) (p. **197**)

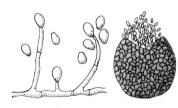

*Also see p. 71, as *Sporothrix schenckii* may fit this description at 25–30°C.

THERMALLY MONOMORPHIC MOULDS

SURFACE: GREENISH, DARK GRAY, OR BLACK
REVERSE: DARK *(continued)*

Having small conidia* (continued)

Scedosporium prolificans
(p. **198**)

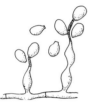

Dactylaria (p. **199**)

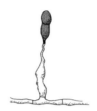

Scopulariopsis brumptii (p. **273**)

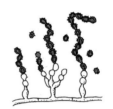

Stachybotrys (p. **214**)

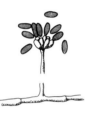

Aureobasidium pullulans
(p. **208**)

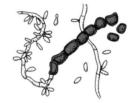

Hormonema dematioides
(p. **210**)

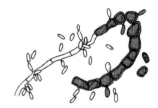

Botrytis (p. **213**)

---

*Also see p. 71, as *Sporothrix schenckii* may fit this description at 25–30°C.

94 GUIDE TO IDENTIFICATION OF FUNGI IN CULTURE

SURFACE: GREENISH, DARK GRAY, OR BLACK
REVERSE: DARK *(continued)*

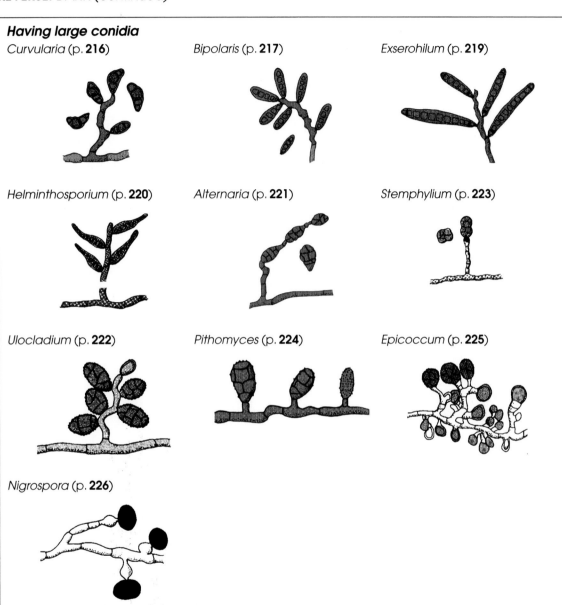

Having large conidia

Curvularia (p. **216**)

Bipolaris (p. **217**)

Exserohilum (p. **219**)

Helminthosporium (p. **220**)

Alternaria (p. **221**)

Stemphylium (p. **223**)

Ulocladium (p. **222**)

Pithomyces (p. **224**)

Epicoccum (p. **225**)

Nigrospora (p. **226**)

THERMALLY MONOMORPHIC MOULDS

SURFACE: GREENISH, DARK GRAY, OR BLACK
REVERSE: DARK *(continued)*

Having arthroconidia

Aureobasidium pullulans
   (p. **208**)

Hormonema dematioides
   (p. **210**)

Scytalidium (p. **211**)

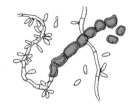
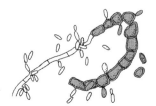
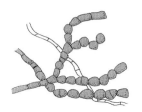

Having only hyphae (with or without chlamydoconidia)

Madurella grisea (p. **205**)

Piedraia hortae (p. **206**)

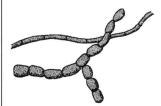
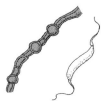

Having large fruiting bodies

Chaetomium (p. **227**)

Phoma (p. **228**)

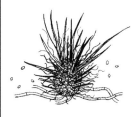
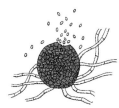

Detailed
Descriptions

Filamentous Bacteria

Introduction

The aerobic actinomycetes resemble fungi in that they form filaments that are well developed and branched (commonly referred to as hyphae). However, the results of cell wall analysis, lack of a membrane-bound nucleus, lack of mitochondria, small size, and susceptibility to antibacterial agents define these organisms as bacteria rather than fungi.

The aerobic actinomycetes are gram positive and have filaments that are 1 μm or less in diameter. Some may be partially acid fast when stained by a modified Kinyoun method (p. 315). These organisms grow on mycology media without antibacterial additives and on routine mycobacteriology media. The colonies are usually gla-brous and often become covered with a chalky or powdery coat. The microscopic morphology is best observed by slide culture on minimal medium, such as cornmeal-Tween 80 agar or 2% plain agar prepared with tap water.

In addition to morphology and staining characteristics, a battery of biochemical tests can be used to differentiate the organisms in this group (see Table 2, p. 103). It is occasionally necessary to confirm an identification by cell wall analysis, which is accomplished with thin-layer chromatography or high-performance liquid chromatography. These procedures are available in some reference laboratories.

The most commonly encountered pathogenic aerobic actinomycetes belong to the genus *Nocardia*; they cause pulmonary, systemic, and cutaneous diseases, including mycetomas. Members of the other genera are etiologic agents of mycetoma; some *Streptomyces* spp. are considered nonpathogenic contaminants.

For a complete review of the aerobic actinomycetes, see
  McNeil and Brown, 1994
  Murray et al. (ed.), 1999, Manual of Clinical Microbiology,
    7th ed., chapter 24

TABLE 2 Differentiation of aerobic actinomycetes[a]

Organism	Colony on Sabouraud dextrose agar	Fragmentation of hyphae[b]	Acid fast (partially)	Decomposition of:[c]						Growth with lysozyme	Acid from:		
				Casein	Tyrosine	Xanthine	Urea	Gelatin	Starch		Lactose	Xylose	Cellobiose
Nocardia asteroides complex[d]	White to pink or orange; glabrous or powdery; wrinkled	+	+	0	0	0	+	0^v	0^v	+	0	0	0
Nocardia brasiliensis	White to pink or orange; glabrous or powdery; wrinkled	+	+	+	+	0	+	+	0^v	+	0	0	0
Nocardia otitidiscaviarum[e]	White to pink or orange; glabrous or powdery; wrinkled	+	+	0	0^v	+	+	0	0^v	+	0	0	0
Nocardiopsis dassonvillei	Yellowish; heaped; wrinkled; chalky or velvety	+	0	+	+	+	+	+	+	0	0	+	+
Actinomadura madurae	White to tan, pink, red, or orange; glabrous; wrinkled; hard; adherent; slow growing	0	0	+	+^v	0	0	+	+	0	V	+	+
Actinomadura pelletieri	Bright red; heaped; glabrous	0	0	+	+	0	0	+	0	0	0	0	0
Streptomyces somaliensis	Cream to brown or black; slow growing; leathery; folded	0	0	+	+	0	0	+	V	0	0	0	0
Streptomyces anulatus (formerly *S.griseus*)	White or grayish, glabrous, chalky, or velvety	0	0 (spores often +)	+	+	+	+	+	+	0	+	+	+
Streptomyces spp. (*S. albus, S. lavendulae, S. rimosus*)	Variety of colors; glabrous, chalky, or velvety	0	0 (spores often +)	+	+	+^v	V	+^v	+^v	V	+^v	V	V

[a]Chromatographic analysis of cell walls or whole cells may be required (performed by reference laboratories). Abbreviations: +, positive; 0, negative; V, variable.

[b]Smears must be made with care to detect spontaneous fragmentation rather than that caused by trauma.

[c]Within 2 weeks at room temperature (25–30°C).

[d]*N. asteroides* complex includes *N. asteroides* sensu stricto (types 1 and IV), *N. nova*, and *N. farcinica*. *N. nova*, and *N. farcinica*. *N. nova* is distinguished by yielding a positive arylsulfatase test (within 14 days) and being susceptible to erythromycin (Kirby-Bauer disk diffusion; 30-μm disk; 48 h at 35°C; zone, ≥30 mm in diameter). *N. farcinica* produces a white opaque area around colonies on Middlebrook agar, and it is resistant to cefotaxime or ceftriaxone (MIC, ≥64 μg/ml).

[e]Formerly *Nocardia caviae*.

Nocardia spp.

PATHOGENICITY: Cause nocardiosis, which symptomatically may be similar to tuberculosis or actinomycosis. Disease may begin as a pulmonary infection and later involve the central nervous system, kidneys, and other organs. Skin lesions or subcutaneous abscesses may be the only manifestation of infection; occasionally mycetomas develop in the extremities. On rare occasions, the eye has been infected. The organisms are ubiquitous in nature and may therefore be encountered as contaminants or colonizers.

RATE OF GROWTH: Moderately rapid; mature in 7–9 days. Optimal growth is at 35–37°C. Grow on Sabouraud dextrose agar (SDA) without antibiotics and also on Lowenstein-Jensen (LJ) and Middlebrook 7H11 media (frequently survive decontamination procedures used for isolation of acid-fast bacilli). Excellent recovery has been reported on nonselective buffered charcoal yeast extract (BCYE) agar and also on Thayer-Martin agar (especially useful for inhibiting other organisms in mixed cultures).

COLONY MORPHOLOGY: Grow aerobically on SDA without antibiotics, forming raised, irregular, folded colonies varying from white to orange, depending on the species. May be glabrous or develop a white chalky coating. (Color Plates 38–41.)

MICROSCOPIC MORPHOLOGY: Delicate, branching, often beaded, intertwining filaments that fragment into bacillary and coccoid forms; best exhibited on slide culture using a minimal medium, such as cornmeal-Tween 80 agar. They are gram positive and often, but not always, partially acid fast (use a modified Kinyoun method [p. 315]). Young primary cultures are usually the most acid fast; acid fastness may be enhanced on Middlebrook 7H11 medium or by growing cultures for 3–4 weeks in a proteinaceous medium, such as litmus milk or bromocresol purple milk.

See Table 2 (p. 103) for differentiation of species.

Nocardia spp. *(continued)*

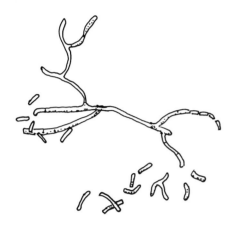

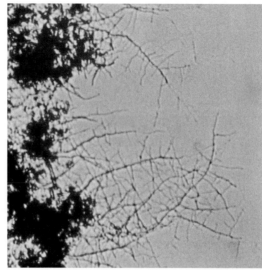

From Joseph Staneck, Aerobic actinomycetes: *Nocardia* and related organisms, ASM Teleconference of 9 August 1994.

For further information, see
   Kwon-Chung and Bennett, 1992, pp. 582–588
   McNeil and Brown, 1994
   Rippon, 1988, pp. 53–68, 94–103
   Wentworth, 1988, pp. 271–302

Streptomyces spp.

PATHOGENICITY: Most *Streptomyces* spp. are considered nonpathogenic contaminants. Other species, such as *S. somaliensis*, cause mycetomas and occasionally other types of infections. *S. anulatus* (formerly *S. griseus*) is the most commonly isolated species, but it only occasionally appears to be an etiologic agent of infection.

RATE OF GROWTH: Rapid or moderate; mature in 4–10 days. Optimum growth occurs at 30°C.

COLONY MORPHOLOGY: Surface is slightly folded, hard, leathery; may develop a fine chalky or powdery aerial mycelium. Many strains have various pigments of gray, orange, rose, red, or occasionally green. (Color plates 42 and 43.) Culture often produces the characteristic odor of freshly tilled soil.

MICROSCOPIC MORPHOLOGY: Hyphae are long, thin (1 μm or less in diameter), and abundantly branching, with filaments which may be straight, wavy, or spiral. Small oblong conidia are produced at distinct points on the filament; this is best observed on slide culture. Some species do not form conidia readily.

See Table 2 (p. 103) for differentiation of aerobic actinomycetes.

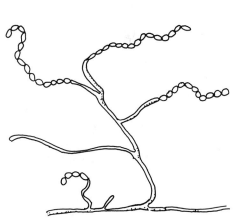
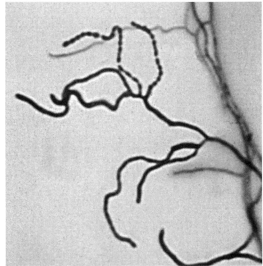

Courtesy of Morris Gordon.

For further information, see
  Kwon-Chung and Bennett, 1992, pp. 584, 588
  McNeil and Brown, 1994
  Rippon, 1988, pp. 97–103
  Wentworth, 1988, pp. 271–302

Actinomadura spp.

PATHOGENICITY: A frequent cause of mycetoma. They have also been isolated from sputum, wounds, blood, and other sites, suggesting the ability to colonize or infect some patients.

RATE OF GROWTH: Usually rapid on Lowenstein-Jensen (LJ) medium; slower on Sabouraud dextrose agar (SDA). Optimum growth is at 35–37°C.

COLONY MORPHOLOGY: Waxy, folded, membranous, or mucoid. May be white, tan, pink, orange, or red. White aerial hyphae may develop after 2 weeks of incubation; best seen on LJ medium.

MICROSCOPIC MORPHOLOGY: Narrow abundantly branched filaments (0.5–1 µm in diameter) that are gram positive, non-acid fast, and nonfragmenting. Short chains of round conidia may be produced from limited portions of the aerial hyphae; this is best observed on slide culture.

See Table 2 (p. 103) for differentiation of aerobic actinomycetes.

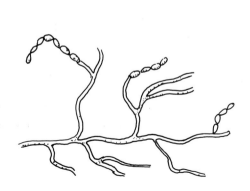 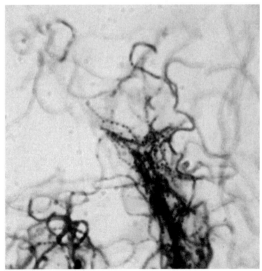

For further information, see
  Kwon-Chung and Bennett, 1992, pp. 582–585
  McNeil and Brown, 1994
  Rippon, 1988, pp. 97–102
  Wentworth, 1988, pp. 289–299

Nocardiopsis dassonvillei

PATHOGENICITY: Considered a potential cause of mycetoma, skin infections, and alveolitis. There have been very few reports of clinical disease.

RATE OF GROWTH: Moderately rapid; mature in 4–10 days.

COLONY MORPHOLOGY: Yellowish, heaped, irregularly wrinkled. Aerial hyphae may develop to form a velvety coating. A newly described species, *Nocardiopsis synnemataformans*, forms a deep pimento-red colony.

MICROSCOPIC MORPHOLOGY: Narrow filaments (1 μm or less in diameter) that are long, extensive, and sometimes branched; they are gram positive and non-acid fast. The filaments fragment into chains of arthroconidia, giving a characteristic zigzag appearance. The total length of the aerial hyphae turns into conidial chains, in contrast to *Actinomadura* spp. and *Streptomyces* spp., which produce conidial chains only at distinct parts of the hyphae.

See Table 2 (p. 103) for differentiation of aerobic actinomycetes.

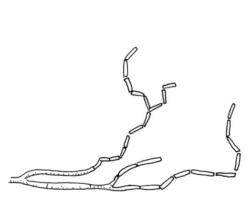
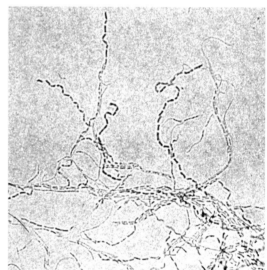

From McNeil and Brown, 1994.

For further information, see
Kwon-Chung and Bennett, 1992, pp. 582–588
McNeil and Brown, 1994
Rippon, 1988, pp. 98, 102

Yeasts and Yeastlike Organisms

Introduction

In this guide, the terms "yeast" and "yeastlike" refer to unicellular organisms that generally reproduce by budding. If the buds (blastoconidia) elongate and remain attached to the parent cell, they form chains known as pseudohyphae. Some of the organisms included here produce true septate hyphae, while others form no hyphal elements of any sort. A few are capable of producing ascospores. Organisms that are actually algae but that grow in a yeastlike manner are traditional members of this group.

Colonies are smooth and glabrous and may be moist or dry; they are usually white to cream colored, but some are tan, pinkish, or orangey.

The ability to produce pseudohyphae, true hyphae, and/or terminal chlamydospores and the shape and arrangement of blastoconidia are used along with other morphologic characteristics and biochemical tests to identify the yeasts to the genus and species levels. A number of commercial systems are available for biochemical testing (see p. 306). Microscopic morphology is studied on agar, such as cornmeal-Tween 80 agar, by using the Dalmau method (p. 335), which ensures the decreased oxygen environment required for the production of structures used for identification.

Yeasts are the most common fungi isolated in the clinical laboratory. They are ubiquitous in our environment and also live as normal inhabitants in our bodies, so it is often difficult to determine the clinical significance of an isolate. Implication of the yeast as the etiologic agent of infection often requires repeated recovery from the site and direct microscopic demonstration of the yeast in infected tissue. The yeasts and yeastlike organisms are considered opportunistic pathogens, causing disease in patients (i) with a breakdown in the body's immune system; (ii) on prolonged treatment with antibiotics, corticosteroids, or cytotoxic drugs; (iii) with intravascular catheters; (iv) with diabetes mellitus; or (v) who are intravenous drug abusers.

Candidiasis (also called candidosis) is by far the most common fungal infection (other than ringworm) seen in humans. Mucocutaneous infections are seen in individuals with defects in cell-mediated immunity, while systemic infections are primarily seen in neutropenic patients. Although *Candida* spp. are often isolated from respiratory specimens, they are seldom of clinical significance.

For further information, see
  Kurtzman and Fell, 2000, The Yeasts, a Taxonomic Study, 4th ed.
  Murray et al. (ed.), 1999, Manual of Clinical Microbiology, 7th ed., chapter 95

Candida albicans

PATHOGENICITY: Most common cause of candidiasis (see p. 52), which is an acute, subacute, or chronic infection involving any part of the body. This organism is found as part of the normal flora in the skin, mouth, vaginal tract, and gastrointestinal tract (therefore, it is often present in stools without significance).

RATE OF GROWTH: Rapid; mature in 3 days.

COLONY MORPHOLOGY: Cream colored, pasty, smooth. On enriched media (e.g., blood agar or chocolate agar), extensions commonly called "feet" develop at the border of the colony. (Color Plate 44.)

MICROSCOPIC MORPHOLOGY: On routine primary media, yeast cells are round to oval (3.5–7 × 4–8 μm). On cornmeal-Tween 80 agar (Dalmau plate, p. 335) at 25°C for 72 h, pseudohyphae (and some true hyphae) form with clusters of round blastoconidia at the septa. Large, thick-walled, usually single terminal chlamydospores are characteristically formed; they are most likely to be seen near the edge of the coverslip. Chlamydospore formation is inhibited at 30–37°C. *C. albicans* gives a positive reaction to the germ tube test (p. 307), as does *Candida dubliniensis*; to differentiate the two species, see Table 5 (p. 118).

Candida stellatoidea is no longer considered a separate species; it is now included in *C. albicans*.

See Table 3 (p. 114) for differentiation of yeastlike genera and Table 4 (p. 116) for characteristics of the most commonly encountered species of *Candida*.

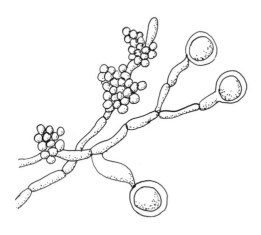

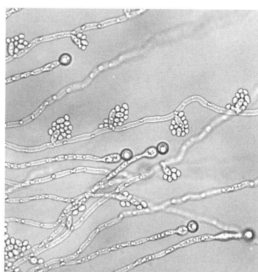

For further information, see
  de Hoog et al., 2000, pp. 184–188
  Kwon-Chung and Bennett, 1992, pp. 310–316
  Rippon, 1988, pp. 536–570

TABLE 3 Characteristics of the genera of clinically encountered yeasts and yeastlike organisms[a]

| Organism | On cornmeal-Tween 80 agar at 25°C | | | | | | | Capsule | Urease | With cycloheximide at 25°C | Growth: | |
	Pseudohyphae	True hyphae	Blastoconidia along hyphae	Arthroconidia	Annelloconidia	Ascospores	Sporangia				On SDA at 37°C	In Sabouraud broth
Candida	+	Few	+	0	0	0	0	0	0^V	V	$+^V$	Some species show surface growth
Rhodotorula	0^R	0		0	0	0	0	V	+	0^V	$+^V$	NSG
Cryptococcus	0^R	0		0	0	0	0	+	+	0	V	NSG
Saccharomyces	V	0		0	0	+	0	0	0	0	+	NSG
Hansenula	0^V	0		0	0	+	0	0	0	0	V	NSG
Malassezia	0^R	0^R		0	0	0	0	0	+	$+^{W,V}$	$+^V$	NSG
Prototheca	0	0		0	0	0	+	0^V	0	0	0^V	Surface growth
Geotrichum	0	+	0	+	0	0	0	0	0	0	0^W	Pellicle forms
Trichosporon	+	+	+	+	0	0	0	0	+	$+^V$	$+^V$	Pellicle forms
Blastoschizomyces	+	+	+	0^V	+	0	0	0	0	+	+	Pellicle forms

[a]Abbreviations: SDA, Sabouraud dextrose agar; +, positive; 0, negative; V, species or strain variation; W, weak; R, rarely few rudimentary forms; NSG, no surface growth.

Candida dubliniensis

PATHOGENICITY: Primarily associated with recurrent erythematous oral candidiasis in human immunodeficiency virus (HIV)-infected patients; it is also known, to a far lesser extent, to cause oral disease in non-HIV-infected individuals. Additionally, it has been involved in cases of disseminated disease in immunocompromised patients who are HIV negative. The organism is widespread throughout the world and has been recovered from a variety of clinical specimens without evidence of infection. Resistance to fluconazole has been found in clinical isolates, and it has been shown that fluconazole-susceptible isolates are able to rapidly develop resistance in vitro.

RATE OF GROWTH: Rapid; mature within 3 days.

COLONY MORPHOLOGY: Cream colored, pasty, smooth. On enriched media (e.g., blood agar or chocolate agar), extensions commonly called "feet" develop at the border of the colony.

MICROSCOPIC MORPHOLOGY: Very similar to that of *Candida albicans*. On cornmeal-Tween 80 agar (Dalmau plate, p. 335) at 25°C for 72 h, forms pseudohyphae, and some true hyphae, with clusters of round blastoconidia at the septa. Large, thick-walled terminal chlamydospores characteristically form in pairs or small clusters (as opposed to *C. albicans*, which usually produces terminal chlamydospores singly). *C. dubliniensis* (like *C. albicans*) yields a positive reaction with the germ tube test (p. 307); to differentiate the two species, see Table 5 (p. 118).

See Table 3 (p. 114) for differentiation of yeastlike genera and Table 4 (p. 116) for characteristics of the most commonly encountered species of *Candida*.

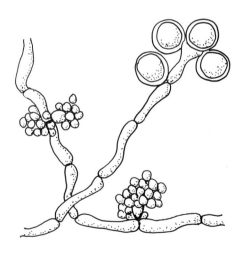

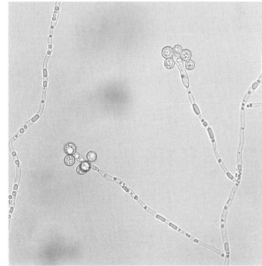

For further information, see
  de Hoog et al., 2000, pp. 194–195;
  Sullivan and Coleman, 1998; Sullivan et al., 1999

TABLE 4 Characteristics of *Candida* spp. most commonly encountered in the clinical laboratory[a]

Organism	Microscopic morphology on cornmeal-Tween 80 agar at 25°C	Growth:				Germ tubes
		In Sabouraud broth	With cycloheximide at 25°C	On SDA at 37°C		
C. albicans C. dubliniensis	Pseudohyphae with terminal chlamydospores; clusters of blastoconidia at septa	NSG	+	+		+
C. tropicalis	Blastoconidia anywhere along pseudohyphae	Narrow surface film with bubbles	0[V]	+		0
C. parapsilosis	Blastoconidia along curved pseudohyphae; giant mycelial cells	NSG	0	+		0
C. lusitaniae	Short chains of elongate blastoconidia along curved pseudohyphae	NSG	0	+		0
C. guilliermondii	Fairly short, fine pseudohyphae; clusters of blastoconidia at septa	NSG	+	+		0
C. kefyr (C. pseudotropicalis)	Elongated blastoconidia resembling "logs in a stream" along pseudohyphae	NSG	+	+		0
C. zeylanoides	Pseudohyphae give feather-like appearance at low power	Pellicle (delayed)	0	0[V]		0
C. glabrata	No pseudohyphae; cells small; terminal budding	NSG	0	+		0
C. krusei	Pseudohyphae with cross-matchsticks or treelike blastoconidia	Wide surface film up sides of tube	0	+		0
C. lipolytica	Elongated blastoconidia in short chains along pseudohyphae	Pellicle (delayed)	+	+		0

[a]Abbreviations: SDA, Sabouraud dextrose agar; +, positive; 0, negative; W, reaction may be weak; V, strain variation; NSG, no surface growth.

[b]Fermentation is demonstrated by the production of *gas* (acid does not indicate fermentation).

Urease (25°C)	Assimilation of:													Fermentation of:[b]						
	Dextrose	Maltose	Sucrose	Lactose	Galactose	Melibiose	Cellobiose	Inositol	Xylose	Raffinose	Trehalose	Dulcitol	KNO_3	Dextrose	Maltose	Sucrose	Lactose	Galactose	Trehalose	Cellobiose
0	+	+	V	0	+	0	0	0	$\frac{+}{0}$	0	$\frac{+}{0^V}$	0	0	+	+	0	0	V	V	0
0	+	+	$+^V$	0	+	0	$+^V$	0	+	0	+	0	0	+	+	$+^V$	0	$+^V$	$+^V$	0
0	+	+	+	0	+	0	0	0	+	0	+	0	0	+	0	0	0	V	0	0
0	+	+	+	0	+	0	+	0	+	0	+	0	0	+	0	V	0	+	V	+
0	+	+	+	0	+	+	+	0	+	+	+	+	0	+	0	$+^W$	0	$+^W$	$+^W$	0
0	+	0	+	+	+	0	+	0	$+^V$	+	0	0	0	+	0	+	+	+	0	0
0	+	0	0	0	0^V	0	0^V	0	0	0	+	0	0	0^W	0	0	0	0	0^V	0
0	+	0	0	0	0	0	0	0	0	0	+	0	0	+	0	0	0	0	$+^V$	0
$+^V$	+	0	0	0	0	0	0	0	0	0	0	0	0	+	0	0	0	0	0	0
+	+	0	0	0	V	0	0	0	0	0	0	0	0	0	0	0	0	0	0	0

TABLE 5 Characteristics that assist in differentiating *Candida dubliniensis* from *Candida albicans*[a]

Organism	Colonies on CHROMagar at 37°C[b]	Growth at 42–45°C at 48 h[c]	Chlamydospores on appropriate agar[d]	Colonies on Staib agar[e]	Assimilation at ≤48 h[f]		
					XYL	MDG	TRE
C. dubliniensis	Usually dark green; most distinct at 72 h	0 or poor	Usually abundant and in pairs or small clusters	Rough; may have hyphal fringe	0	0	0[v]
C. albicans	Usually light green or light bluish green	+[v]	Usually single; very occasionally in pairs or small clusters	Smooth; shiny	+[v]	+[v]	+

[a]Variability has been reported in all of the tests; there is no single phenotypic test that can reliably discriminate *C. dubliniensis* from *C. albicans*. It is advisable to perform several of the tests simultaneously. Abbreviations: +, positive; 0, negative; V, variable; XYL, xylose; MDG, α-*methyl*-D-glucoside; TRE, trehalose.

[b]CHROMagar Candida (BBL, p. 334) must be incubated at 37°C (not 25–30°C) for clearest results. The ability of *C. dubliniensis* to produce dark-green colonies on CHROMagar is best observed upon primary isolation of the organism; the property has been found to be unstable following subculture or storage of the isolate.

[c]Inoculate isolate onto two Sabouraud dextrose agar slants or plates; incubate one at 42–45°C and the other at 37°C (as a comparative growth control). *C. albicans* grows well at the higher temperatures, but often at a slower rate. It is essential that the temperature of the incubator be carefully controlled to ensure accuracy.

[d]Media used for the production of chlamydospores (room temperature): cornmeal-Tween 80 agar, Tween 80-oxgall-caffeic acid agar, or rice agar Tween. Clusters of chlamydospores are best seen on primary isolates; storage of isolate may diminish chlamydospore production.

[e]Inoculate a Staib agar (p. 332) plate for isolated colonies, and incubate it at 30°C for 48–72 h.

[f]Assimilation results refer only to commercial rapid miniature systems, not to the conventional Wickerham tube method. Commercial databases may not be updated to include findings of recent studies; therefore, the individual significant substrate reactions must be examined. For further information on the various commercial systems and their abilities to identify *C. dubliniensis*, see Pincus et al., 1999.

Candida tropicalis

PATHOGENICITY: As is true of many species of *Candida* and other yeasts, *C. tropicalis* is known to cause infection, especially in immunocompromised, predisposed patients, as discussed on p. 111. It appears to be especially virulent in patients with leukemia or similar malignancies. It is also found without evidence of disease.

RATE OF GROWTH: Rapid; mature in 3 days.

COLONY MORPHOLOGY: Creamy; near the edge it may be wrinkled or have a slight mycelial fringe. (Color Plate 47.)

MICROSCOPIC MORPHOLOGY: On routine primary media, yeast cells are round to oval (3.5.–7 × 5.5–10 μm). On cornmeal-Tween 80 agar at 25°C for 72 h, *C. tropicalis* forms blastoconidia singly or in very small groups all along graceful, long pseudohyphae. True hyphae may also be present. A few teardrop-shaped chlamydospores may rarely be produced.

See Table 3 (p. 114) for differentiation of yeastlike genera and Table 4 (p. 116) for characteristics of the most commonly encountered species of *Candida*.

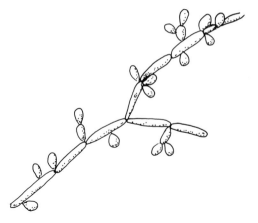 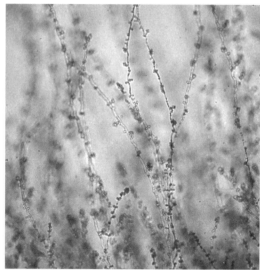

For further information, see
  de Hoog et al., 2000, pp. 220–222
  Kwon-Chung and Bennett, 1992, pp. 319–321

YEASTS AND YEASTLIKE ORGANISMS

Candida parapsilosis

PATHOGENICITY: Known to cause infections in particularly susceptible individuals, as discussed on p. 111. It is a relatively frequent cause of candidal endocarditis.

RATE OF GROWTH: Rapid; mature in 3 days.

COLONY MORPHOLOGY: Creamy, sometimes developing a lacy appearance.

MICROSCOPIC MORPHOLOGY: On routine primary media, yeast cells are ovoid (3–4 × 5–8 μm). On cornmeal-Tween 80 agar at 25°C for 72 h, blastoconidia, singly or in small clusters, are seen along the pseudohyphae. Outstanding characteristics are the crooked or curved appearance of relatively short pseudohyphae (compared to those of *Candida tropicalis*) and the occasional presence of large hyphal elements called giant cells.

See Table 3 (p. 114) for differentiation of yeastlike genera and Table 4 (p. 116) for characteristics of the most commonly encountered species of *Candida*.

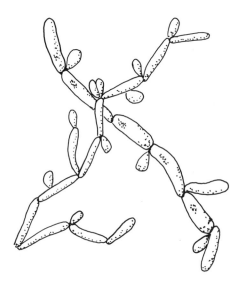
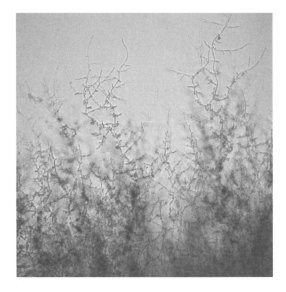

For further information, see
  de Hoog et al., 2000, pp. 212–214
  Kwon-Chung and Bennett, 1992, pp. 319–320

Candida lusitaniae

PATHOGENICITY: Encountered as an opportunistic pathogen in immunocompromised patients. Resistance to amphotericin B has frequently been reported.

RATE OF GROWTH: Rapid; mature in 3 days.

COLONY MORPHOLOGY: Cream colored, smooth, glistening.

MICROSCOPIC MORPHOLOGY: On routine primary media, yeast cells are round to oval (2–6 × 3–10 μm). On cornmeal-Tween 80 agar at 25°C for 72 h, pseudo-hyphae are slender, branched, and curved with short chains of elongate blastoconidia. Morphologically *C. lusitaniae* resembles *Candida tropicalis* and *Candida parapsilosis* but differs in its ability to ferment cellobiose and usually to assimilate rhamnose.

See Table 3 (p. 114) for differentiation of yeastlike genera and Table 4 (p. 116) for characteristics of the most commonly encountered species of *Candida*.

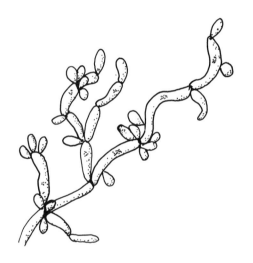
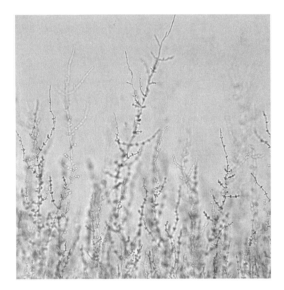

For further information, see
  Blinkhorn et al., 1989
  de Hoog et al., 2000, pp. 209–210
  Kwon-Chung and Bennett, 1992, pp. 318–319

PATHOGENICITY: Known to cause infections in particularly susceptible individuals, as discussed on p. 111. It is considered innately resistant to fluconazole.

RATE OF GROWTH: Rapid; mature in 3 days.

COLONY MORPHOLOGY: Flat, dry, dull, developing a mycelial fringe. Cream colored. (Color Plates 48 and 49.)

MICROSCOPIC MORPHOLOGY: On routine primary media, yeast cells are round to oval or elongate (2–6 × 4–10 μm). On cornmeal-Tween 80 agar at 25°C for 72 h, *C. krusei* forms pseudohyphae with elongate blastoconidia forming a cross-matchsticks or treelike appearance. The formations may be confused with the annellides of *Blastoschizomyces capitatus* (p. 142); see Table 7 (p. 123) for the differentiation of these two yeasts.

Although the biochemical profile of *Candida inconspicua* is extremely similar to that of *C. krusei*, they can each be identified by the characteristics in Table 6 (p. 123).

See Table 3 (p. 114) for differentiation of yeastlike genera and Table 4 (p. 116) for characteristics of the most commonly encountered species of *Candida*.

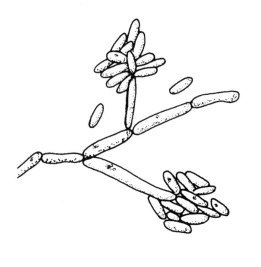
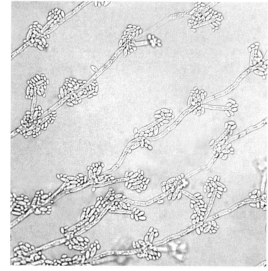

For further information, see
  de Hoog et al., 2000, pp. 206–207
  Kwon-Chung and Bennett, 1992, pp. 316–318

TABLE 6 Differentiating characteristics of *Blastoschizomyces capitatus* vs *Candida krusei*[a]

Organism	Growth with cycloheximide	Galactose assimilation	Dextrose fermentation	Urease	Conidia
B. capitatus	+	+	0	0	Annelloconidia
C. krusei	0	0	+	+[V]	Blastoconidia

[a]Abbreviations: +, positive; 0, negative; V, variable.

TABLE 7 Differentiating characteristics of *Candida krusei* vs *Candida inconspicua*

Organism	Pseudohyphae on cornmeal-Tween 80 agar	Fermentation of dextrose	Growth on *Trichophyton* agar no. 1[a]
C. krusei	+	+	+
C. inconspicua	0 Short chains of oval cells may form	0	0[b]

[a]Vitamin-free medium.
[b]May grow after an initial lag period.

Candida kefyr (formerly *Candida pseudotropicalis*)

PATHOGENICITY: Usually considered nonpathogenic but sometimes causes infection in particularly susceptible individuals, as discussed on p. 111.

RATE OF GROWTH: Rapid; mature in 3 days.

COLONY MORPHOLOGY: Creamy, smooth.

MICROSCOPIC MORPHOLOGY: On routine primary media, yeast cells are round to oval (3–8 × 5–12 μm). On cornmeal-Tween 80 agar at 25°C for 72 h, *C. kefyr* forms pseudohyphae with elongate blastoconidia that characteristically line up in parallel, giving the appearance of "logs in a stream."

See Table 3 (p. 114) for differentiation of yeastlike genera and Table 4 (p. 116) for characteristics of the most commonly encountered species of *Candida*.

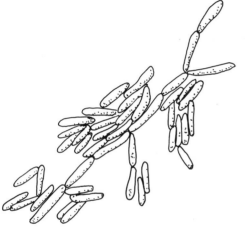
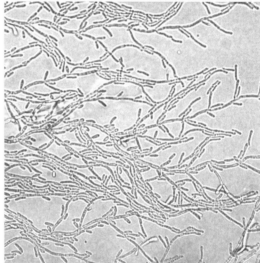

For further information, see
  de Hoog et al., 2000, pp. 204–205
  Kwon-Chung and Bennett, 1992, pp. 316–317

Candida guilliermondii

PATHOGENICITY: Usually considered nonpathogenic, but has been known to cause infection in particularly susceptible individuals, as described on p. 111.

RATE OF GROWTH: Rapid; mature in 3 days.

COLONY MORPHOLOGY: Flat, glossy, smooth edged, and usually cream colored but may become tan or pinkish with age.

MICROSCOPIC MORPHOLOGY: On routine primary media, yeast cells are ovoid to elongate (2–5 × 3–12 μm). On cornmeal-Tween 80 agar at 25°C for 72 h, *C. guilliermondii* forms clusters of yeast cells with relatively few, short pseudohyphae often having small groups of blastoconidia at the septa. True hyphae are not produced.

See Table 3 (p. 114) for differentiation of yeastlike genera and Table 4 (p. 116) for characteristics of the most commonly encountered species of *Candida*.

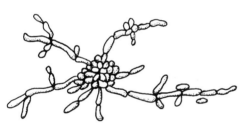

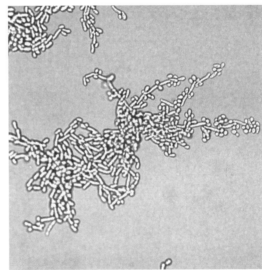

For further information, see
de Hoog et al., 2000, pp. 200–201
Kwon-Chung and Bennett, 1992, p. 315

Candida lipolytica

PATHOGENICITY: An emerging opportunistic pathogen; may cause disease in the immunocompromised patient, as discussed on p. 111.

RATE OF GROWTH: Rapid; mature in 5 days.

COLONY MORPHOLOGY: Creamy, smooth; may be delicately wrinkled.

MICROSCOPIC MORPHOLOGY: On routine primary media, yeast cells are round to oval (3–6 × 4–16 μm). On cornmeal-Tween 80 agar at 25°C for 72 h, pseudohyphae and septate true hyphae bearing elongate blastoconidia in short chains form and produce a stark, branching appearance. Arthroconidia may be present. *C. lipolytica* physiologically resembles *Candida krusei* but clearly differs by growing in the presence of cycloheximide and not fermenting dextrose (in addition to the morphologic differences).

See Table 3 (p. 114) for differentiation of yeastlike genera and Table 4 (p. 116) for characteristics of the most commonly encountered species of *Candida*.

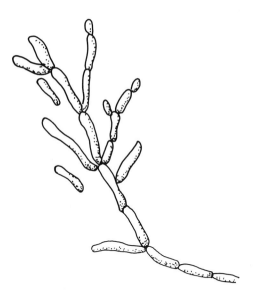
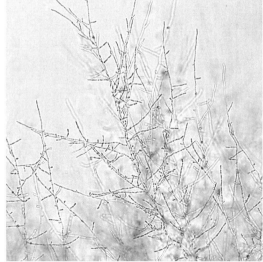

For further information, see
de Hoog et al., 2000, pp. 236–237
Kurtzman and Fell, 2000, pp. 420–421

Candida zeylanoides

PATHOGENICITY: Rarely reported as cause of fungemia, arthritis, and skin and nail infections.

RATE OF GROWTH: Rapid; mature in 3 days at 25–30°C; variable growth at 35–37°C.

COLONY MORPHOLOGY: Smooth, dull, cream colored to yellowish.

MICROSCOPIC MORPHOLOGY: On routine primary media, yeast cells are oval to elongate (3–5 × 6–11 μm). On cornmeal-Tween 80 agar at 25°C for 72 h, pseudo-hyphae consist of cells that are frequently curved and bear oval or elongate blasto-conidia singly and in small clusters and short chains. More blastoconidia are formed at the beginnings of the pseudohyphae than at the distal ends, creating a feather-like appearance at low power.

See Table 3 (p. 114) for differentiation of yeastlike genera and Table 4 (p. 116) for characteristics of the most commonly encountered species of *Candida*.

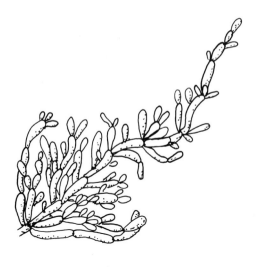
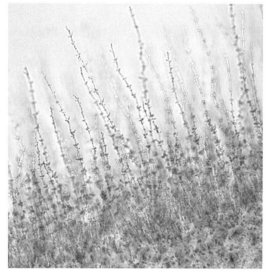

For further information, see
  de Hoog et al., 2000, pp. 225–226
  Kurtzman and Fell, 2000, pp. 571–572
  Levenson et al., 1991

Candida glabrata (formerly *Torulopsis glabrata*)

PATHOGENICITY: Causes infections usually occurring in the bloodstream or urogenital tract and occasionally in the lung and other sites. A significant number of clinical isolates have shown emerging resistance to amphotericin B and fluconazole. The organism is also found in healthy individuals and appears to cause infection only in particularly susceptible persons, as discussed on p. 111.

RATE OF GROWTH: Rapid; mature in 3–5 days; grows a bit more slowly than the other species of *Candida*.

COLONY MORPHOLOGY: Small yeastlike colonies, pasty, smooth, white to cream. (Color Plate 50.)

MICROSCOPIC MORPHOLOGY: On cornmeal-Tween 80 agar at 25°C for 72 h, only small (2–3 × 3.5–4.5 μm) oval yeast cells with single terminal budding are seen. No pseudohyphae are formed; occasionally a few short chains of ovoid cells are seen.

See Table 3 (p. 114) for differentiation of yeastlike genera and Table 4 (p. 116) for characteristics of the most commonly encountered species of *Candida*. *C. glabrata* can be quickly identified by the rapid assimilation of trehalose (RAT) test (p. 341). (Color Plate 51.)

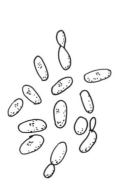
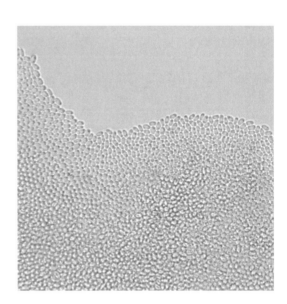

For further information, see
de Hoog et al., 2000, pp. 198–199
Kwon-Chung and Bennett, 1992, pp. 309–310, 314
McGinnis, 1980, p. 398
Rippon, 1988, p. 571

Cryptococcus neoformans

PATHOGENICITY: Causes cryptococcosis, a subacute or chronic infection most frequently involving the tissue of the central nervous system but occasionally producing lesions in the skin, bones, lungs, or other internal organs. Cryptococcal meningitis is extremely common in AIDS patients. The other species of this genus are commonly considered nonpathogenic but may occasionally cause disease in severely immunosuppressed patients.

RATE OF GROWTH: Rapid; mature in 3 days.

COLONY MORPHOLOGY: Colonies are flat or slightly heaped, shiny, moist, and usually mucoid, with smooth edges. Color is cream at first, later becoming tannish. Usually grows equally well at 25 and 37°C, whereas some of the other species of the genus will not grow well, if at all, at 37°C. (Color Plate 52.)

MICROSCOPIC MORPHOLOGY: On cornmeal-Tween 80 agar at 25°C for 72 h, cells (4–8 μm in diameter) are round, dark walled, and budding. Usually no hyphae are seen. Capsules are often discernible on cornmeal-Tween 80 by the spaces (due to capsular material) between the yeast cells. The capsules are best demonstrated with an India ink preparation (p. 299). Production of capsular material may be increased by growth in 1% peptone solution. Some strains of *C. neoformans*, as well as other cryptococci, may not produce apparent capsules in vitro.

See Table 3 (p. 114) for differentiation of yeastlike genera and Table 8 (p. 130) for characteristics of the most commonly encountered species of *Cryptococcus*. *C. neoformans* can be rapidly differentiated from other species of *Cryptococcus* by the caffeic acid test (p. 308). (Color Plate 54.)

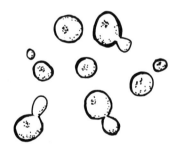
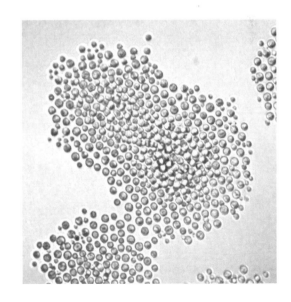

For further information, see
de Hoog et al., 2000, pp. 139–143
Kwon-Chung and Bennett, 1992,
pp. 397–446
McGinnis, 1980, pp. 389–392
Rippon, 1988, pp. 582–609

TABLE 8 Characteristics of *Cryptococcus* spp.[a]

Organism	Color on birdseed agar[b]	Growth at 37°C on SDA	Growth with cycloheximide at 25°C	Pseudo-hyphae (short)	Urease (25°C; 4 days)	Assimilation of:													Fermentation
						Dextrose	Maltose	Sucrose	Lactose	Galactose	Melibiose	Cellobiose	Inositol	Xylose	Raffinose	Trehalose	Dulcitol	KNO₃	
C. neoformans	Brown	+	0	0^R	+	+	+	+	0	+	0	+^V	+	+	+^V	+	+	0	
C. uniguttulatus	White	0	0	0	+	+	+	+	0	0^V	0	0^V	+	+	+^V	+^V	0	0	
C. albidus var. *albidus*	White	0^V	0	+^V	+	+	+	+	+^V	+^V	0^V	+	+	+	+^W	+^V	+^V	+	
C. albidus var. *diffluens*	White	+^V	0	0^V	+	+	+	+	0	0^V	+^V	+	+	+	+^W	+	+^V	+	All species of *Cryptococcus* lack fermentative ability
C. laurentii	White or greenish	+	0^V	0	+	+	+	+	+	+	+^V	+	+	+	+^V	+^V	+	0	
C. luteolus	White	0	0	0	+	+	+	+	0^V	+	+	+	+	+	+	+	+^V	0	
C. terreus	White	+	0	0^V	+	+	+^V	0^V	0^V	+^V	0	+	+	+	0	+^V	+^V	+	
C. gastricus	White	0	0	0	+	+	+	0^V	0^V	+	0	+	+	+	0	+	0	0	

[a]Abbreviations: SDA, Sabouraud dextrose agar; +, positive; 0, negative; V, strain variation; R, occur rarely; W, reaction may be weak.

[b]The caffeic acid disk test (p. 308) is a rapid and sensitive alternative to birdseed agar.

TABLE 9 Characteristics of yeasts and yeastlike organisms other than *Candida* spp. and *Cryptococcus* spp.[a]

Organism	Microscopic morphology on cornmeal-Tween 80 agar at 25°C	Growth of SDA at 37°C	Ascospores	Urease (25°C; 4 days)	Assimilation of:													Fermentation of:						
					Dextrose	Maltose	Sucrose	Lactose	Galactose	Melibiose	Cellobiose	Inositol	Xylose	Raffinose	Trehalose	Dulcitol	KNO₃	Dextrose	Maltose	Sucrose	Lactose	Galactose	Trehalose	Cellobiose
Saccharomyces cerevisiae	Occasional short pseudohyphae	V	+	0	+	+V	+	0	+V	V	0	0	0	+	+V	0	0	+	V	+	0	V	+V	0
Pichia (Hansenula) anomala	May form pseudohyphae	V	+	0	+	+	+	0	+V	0	+	0	+V	+V	+	0	+	+	+V	+	0	+V	+	V
Geotrichum candidum	True hyphae, arthroconidia; no blastoconidia	0	0	0	+	0	0	0	+	0	0	0	+	0	0	0	0	0	0	0	0	0	0	0
Blastoschizomyces capitatus[b]	Pseudohyphae and true hyphae; annelloconidia; few arthroconidia	+	0	0	+	0	0	0	+	0	0	0	0	0	0	0	0	0	0	0	0	0	0	0
Trichosporon spp.	Pseudohyphae and true hyphae; arthroconidia; blastoconidia	+V	0	+	+	+V	+V	+	+V	+V	+V	+V	+V	+V	+V	+V	0	0	0	0	0	0	0	0
Rhodotorula mucilaginosa	Usually no pseudohyphae	+V	0	+	+	V	+	0	V	0	V	0	+	+	+	0	0	0	0	0	0	0	0	0
Rhodotorula glutinis	Usually no pseudohyphae	+V	0	+	+	+	+	0	V	0	V	0	V	+V	+	0	+	0	0	0	0	0	0	0
Sporobolomyces salmonicolor	Ballistoconidia; various amounts of true and pseudohyphae	V	0	+	+	0V	+	0	+	0V	0V	0	+	V	+	0	+	0	0	0	0	0	0	0
Malassezia pachydermatis	Usually no hyphae	+	0	+	+	0	0	0	0	0	0	0	0	0	0	0	0	0	0	0	0	0	0	0
Prototheca wickerhami		+V	0	0	+	0	0	0	+V	0	0	0	0	0	+	+	0	0	0	0	0	0	0	0
Prototheca zopfii	Sporangia; no hyphae	+V	0	0	+	0	0	0	0V	0	0	0	0	0	0	0	0	0	0	0	0	0	0	0
Prototheca stagnora		0	0	0	+	0	V	V	+	0	0	0	0	0	0	0	0	0	0	0	0	0	0	0

[a] Abbreviations: SDA, Sabouraud dextrose agar; +, positive; 0, negative; V, strain variation.
[b] Annelloconidia forming clusters at the ends of hyphae of *B. capitatus* may resemble the elongated blastoconidia of *Candida krusei*.

131

Rhodotorula spp.*

PATHOGENICITY: Commonly known as contaminants. When isolated from specimens, the clinical significance is often uncertain. Their presence in terminal stages of debilitating diseases, such as carcinoma and bacterial endocarditis, may indicate an ability to colonize and infect particularly susceptible individuals.

RATE OF GROWTH: Rapid; mature in 4 days.

COLONY MORPHOLOGY: Usually pink to coral, but can also be more orange to red. Colony is yeastlike, soft, smooth, moist, and sometimes mucoid. (Color Plate 55.)

MICROSCOPIC MORPHOLOGY: On cornmeal-Tween 80 agar at 25°C for 72 h, budding cells are round or oval (2.5–5 × 3–10 μm); occasionally a few rudimentary pseudohyphae are seen. A faint capsule is sometimes formed.

See Tables 3 (p. 114) and 9 (p. 131) for differentiation of yeastlike fungi.

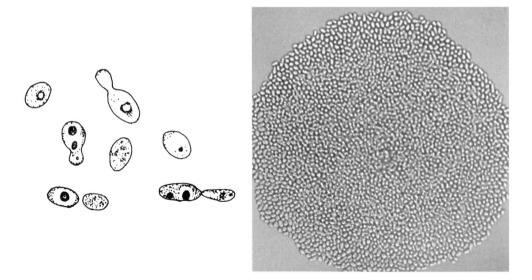

For further information, see
de Hoog et al., 2000, pp. 156–161
Kwon-Chung and Bennett, 1992, pp. 770–773
Rippon, 1988, pp. 610–611

Rhodotorula mucilaginosa is the accepted name for the species previously known as *Rhodotorula rubra*.

Sporobolomyces salmonicolor

PATHOGENICITY: Most commonly isolated from environmental sources. Very rarely reported as the cause of infection in immunocompromised patients.

RATE OF GROWTH: Rapid, mature in 5 days. Best growth is at 25–30°C; may not grow well at 35–37°C.

COLONY MORPHOLOGY: Smooth to slightly rough; characteristic salmon pink/coral color resembles that of *Rhodotorula* spp. (p. 132). Satellite colonies eventually form around the original colonies due to production of ballistoconidia. Ballistoconidia can be best demonstrated by taping an inoculated cornmeal agar plate face to face to an uninoculated cornmeal plate. After extended incubation at 25°C, with the inoculated plate on top, the ballistoconidia that are shot off the inoculated plate will form a mirror image of the colonies on the other plate. (Color Plates 56–58.)

MICROSCOPIC MORPHOLOGY: On cornmeal-Tween 80 agar at 25°C, oval to elongate yeastlike cells (2–12 × 3–35 μm) are seen; pseudohyphae and true hyphae may be absent or abundant. Kidney-shaped ballistoconidia (3–5 × 5–12 μm) are produced on denticles; they are forcibly discharged, forming the satellite colonies.

See Tables 3 (p. 114) and 9 (p. 131) for differentiation of yeasts and yeastlike fungi.

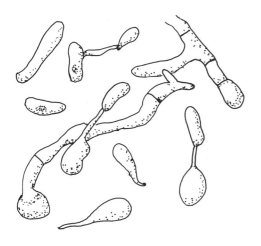
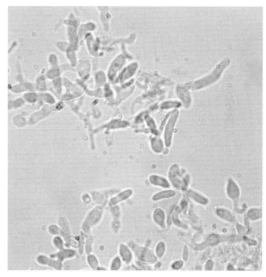

For further information, see
de Hoog et al., 2000, pp. 162–163
McGinnis, 1980, pp. 397–398

Saccharomyces cerevisiae

PATHOGENICITY: Usually considered nonpathogenic but has been implicated in various infections in predisposed individuals.

RATE OF GROWTH: Rapid; mature in 3 days.

COLONY MORPHOLOGY: Smooth colonies, moist, white to cream colored.

MICROSCOPIC MORPHOLOGY: On cornmeal-Tween 80 agar at 25°C for 72 h, oval to round yeast cells (3–8 × 5–10 μm) with multilateral budding are seen. A few very short pseudohyphae may form.

Note: Characteristic roundish ascospores (1 to 4 per ascus) are best demonstrated when the organism is grown on a special medium, such as V-8 medium, acetate ascospore agar, or Gorodkowa medium (p. 327), and stained with ascospore stain (p. 316) or Kinyoun stain (p. 316). (Color Plate 59.) In addition, ascospores are gram negative, while vegetative cells are gram positive.

See Tables 3 (p. 114) and 9 (p. 131) for differentiation of yeasts and yeastlike organisms.

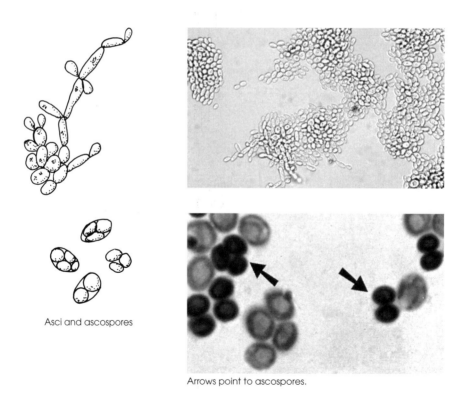

Asci and ascospores

Arrows point to ascospores.

For further information, see de Hoog et al., 2000, pp. 234–235; Kwon-Chung and Bennett, 1992, pp. 772–773; McGinnis, 1980, p. 379

*Pichia anomala** (formerly *Hansenula anomala*)

PATHOGENICITY: Commonly considered a saprophyte; occasionally causes infection in predisposed patients.

RATE OF GROWTH: Rapid; mature in 3 days.

COLONY MORPHOLOGY: Smooth, moist, cream colored.

MICROSCOPIC MORPHOLOGY: On cornmeal-Tween 80 agar at 25°C for 72 h, budding yeast cells are seen (2–4 × 2–6 μm). Pseudohyphae form in some species. When cultured on ascospore medium (p. 327) and stained with Kinyoun (p. 316) or ascospore (p. 316) stain, 1 to 4 ascospores per ascus are seen. There is a brim that turns downward around each ascospore, giving the impression of a helmet or hat. (Color Plate 60.)

See Tables 3 (p. 114) and 9 (p. 131) for identification of yeasts and yeastlike fungi.

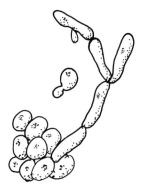

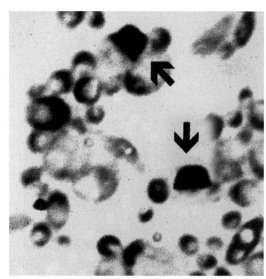

Arrows point to ascospores.

Ascospores

For further information, see
de Hoog et al., 2000, pp. 215–216
Kwon-Chung and Bennett, 1992, pp. 778–779
McGinnis, 1980, p. 377

*The asexual form of this organism is *Candida pelliculosa*.

Malassezia furfur

PATHOGENICITY: Etiologic agent of pityriasis (tinea) versicolor, a superficial infection characterized by pale or dark patches of skin; medical attention is usually sought for cosmetic reasons. Folliculitis, resembling acne, occasionally occurs. Catheter-associated sepsis due to this organism is commonly seen in neonates and adults receiving prolonged intravenous lipids; pneumonia may develop in these patients. The organism has been reported to cause peritonitis in patients receiving continuous peritoneal dialysis; it has also rarely been found in cases of septic arthritis, mastitis, sinusitis, and obstruction of the tear duct. *M. furfur* is part of the normal skin flora in over 90% of adults.

RATE OF GROWTH: Rapid; mature in 5 days at 30–37°C. Grows poorly at 25°C. The organism requires long-chain fatty acids for growth; solid medium overlaid with a thin film of olive oil is the most common method used.* Blood for culture must be taken through the lipid infusion catheter for best recovery of the organism; lysis-centrifugation (ISOLATOR tubes, Wampole Laboratories) is advised as a result of many comparative studies.

COLONY MORPHOLOGY: Smooth, cream to yellowish brown; often becomes dry, dull, and lightly wrinkled with age.

MICROSCOPIC MORPHOLOGY: Yeastlike cells (1.5–4.5 × 2.0–6.5 μm) are actually phialides with small collarettes; the collarettes are very difficult to discern with a routine light microscope. The cells of this genus are unique in being round at one end and bluntly cut off at the other, where wide budlike structures form singly on a broad base. There is no constriction at the point of conidiation. Staining with safranin and examining under oil immersion is a simple and effective way to observe the shape of the organism; also, Calcofluor White allows for very clear delineation of the cell wall and shape. (Color Plate 61.) Hyphal elements are usually absent, but sparse rudimentary forms may occasionally develop.

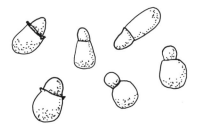
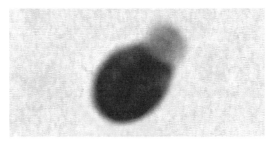

For further information, see
  de Hoog et al., 2000, pp. 145–146
  Kwon-Chung and Bennett, 1992, pp. 170–182
  Marcon and Powell, 1992

---

*Olive oil-saturated disks (p. 309) can be used in place of the overlay method. *M. furfur* can have its lipid requirement supplied by oleic acid or Tween 80; *Malassezia sympodialis* cannot. This serves to distinguish *M. furfur* from the seldom-encountered *M. sympodialis*.

Malassezia pachydermatis

PATHOGENICITY: More often found in lower animals than in humans, it has been associated with inflammation of the ears of dogs. Occasionally reported to cause human infection, particularly in premature neonates receiving intravenous lipid emulsions.

RATE OF GROWTH: Rapid; mature in 5 days. Best growth is at 35–37°C; weak growth is seen at 25°C.

COLONY MORPHOLOGY: Creamy, dull, smooth; at first it is cream colored, becoming buff to orange-beige with age. Addition of fatty acids to the medium is NOT required for growth.

MICROSCOPIC MORPHOLOGY: Yeast cells are similar to *Malassezia furfur* (p. 136); they are round to oval (2.5–5.5 × 3.0–6.5 μm); conidia are produced on a broad base at one pole, which develops a collarette. Pseudohyphae and true hyphae are usually absent, occasionally sparsely present. Biochemical yeast identification systems may misidentify this organism as *Candida lipolytica*; examination of microscopic morphology is essential.

See Tables 3 (p. 114) and 9 (p. 131) for differentiation of yeastlike fungi.

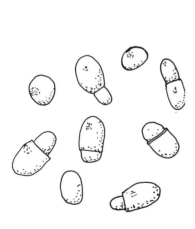 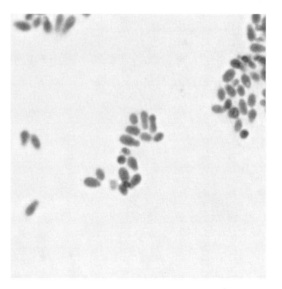

For further information, see
de Hoog et al., 2000, pp. 150–151
Kwon-Chung and Bennett, 1992, p. 179
Marcon and Powell, 1992

Ustilago sp.

PATHOGENICITY: Parasitic on seeds and flowers of many cereals and grasses. May cause contamination in cultures. It has seldom been implicated in human disease but may be inhaled and subsequently isolated from sputum specimens.

RATE OF GROWTH: Varies; mature in 5–20 days.

COLONY MORPHOLOGY: At first white, moist, pasty, and yeastlike; later it becomes tan to brown, wrinkled, raised, membranous, or velvety. Reverse is light in color.

MICROSCOPIC MORPHOLOGY: Elongate (2–3 × 9–30 μm), irregular, spindle-shaped or beanpod-shaped yeastlike cells. Short hyphae with clamp connections are sometimes observed.

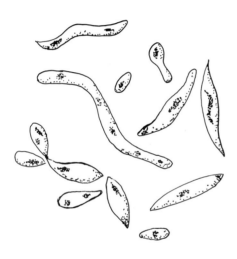
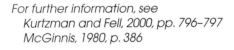
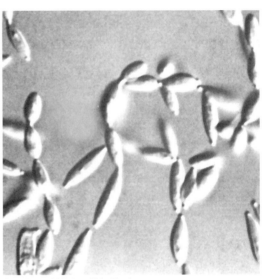

Courtesy of Michael McGinnis.

For further information, see
  Kurtzman and Fell, 2000, pp. 796–797
  McGinnis, 1980, p. 386

Prototheca spp.

(Commonly classified as achlorophyllous algae; included in this guide because they cause mycosis-like infections and are often mistaken for yeasts)

PATHOGENICITY: Cause prototothecosis, which may be cutaneous, subcutaneous, or systemic. Infection may arise through traumatic implantation into subcutaneous tissue. The organisms have also been isolated from clinical specimens in the absence of disease.

RATE OF GROWTH: Rapid; mature in 3 days.

COLONY MORPHOLOGY: Dull white to cream colored; yeastlike in consistency.

MICROSCOPIC MORPHOLOGY: Sporangia of various sizes (7–25 μm in diameter) containing sporangiospores (endospores). Budding does not occur and no hyphae are produced. The cells of *P. wickerhamii* are somewhat smaller (7–13 μm in diameter) than those of *P. zopfii* (14–25 μm in diameter), but the size may depend on the substrate and environmental conditions. *P. stagnora* produces a capsule.

See Tables 3 (p. 114) and 9 (p. 131) for identification of yeastlike organisms.
For further information, see

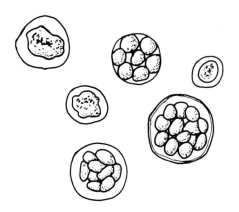 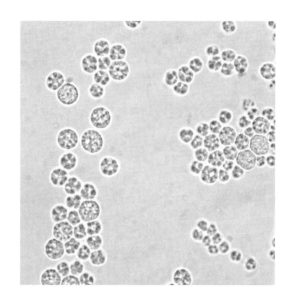

Kurtzman and Fell, 2000, pp. 883–887
Kwon-Chung and Bennett, 1992, pp. 785–794
McGinnis, 1980, p. 394
Rippon, 1988, pp. 723–728

The genus *Trichosporon* has undergone taxonomic revision. Until recently, most clinical isolates were identified (on the basis of many characteristics that were deemed "variable") as *T. beigelii* or, before that, *T. cutaneum*. Extensive studies have shown that the genus consists of numerous distinct species, but only five are of clinical significance.

PATHOGENICITY: *Trichosporon* is increasingly involved in invasive localized and disseminated disease. Immunocompromised patients with neutropenia are especially susceptible. Some species cause white piedra, a superficial infection of the hair characterized by relatively soft, white nodules located along the shafts of hair. (Black piedra is caused by *Piedraia hortae*, p. 206.) The type and site of infection is somewhat predictive of the involved species (Table 10, p. 141). The organisms are also found as normal flora in the skin, nails, and mouth.

RATE OF GROWTH: Moderately rapid; mature in 5–7 days.

COLONY MORPHOLOGY: Yeastlike; at first cream colored, moist, and soft. The surface becomes irregularly wrinkled, rather powdery or crumb-like; the center may become heaped, and the colony may adhere to, and crack, the agar. The color often darkens to yellowish gray.

MICROSCOPIC MORPHOLOGY: On cornmeal-Tween 80 agar at 25°C for 72 h, true hyphae and pseudohyphae with blastoconidia singly or in short chains are seen. Arthroconidia (2–4 × 3–9 μm) form on older cultures. The presence of blastoconidia along the hyphae differentiates *Trichosporon* from *Geotrichum* spp.

See Tables 3 (p. 114) and 9 (p. 131) for further differentiation of yeastlike organisms.

See Table 10 (p. 141) for key characteristics of clinically encountered *Trichosporon* spp.

See Table 21 (p. 260) for differential characteristics of fungi in which arthroconidia predominate.

Note: Because of shared antigens, sera from patients with disseminated *Trichosporon* infection may give positive reactions with the cryptococcal antigen latex test.

Trichosporon spp. *(continued)*

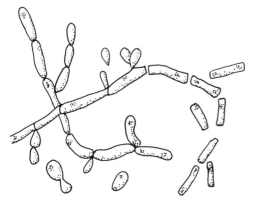

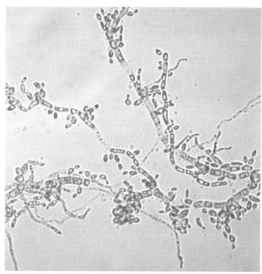

For further information, see
de Hoog et al., 2000, pp. 164–175
Guého et al., 1992, 1994

TABLE 10 Key characteristics of clinically encountered *Trichosporon* spp.[a]

Species	Infections	Urease	Growth at 37°C	Assimilation		
				Inos	Arab	Sorb
T. asahii	Systemic with predilection for hematogenous dissemination	+	+	0	+	0
T. mucoides	Systemic with preference for central nervous system	+	+	+	+	+
T. cutaneum	Rarely skin lesions and white piedra of underarm hairs	+	0	+	+	+
T. inkin	Mostly white piedra of pubic hairs; occasionally systemic	+	+	+	0	0
T. ovoides	White piedra of head hairs; occasional skin lesions	+	V	0	V	0

[a]Abbreviations: +, positive; 0, negative; V, strain variation; Inos, inositol; Arab, L-arabinose; Sorb, sorbitol.

YEASTS AND YEASTLIKE ORGANISMS

*Blastoschizomyces capitatus** (formerly *Trichosporon capitatum*)

PATHOGENICITY: Infrequent cause of invasive, systemic infection in immunocompromised hosts, most commonly in neutropenic leukemia patients. Lesions have occurred in the lung, kidney, liver, spleen, brain, and other organs; it has also caused endocarditis. The organism is distributed in nature and may be found as normal flora of the skin, respiratory tract, and gastrointestinal tract.

RATE OF GROWTH: Rapid; mature in 5 days.

COLONY MORPHOLOGY: Yeastlike, smooth to wrinkled, radiating edges, developing short aerial hyphae with age; white to cream colored.

MICROSCOPIC MORPHOLOGY: On cornmeal-Tween 80 agar, round to oval budding yeastlike cells, hyphae and pseudohyphae; few arthroconidia and many annelloconidia are seen. Annellides form along the hyphae or at the ends of hyphal branches; annelloconidia are elongate (2.5–3.5 × 7–10 µm) and flattened at the base and accumulate in clusters at the tips of the annellides. It is difficult to determine that the conidia are annelloconidia and not arthroconidia or blastoconidia; this may account for its confusion with (and sometimes misidentification as) *Trichosporon* sp. or *Candida krusei*. Careful attention to biochemical test results is required to differentiate these organisms.

See Table 3 (p. 114) and Table 9 (p. 131) for differentiation of yeastlike fungi.

See Table 7 (p. 123) for comparison with *C. krusei*.

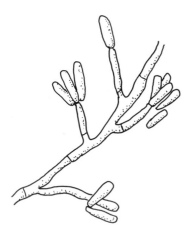
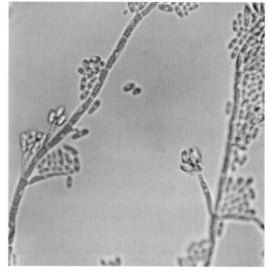

For further information, see
  Kwon-Chung and Bennett, 1992, pp. 768–771; Polacheck et al., 1992; Salkin et al., 1985a

*Some mycologists maintain that the proper name of this organism is *Geotrichum capitatum*.

Geotrichum candidum

PATHOGENICITY: *G. candidum* has been isolated from a variety of specimens (lungs, blood, mouth, intestines, vagina, and skin), but its role in infection is dubious. *Geotrichum* is found as normal flora in humans and seems to cause disease (primarily of the lungs) only in severely compromised hosts.

RATE OF GROWTH: Rapid; mature in 4 days.

COLONY MORPHOLOGY: At 25°C, young colonies are white, moist, yeastlike, and easily picked up. Submerged hyphae are later seen at the periphery, giving the appearance of ground glass. Some strains develop a short, white, cottony aerial mycelium. Many strains do not grow at 37°C, but some may have a small amount of surface growth and extensive subsurface growth at this temperature. (Color Plates 62, 63.)

MICROSCOPIC MORPHOLOGY: Coarse true hyphae (no pseudohyphae) that segment into rectangular arthroconidia which vary in length (4–10 μm) and in the roundness of their ends. Some may become quite round. The rectangular cells characteristically germinate from one corner. The biochemical characteristics and the absence of blastoconidia along the hyphae differentiate this organism from *Trichosporon* spp. (p. 140); the consecutive formation of the arthroconidia (not alternating with empty cells) serves to separate it from *Coccidioides immitis* (p. 259), *Malbranchea* (p. 261), and *Geomyces* (p. 262); and the absence of conidiophores distinguishes it from *Arthrographis* (p. 263).

See Tables 3 (p. 114) and 9 (p. 131) for differentiation of yeastlike organisms.

See Table 21 (p. 260) for differential characteristics of fungi with predominating arthroconidia.

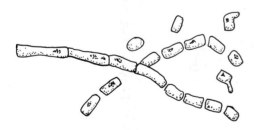

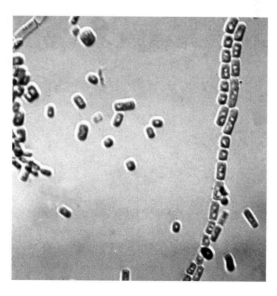

For further information, see
de Hoog et al., 2000, pp. 228–230
Kwon-Chung and Bennett, 1992,
pp. 740–743
McGinnis, 1980, pp. 221–225
Rippon, 1988, pp. 714–718

Thermally Dimorphic Fungi

Introduction

The fungi included here are unique in that they grow as filamentous moulds in the environment or when cultured on routine mycology agar (e.g., Sabouraud dextrose agar) at 25–30°C and are yeastlike in tissue or when cultured on an enriched medium (e.g., brain heart infusion agar) at 35–37°C. All of them are known to be pathogenic.

Coccidioides immitis (often placed with these organisms in other texts) does NOT produce yeastlike colonies or cells at 35–37°C on routine mycology agar; therefore, in this guide it is placed wth the hyaline hyphomycetes (p. 259).

Cokeromyces recurvatus is thermally dimorphic, but because of its zygomycetous properties, it has been placed with that class (p. 173).

For further information, see
> Murray et al. (ed.), 1999, Manual of Clinical Microbiology, 7th ed.,
> chapter 99 for Histoplasma, Blastomyces, and Paracoccidioides;
> chapter 101 for Sporothrix schenckii; chapter 97 for Penicillium
> marneffei

Sporothrix schenckii

PATHOGENICITY: Causes sporotrichosis, a chronic infection that frequently begins as a lesion of the skin and subcutaneous tissue and then involves the lymphatic channels and lymph nodes draining the area. Initial introduction into the body is usually due to a puncture by contaminated plant material (e.g., wood splinters, thorns, sphagnum moss, or hay). Primary pulmonary sporotrichosis may develop in predisposed individuals after inhaling the fungus. On rare occasions, the infection has disseminated and been fatal.

RATE OF GROWTH: Rapid; mature within 5 days.

COLONY MORPHOLOGY: Thermally dimorphic. At 25–30°C the colonies are at first small and white with no cottony aerial hyphae. Later, the colonies become moist, wrinkled, leathery, or velvety and often darken to a salt-and-peppery brown or black with a narrow white border. Some isolates are black from the beginning; stock cultures may become, and remain, nonpigmented. Colonies with a dark surface have a reverse that is commonly dark in the center and light at the periphery. (Color Plates 65 and 66.)

At 35–37°C, colonies are cream or tan, smooth, and yeastlike. It is best to use brain heart infusion agar and transfer several generations to obtain a good yeast phase (p. 309).

MICROSCOPIC MORPHOLOGY: At 25–30°C, hyphae are narrow (1–2 μm in diameter), septate, and branching, with slender, tapering conidiophores rising at right angles. The apex of the conidiophore is often slightly swollen and bears many small tear-shaped or almost round conidia (2–3 × 3–6 μm) on delicate threadlike denticles, forming a "rosette-like" cluster in young cultures; conidia also form singly along the hyphae.

At 35–37°C, round, oval, and fusiform budding cells of various sizes (1–3 × 3–10 μm), commonly called cigar bodies, are seen.

The conversion of the mycelial form to the yeastlike form is essential for confirmation of identification (see p. 309).

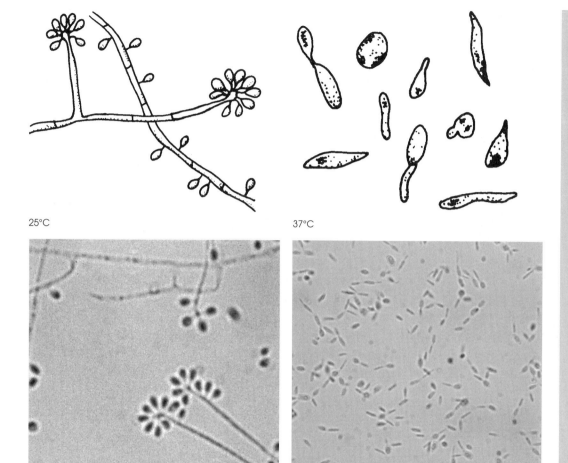

25°C

37°C

25°C on SDA.

37°C on BHI agar.

For further information, see
de Hoog et al., 2000, pp. 925–927
Kwon-Chung and Bennett, 1992, pp. 707–729
McGinnis, 1980, pp. 278–279, 514–515
Rippon, 1988, pp. 325–352
Wentworth, 1988, pp. 99–106

Histoplasma capsulatum*

PATHOGENICITY: Causes histoplasmosis, which may be an acute, benign pulmonary disease or may be chronic or progressive and fatal. It may be localized or cause a disseminated, life-threatening infection (primarily of the reticuloendothelial system) and involve various tissues and organs of the body. The organism is primarily found in bird and bat droppings and is endemic in the Ohio and Mississippi river valleys as well as in other regions of the world, both temperate and tropical.

RATE OF GROWTH: Slow; mycelial forms usually mature within 15–20 days but may take up to 8 weeks. (The organism does not survive well in clinical specimens, so when histoplasmosis is suspected, the specimen must be processed immediately.)

COLONY MORPHOLOGY: Thermally dimorphic. At 25–30°C on Sabouraud dextrose agar (SDA), it is white to brown, or pinkish, with a fine, dense cottony texture. The reverse is white, sometimes yellow or orange-tan. An enriched agar may be the best growth medium, but characteristic morphology of the mould phase is seen on SDA or similar media. (Color Plate 67.)

At 35–37°C on brain heart infusion (BHI) agar, moist, white, yeastlike colonies may eventually form, often requiring many generations. The yeast phase is inhibited by cycloheximide.

MICROSCOPIC MORPHOLOGY: At 25–30°C in young cultures, septate hyphae are seen bearing round to pear-shaped, smooth or occasionally spiny microconidia (2–5 μm in diameter) on short branches or directly on the sides of the hyphae. At this early stage, *H. capsulatum* can be confused with *Blastomyces dermatitidis* (p. 152). After several weeks, large, thick-walled, round macroconidia (7–15 μm in diameter) form; they are tuberculate, knobby, or have short cylindrical projections; occasionally they may be smooth. The macroconidia greatly resemble those of *Sepedonium* sp. (p. 288), but *Sepedonium* sp. does not produce microconidia and grows poorly or not at all at 37°C.

At 35–37°C, small round or oval budding cells (2–3 × 4–5 μm) and occasional abortive hyphae may be seen.

The conversion of the mycelial form to the yeast phase has been required in the past for morphologic identification (see p. 309) but is not always possible in vitro. A test for specific exoantigen or use of the commercially available DNA probe can more readily confirm the identification.

---

*There are two major varieties of *H. capsulatum*. The variety *duboisii* is endemic only in tropical central Africa. It differs from the variety *capsulatum* by producing larger yeast cells (8–15 μm in length); in other morphologic aspects they are identical.

Histoplasma capsulatum *(continued)*

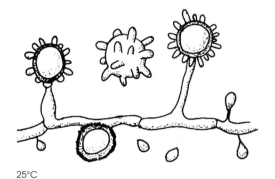

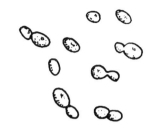

25°C

37°C

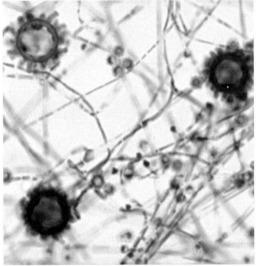

25°C on SDA.

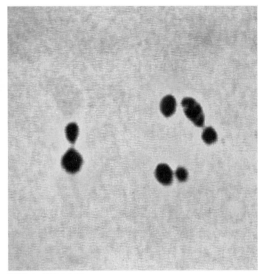

37°C on BHI agar.

For further information, see
de Hoog et al., 2000, pp. 708–711
Kwon-Chung and Bennett, 1992, pp. 464–513
McGinnis, 1980, pp. 229–231, 500–504
Rippon, 1988, pp. 381–423
Wentworth, 1988, pp. 206–215

Blastomyces dermatitidis

PATHOGENICITY: Causes blastomycosis, which is a chronic infection characterized by suppurative and granulomatous lesions in any part of the body; it most commonly begins in the lungs and is disseminated to the skin and bones.

RATE OF GROWTH: Slow; mycelial forms mature within 14 days. Some strains are slower; cultures should be held for 8 weeks if blastomycosis is suspected. (Organism does not survive well in specimens and must therefore be cultured immediately.)

COLONY MORPHOLOGY: Thermally dimorphic. At 25–30°C on Sabouraud dextrose agar (SDA), it is at first yeastlike, then prickly, and finally very cottony with a white aerial mycelium; it turns tan or brown with age. Reverse is tan. (Color Plate 68.)

At 35–37°C, it is cream to tan in color, heaped or wrinkled, and waxy in appearance; it is best seen on brain heart infusion (BHI) agar. Yeast phase is inhibited by cycloheximide.

MICROSCOPIC MORPHOLOGY: At 25–30°C on SDA, forms septate hyphae with short or long conidiophores; round or pear-shaped conidia (2–10 μm in diameter) develop at the apex of the conidiophore (causing a lollipop-like appearance) or directly on the hyphae. It may resemble *Scedosporium apiospermum* (p. 196) or *Chrysosporium* spp. (p. 284). Older cultures have thick-walled chlamydoconidia.

At 35–37°C on BHI agar, forms yeastlike cells (usually 8–15 μm in diameter) that bud on a broad base (4–5 μm wide) and appear to be thick walled and double contoured; the bud often remains attached until it becomes the same size as the parent cell.

Confirmation of identification is essential; it can be accomplished by culture conversion from the mould to yeast phase (p. 309) or more rapidly by testing for specific exoantigen or by using the commercially available DNA probe (performed by most reference laboratories).

Blastomyces dermatitidis (continued)

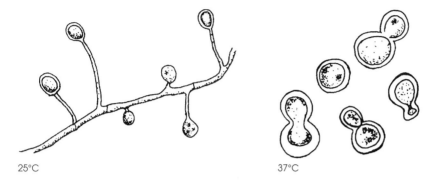

25°C

37°C

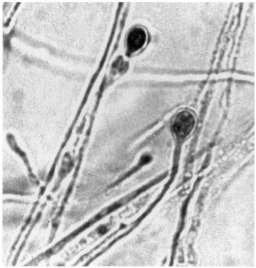

25°C on SDA.

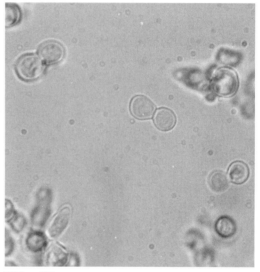

37°C on BHI agar.

For further information, see
   de Hoog et al., 2000, pp. 535–536
   Kwon-Chung and Bennett, 1992, pp. 248–279
   McGinnis, 1980, pp. 187–192, 477–480
   Rippon, 1988, pp. 474–505
   Wentworth, 1988, pp. 183–196

THERMALLY DIMORPHIC FUNGI

Paracoccidioides brasiliensis

PATHOGENICITY: Causes paracoccidioidomycosis (South American blastomycosis), a chronic granulomatous disease characteristically beginning in the lungs and spreading to the mucous membranes of the nose, mouth, and occasionally the gastrointestinal tract. Dissemination to skin, lymph nodes, and other internal organs is common.

RATE OF GROWTH: Very slow; mycelial forms mature within 21 days.

COLONY MORPHOLOGY: Thermally dimorphic. At 25–30°C on Sabouraud dextrose agar (SDA), colony is white, heaped, compact, usually folded, and almost glabrous or with a short nap of white aerial mycelium that often turns brown with age. Reverse is light or brownish.

At 35–37°C on brain heart infusion (BHI) agar, colony is heaped, cream to tan, moist, and soft, becoming waxy and yeastlike.

MICROSCOPIC MORPHOLOGY: At 25–30°C on SDA, usually forms only septate, branched hyphae with some intercalary and terminal chlamydospores; a few microconidia are sometimes observed along the hyphae.

At 35–37°C on BHI agar, large, round, fairly thick-walled cells (5–50 μm in diameter) with single and multiple buddings (2–10 μm in diameter) are seen. The buds are attached to the mother cell by narrow connections and may almost completely surround the cell, giving the characteristic "ship's wheel" appearance. Care must be taken not to confuse single-budding cells with *Blastomyces dermatitidis*.

Conversion of the mould form to the yeast phase is essential for identification (see p. 309).

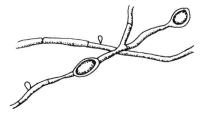

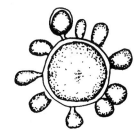

25°C

37°C

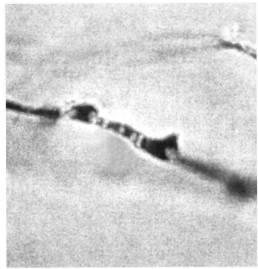

25°C on PDA. From Walsh et al., *Manual of Clinical Microbiology*, 6th ed.

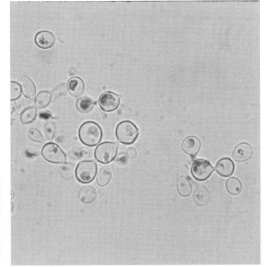

37°C on BHI agar.

For further information, see
   de Hoog et al., 2000, pp. 812–813
   Kwon-Chung and Bennett, 1992, pp. 594–619
   McGinnis, 1980, pp. 248–251, 509–510
   Rippon, 1988, pp. 506–531
   Wentworth, 1988, pp. 215–219

PATHOGENICITY: Causes deep-seated infection that can be focal or disseminated, predominantly in immunocompromised (human immunodeficiency virus [HIV]-positive) patients and occasionally in immunocompetent individuals who live in, or have traveled in, areas of Southeast Asia where *P. marneffei* is endemic. The organism has been isolated from blood, bone marrow, skin, lung, mucosa, lymph nodes, urine, stool, cerebrospinal fluid, and various internal organs.

RATE OF GROWTH: Rapid; mature within 3 days at 25–30°C. Yeastlike form develops more slowly at 35–37°C. Sabouraud dextrose agar (SDA) supports growth at 25–37°C and demonstrates thermal dimorphism. Cycloheximide inhibits growth.

COLONY MORPHOLOGY: Thermally dimorphic. At 25–30°C on SDA, colony is flat, powdery to velvety, and tan, later becoming reddish yellow with a yellow or white edge; it is often bluish gray-green in the center. A deep-reddish soluble pigment diffuses into the medium after 3–7 days; this is best seen on potato dextrose agar (PDA). Other species of *Penicillium* may also produce a red pigment but will not convert to a yeastlike form at 35–37°C. Reverse is brownish red. (Color Plates 69–71.)

At 35–37°C on SDA, inhibitory mould agar (IMA), or brain heart infusion (BHI) agar, colony is soft, white to tan, dry, and yeastlike. Conversion from the mould to yeast-like form may take up to 14 days; it is most rapidly accomplished (in approximately 4 days) by culturing in BHI broth on a shaker; the next-best method is on 5% sheep blood agar.

MICROSCOPIC MORPHOLOGY: At 25–30°C, structures typical of the genus *Penicillium* (p. 269) develop, i.e., smooth conidiophores with 4 to 5 terminal metulae, each metula bearing 4 to 6 phialides. Conidia are smooth or slightly rough and oval (2–3 × 2.5–5 μm) and form chains; short, narrow extensions connect the conidia.

When conidia are incubated at 35–37°C, they form hyphal elements that eventually fragment at the septa, producing single-celled round to oval arthroconidia (3–5 μm in diameter); this is the form commonly referred to as yeastlike cells; buds are not produced. The arthroconidia continue to reproduce by fission and in so doing may elongate to 8–9 μm.

Penicillium marneffei *(continued)*

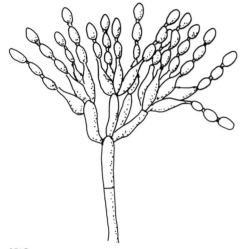

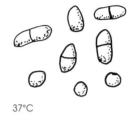

37°C

25°C

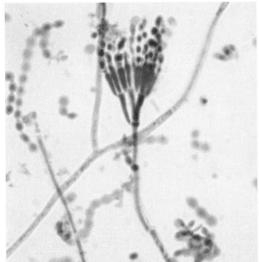

25°C on SDA. Courtesy of William Merz.

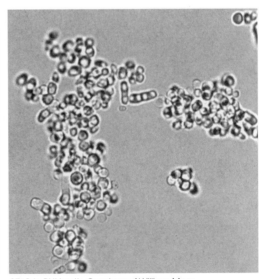

37°C in BHI broth. Courtesy of William Merz.

For further information, see
  Cooper and Haycocks, 2000
  Kwon-Chung and Bennett, 1992, pp. 755–758
  Supparatpinyo et al., 1994
  Vossler, 2001

Thermally Monomorphic
Moulds

Thermally monomorphic moulds are fungi that are filamentous at whatever temperatures they are able to grow (25–35°C). Some do not grow at 35–37°C but are filamentous at 25–30°C.

Zygomycetes

Introduction

Zygomycetes are a class of fungi that have broad hyphae (6–15 μm wide) and are almost nonseptate. Septa are most often seen on sporangiophores just below the sporangia and elsewhere in older cultures. Asexual reproduction occurs in a sac-like structure called a sporangium, in which the internal contents are cleaved into spores.

Most zygomycetes that are encountered in the clinical laboratory belong to the order Mucorales. These are easily recognized by their grayish, very fluffy colonies that rapidly fill the tube or petri plate in a cotton candy-like fashion. The differentiation of the various genera is based on

- The presence and location (or absence) of rhizoids (rootlike structures along the vegetative hyphae)
- The branching or unbranched nature of the sporangiophores (the stalks bearing the sac-like sporangia)
- The shape of the columella (the small dome-like area at the apex of the sporangiophore)
- The appearance of an apophysis (a broadening near the apex of the sporangiophore, just below the columella)
- The size and shape of the sporangia

See labeled diagram, p. 169.

A few genera (e.g., *Apophysomyces* and *Saksenaea*) require special media (p. 310) to enhance sporulation.

Some of the zygomycetes in the order Mucorales can cause severe disease (zygomycosis), predominantly in patients who are predisposed by diabetes, leukopenia, immunosuppression, AIDS, severe burns, intravenous drug abuse, malnutrition, etc. Infections have been reported from a wide range of anatomic sites but are most commonly rhinocerebral, pulmonary, cutaneous, and disseminated. The organisms are known for their disastrous ability to invade and block blood vessels.

The other order of zygomycetes, the Entomophthorales, are less commonly encountered. Their colonies are flat and buff to grayish brown with a waxy texture, and they develop short aerial hyphae and darken with age. They have broad hyphae and unique microscopic structures. Two genera of Entomophthorales (*Basidiobolus* and *Conidiobolus*) cause tropical subcutaneous mycoses and are discussed in the latter portion of this section.

For further information, see
Murray et al. (ed.), 1999, Manual of Clinical Microbiology, 7th ed., chapter 98
Ribes et al., 2000

TABLE 11 Differential characteristics of similar organisms in the class Zygomycetes[a]

Genus	Rhizoids	Sporangiophores	Apophysis	Columellae	Sporangia	Maximum growth temp (°C)
Rhizopus	Present	Single or in tufts; usually unbranched; mostly brown	Mostly inconspicuous	Almost round or slightly elongated	Round	~45
Rhizomucor	Present	Branched; dark brown	Absent (or very tiny)	Almost round	Round	~54
Mucor	Absent	Branched or unbranched; mostly hyaline	Absent	Various shapes	Round	<37
Absidia	Present, but often indistinct	Finely branched; almost hyaline	Conspicuous; conical	Semicircle: may have projection at top	Pyriform (pear shaped)	~45
Apophysomyces	Present	Generally single and unbranched; grayish brown	Conspicuous; bell shaped	Semicircle: may be elongated	Pyriform	≥42

[a]Adapted from Scholer et al., 1983, with additions.

TABLE 12 Differential characteristics of the clinically encountered *Rhizopus* spp.[a]

Organism	Pathogenic	Maximum growth temp (°C)	Rhizoid length (μm)	Sporangiophore length (μm)	Sporangium diameter (μm)	Columellae	Sporangiospores
R. oryzae (arrhizus) (most common agent of zygomycosis)	+	40–46	150–300	500–3,500	50–250	Almost round	Variable size; average length, 6–8 μm; striated; elongate to lemon shaped
R. microsporus var. rhizopodiformis	+	50–52	100–120	200–1,000	40–130	Slightly elongated; distinct apophysis	Equal in size; average length, 4–6 μm; smooth to slightly striated, almost round to slightly elongated
R. stolonifer	0	30–32	300–350	1,500–4,000	150–350	Almost round	Variable in size; average length, 9–11 μm; very striated; elongate to polyhedric

[a]Abbreviations: +, positive; 0, negative.

Rhizopus spp.

PATHOGENICITY: The most common etiologic agents of zygomycosis (see p. 35 for a description of the disease). They are also found as common contaminants.

RATE OF GROWTH: Rapid; mature within 4 days. The pathogenic species grow well at 37°C. Growth is inhibited by cycloheximide.

COLONY MORPHOLOGY: Quickly covers agar surface with dense growth that is cotton candy-like; colonies are white at first and then gray or yellowish brown. Reverse is white. (Color Plate 72.)

MICROSCOPIC MORPHOLOGY: Broad hyphae (6–15 μm in diameter) have no, or very few, septa. Numerous stolons run among the mycelia, connecting groups of long sporangiophores that usually are unbranched. At the point where the stolons and sporangiophores meet, rootlike hyphae (rhizoids) are produced. The sporangiophores are long (up to 4 mm) and terminate with a dark, round sporangium (40–350 μm in diameter) containing a columella and many oval, colorless or brown spores (4–11 μm in diameter). No collarette remains when the sporangial wall dissolves. This genus is differentiated from *Mucor* spp. (p. 167) by the presence of stolons, rhizoids, and usually unbranched sporangiophores. It is differentiated from *Absidia* spp. (p. 169) by the location of the rhizoids in relation to the sporangiophores and by the shape of the sporangia.

See Table 11 and Table 12 (p. 165) for identification of genus and species.

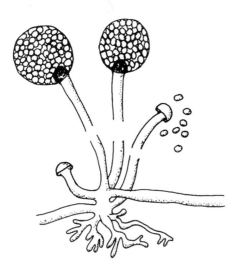
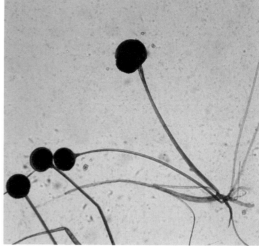

For further information, see
   de Hoog et al., 2000, pp. 101–111
   Kwon-Chung and Bennett, 1992, pp. 541–545
   McGinnis, 1980, pp. 323–325, 518–522
   Rippon, 1988, pp. 702–705, 748–750

Mucor spp.

PATHOGENICITY: Occasionally the etiologic agent of zygomycosis (for a description of the disease, see p. 35). These fungi are also known as common contaminants.

RATE OF GROWTH: Rapid; mature within 4 days. Growth is inhibited by cycloheximide. Most species do not grow well at 37°C.

COLONY MORPHOLOGY: Quickly covers agar surface with fluff resembling cotton candy; white, later turns gray or grayish brown. Reverse is white.

MICROSCOPIC MORPHOLOGY: Hyphae are wide (6–15 μm) and practically nonseptate. Sporangiophores are long and often branched and bear terminal round, spore-filled sporangia (50–300 μm in diameter). The sporangial wall dissolves, scattering the round or slightly oblong spores (4–8 μm in diameter), revealing the columella and sometimes leaving a collarette at the base of the sporangium. There is no apophysis. No rhizoids are formed.

See Table 11 (p. 165) for differentiation of similar organisms in the class Zygomycetes.

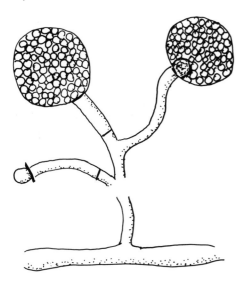 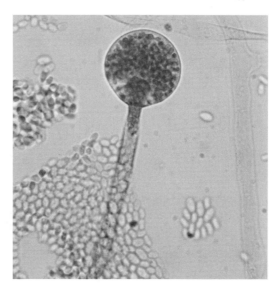

For further information, see
  de Hoog et al., 2000, pp. 81–93
  Kwon-Chung and Bennett, 1992, pp. 547–549
  McGinnis, 1980, pp. 316–320, 518–522
  Rippon, 1988, pp. 705–706, 748–749

THERMALLY MONOMORPHIC MOULDS: Zygomycetes

Rhizomucor spp.

PATHOGENICITY: An occasional etiologic agent of zygomycosis (for a description of the disease, see p. 35), primarily in leukemic patients. Incidence in the clinical laboratory is uncertain, as isolates may have been misidentified in the past.

RATE OF GROWTH: Rapid; mature within 4 days. Members of the genus are thermophilic; maximum growth temperature is 54–58°C. Growth is inhibited by cycloheximide.

COLONY MORPHOLOGY: Very fluffy growth with texture of cotton candy; gray, becoming dark brown with age. Reverse is white.

MICROSCOPIC MORPHOLOGY: Appears to be intermediate between *Rhizopus* (p. 166) and *Mucor* (p. 167) spp. Sporangia are round and are usually 60–100 μm in diameter. A few primitive, short, irregularly branched rhizoids are formed, differentiating the organism from *Mucor* spp. It differs from *Rhizopus* spp. by having branched sporangiophores and by the location of the rhizoids (at points on the stolon between the sporangiophores).

See Table 11 (p. 165) for differentiation of similar organisms in the class Zygomycetes.

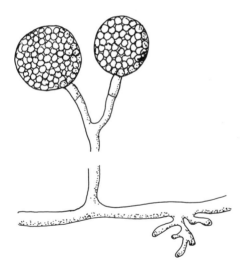
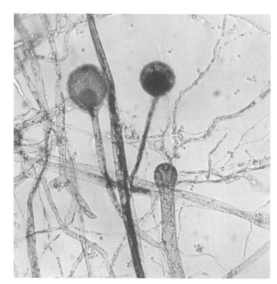

For further information, see
  de Hoog et al., 2000, pp. 94–100
  Kwon-Chung and Bennett, 1992, pp. 546, 549
  McGinnis, 1980, pp. 321–322, 518–522
  Rippon, 1988, p. 706

Absidia corymbifera

PATHOGENICITY: An infrequent etiologic agent of zygomycos[is] of the disease, see p. 35). The organism is ubiquitous and may [be a con]taminant in cultures.

RATE OF GROWTH: Rapid; mature within 4 days. Growth is inh[ibited by cyclohex]imide.

COLONY MORPHOLOGY: Coarse woolly gray surface; rapidly [growing] with fluff resembling gray cotton candy. Reverse is white. (Color P[late])

MICROSCOPIC MORPHOLOGY: Hyphae are wide (6–15 μm in diameter) and nonseptate (or almost so). It is similar in structure to *Rhizopus* spp. (p. 166) except that the sporangiophores of *Absidia* arise at points on the stolon that are between the rhizoids and not opposite them. Also, the sporangiophores (up to 450 μm long) are branched and widen, forming a conical apophysis just below the columella. The columella is typically shaped like a semicircle with a small projection on top. The sporangia are relatively small (20–120 μm in diameter) and slightly pear shaped instead of spherical. When the sporangial wall dissolves, a short collarette often remains where the wall met the sporangiophore. The sporangiospores are round to oval (3–4.5 μm in diameter).

Note: The rhizoids may be difficult to find and are best observed by using a dissecting microscope to examine colonies on an agar surface.

See p. 170 for differentiation from *Apophysomyces elegans*, which it closely resembles.

See Table 11 (p. 165) for differentiation of similar organisms in the class Zygomycetes.

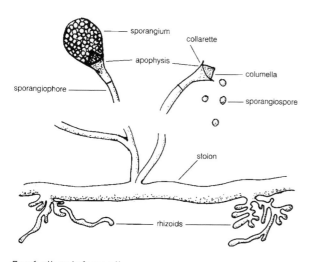

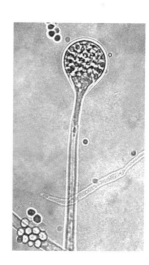

For further information, see
de Hoog et al., 2000, pp. 62–67; Kwon-Chung and Bennett, 1992, pp. 544–548;
McGinnis, 1980, pp. 304–306, 518–522; Rippon, 1988, pp. 706–707, 751–752

PATHOGENICITY: Occasional agent of zygomycosis (for a description of the disease, see p. 35). Infection is usually acquired by traumatic implantation, such as accidental injuries, surgery, insect bites, and contamination of burns. Systemic cases have also been reported. Some infected patients appear to be otherwise immunocompetent. The organism is found in soil.

RATE OF GROWTH: Rapid; growth fills plate or tube within 4 days; grows at temperatures up to 42°C. It grows on media containing cycloheximide (in contrast to other zygomycetes).

COLONY MORPHOLOGY: Fluffy cottony growth that fills tube or plate; surface is white when young, becoming cream to yellow or brownish gray with age. Reverse is white to pale yellow.

MICROSCOPIC MORPHOLOGY: Sporulation does not occur on routine media; only broad, almost nonseptate hyphae form. A special culture method (p. 310) is required to induce sporulation. Hyphae are generally nonseptate and branched (4–8 μm in diameter). Sporangiophores are long (up to 530 μm) and unbranched and arise singly from a hyphal segment that resembles the foot cells seen in *Aspergillus* spp. (p. 268); the apex of the sporangiophore widens to form a funnel-shaped or bell-shaped apophysis (11–40 μm in diameter at the widest part). The columella is a half circle. Sporangia are pear shaped, or pyriform (20–58 μm in diameter), and upon dissolution may leave a small collar at the base of the columella. The sporangiospores are smooth and mostly oblong (5–8 μm in length) and may appear pale brown in mass. Rhizoids may be between the points of origin of the sporangiophores or opposite the sporangiophore, depending on the medium.

Apophysomyces is similar to *Absidia* but differs by having
- A more pronounced apophysis, which is bell shaped rather than conical
- A "foot cell" at the base of the sporangiophore
- Sporangiophores developing opposite rhizoids on plain agar
- Darkening and thickening of the sporangiophore wall below the apophysis
- Failure to sporulate readily with routine culture methods
- Resistance to cycloheximide

See Table 11 (p. 165) for differentiation of similar organisms in the class Zygomycetes.

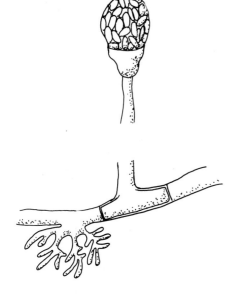

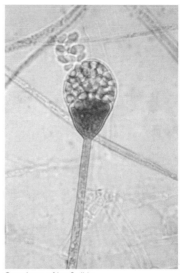

Courtesy of Ira Salkin.

For further information, see
de Hoog et al., 2000, pp. 68–69
Kimura et al., 1999
Kwon-Chung and Bennett, 1992, p. 500
Misra et al., 1979

Saksenaea vasiformis

PATHOGENICITY: Occasionally an agent of zygomycosis (for a description of the disease, see p. 35). Cases are usually preceded by traumatic implantation. Infections reported have been cutaneous and subcutaneous, osteomyelitic, rhinocerebral, and cranial; systemic infection is often fatal. Many of the patients appear to be otherwise immunocompetent.

RATE OF GROWTH: Rapid; growth fills plate or tube within 4 days. Maximum growth temperature is 44°C.

COLONY MORPHOLOGY: Very cottony, fluffy white surface. Reverse is white.

MICROSCOPIC MORPHOLOGY: On routine media the organism does not sporulate; only broad, mostly nonseptate, branched, hyaline hyphae form. A special procedure (p. 310) is required for stimulation of sporulation. Sporangiophores (24–64 μm long) bear sporangia that are flask shaped (50–150 μm long), having a swollen portion near the base and a long neck that broadens at the apex. Sporangiospores are elongate (3–4 μm long) and smooth. Rhizoids form near the base of the sporangiophore, are dichotomously branched, and darken with age.

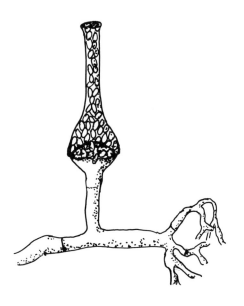
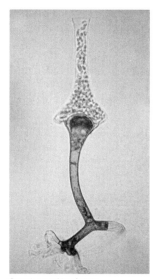

Courtesy of Ira Salkin.

For further information, see
   de Hoog et al., 2000, p. 112
   Kwon-Chung and Bennett, 1992, pp. 528, 534–535, 551

Cokeromyces recurvatus

PATHOGENICITY: The organism has been recovered several times from genitourinary sites (cervix, vagina, and bladder), but there was no tissue invasion demonstrated. It appears to have a predilection for colonization of those sites. It has very rarely been reported in infections at other sites; its possible role as an etiologic agent of mycotic disease is uncertain.

RATE OF GROWTH: Moderate; mature in 5–10 days.

COLONY MORPHOLOGY: At 25–30°C on Sabouraud dextrose agar, thermally dimorphic colonies are at first cream to tan, thin, feltlike or powdery, and radially folded; the central area later becomes heaped and dark; entire colony may become brown with age. Reverse is tan to brown. (Color Plate 74.)

At 35–37°C on enriched medium such as brain heart infusion agar, preferably in 5–7% CO_2, tan to gray, slightly wrinkled yeastlike colonies develop in 2 days.

MICROSCOPIC MORPHOLOGY: At 25–30°C, broad, sparsely septate hyphae are seen. Sporangiophores (100–500 μm long) terminate in a round vesicle that produces recurving stalks, each bearing a round sporangiole (9–13 μm in diameter). The sporangiole contains 12–20 sporangiospores that are smooth walled and of variable size and shape, mostly oval (average, 2.5 × 4.5 μm). No rhizoids are formed. Zygospores are abundantly produced between pairs of hyphal segments, sporangiophores, or suspensors of mature zygospores. Mature zygospores are round (35–55 μm in diameter), brown, and rough walled; the organism is homothallic, i.e., it requires only one thallus for production of sexual spores.

At 35–37°C in 5–7% CO_2, thin-walled, round yeast cells (15–90 μm in diameter) develop, with single or multiple budding that may resemble the "ship's wheel" appearance of *Paracoccidioides brasiliensis* (p. 154).

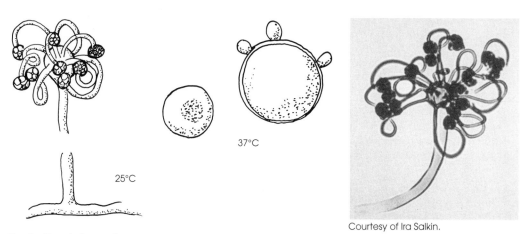

37°C

25°C

Courtesy of Ira Salkin.

For further information, see
de Hoog et al., 2000, pp. 72–73; Kemna et al., 1994; McGough et al., 1990

Cunninghamella bertholletiae

PATHOGENICITY: Commonly considered a contaminant, but has been involved in a few disseminated and pulmonary infections in compromised hosts.

RATE OF GROWTH: Rapid; mature within 4 days. Growth is inhibited by cycloheximide.

COLONY MORPHOLOGY: Very fluffy, like cotton candy; white, then gray. Reverse is white. (Color Plate 75.)

MICROSCOPIC MORPHOLOGY: Broad hyphae, almost nonseptate. Sporangiophores are long, branched, ending in swollen vesicles (30–65 μm in diameter); vesicles on lateral branches are smaller (14–35 μm in diameter). The vesicles are covered with spinelike denticles, each supporting a round to oval sporangiolum (5–8 × 6–14 μm; each sporangiolum contains one spore). The walls of the sporangiola are often encrusted with needlelike crystals. Rhizoids may be seen.

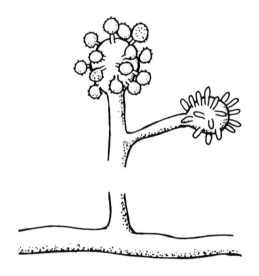 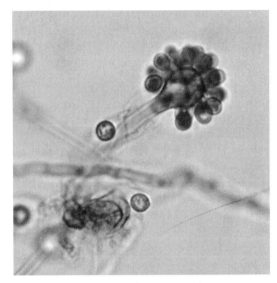

For further information, see
    de Hoog et al., 2000, pp. 74–75
    Kwon-Chung and Bennett, 1992, pp. 550–551, 802
    McGinnis, 1980, pp. 313, 315, 318
    Rippon, 1988, pp. 684, 752, 754

Syncephalastrum racemosum

PATHOGENICITY: Considered a contaminant; very rarely involved in infection.

RATE OF GROWTH: Rapid; mature within 3 days.

COLONY MORPHOLOGY: Quickly fills petri plate with white cotton candy-like fluff, then turns dark gray to almost black. Reverse is white. (Color Plate 76.)

MICROSCOPIC MORPHOLOGY: Hyphae are broad (4–10 μm in diameter) and almost nonseptate (irregular septa may form with age). Sporangiophores are rather short and branched and terminate in a round vesicle. On the vesicle are chains of round spores enclosed in fingerlike tubular sporangia (4–6 × 9–60 μm). Rhizoids are usually formed. This organism may at first resemble *Aspergillus niger* (p. 266), but careful examination reveals the tubular sporangia and the absence of phialides.

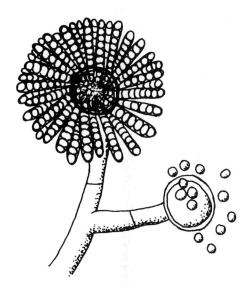 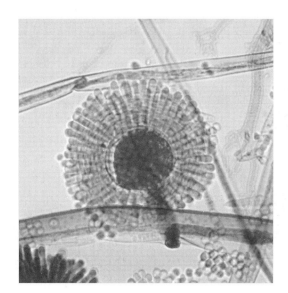

For further information, see
  de Hoog et al., 2000, pp. 113–114
  Kwon-Chung and Bennett, 1992, pp. 551–552, 807
  McGinnis, 1980, pp. 324–326
  Rippon, 1988, p. 751

Basidiobolus sp.

PATHOGENICITY: Etiologic agent of entomophthoromycosis basidiobolae (subcutaneous zygomycosis), which is a chronic inflammatory or granulomatous disease generally restricted to the limbs, chest, back, or buttocks. The lesions are characteristically huge, palpable, hard, nonulcerating subcutaneous masses. Gastrointestinal infections are also known to occasionally occur.

RATE OF GROWTH: Rapid; mature within 5 days.

COLONY MORPHOLOGY: Thin, flat, waxy; buff to gray. Becomes heaped up or radially folded, grayish brown, and covered with white aerial hyphae. Reverse is white. Some strains have an earthy odor similar to that of *Streptomyces* spp.

MICROSCOPIC MORPHOLOGY: Wide (8–20 μm) hyphae having occasional septa that become numerous with the production of spores. Short sporophores enlarge apically to form a swollen area from which a single-celled spore and a fragment of the sporophore are forcibly discharged. Other sporophores (not swollen) passively release club-shaped spores having a knob-like tip; these spores can function as sporangia, producing more sporangiospores. The organism also produces many round intercalary zygospores (20–50 μm in diameter) with smooth (occasionally rough), thick walls and a prominent beak-like appendage (remnant of a copulatory tube) on one side.

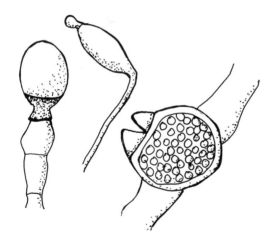
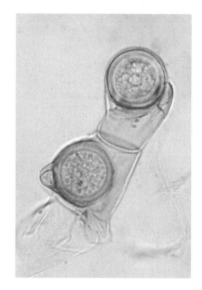

For further information, see
  de Hoog et al., 2000, pp. 116–117
  Kwon-Chung and Bennett, 1992, pp. 447–463
  McGinnis, 1980, pp. 306–309, 517
  Rippon, 1988, pp. 692–693, 708–709
  Wentworth, 1988, pp. 151–157, 225–227

Conidiobolus coronatus

PATHOGENICITY: Etiologic agent of entomophthoromycosis conidiobolae, which is a chronic inflammatory or granulomatous disease usually restricted to the nasal mucosa; it can spread to adjacent subcutaneous tissue and cause disfigurement of the face. The disease is characterized by polyps or palpable subcutaneous masses. On rare occasions, this and other species of the genus have caused deeply invasive, life-threatening infections.

RATE OF GROWTH: Rapid; mature within 5 days.

COLONY MORPHOLOGY: Flat, waxy; buff or gray, becoming sparsely covered with short white aerial hyphae. With age, colony becomes tan to brown. Reverse is white. Sides of culture tube or plate become covered with spores forcibly discharged by the sporophores.

MICROSCOPIC MORPHOLOGY: Hyphae have few septa; unbranched sporophores bear single-celled round spores (10–30 μm in diameter). At maturity, the spores are forcibly ejected and bear a broad, tapering projection at the site of former attachment. The spores may germinate and produce long hyphal tubes that become sporophores, each bearing another spore. A spore may also develop a number of short extensions that give rise to a corona of secondary spores. Spores may produce short, hairlike appendages.

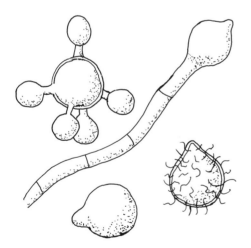

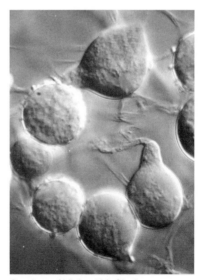

Courtesy of Michael McGinnis.

For further information, see
de Hoog et al., 2000, pp. 119–124; Kwon-Chung and Bennett, 1992, pp. 447–463;
McGinnis, 1980, pp. 310–313, 516–517; Rippon, 1988, pp. 690–692, 709–710;
Walsh et al., 1994; Wentworth, 1988, pp. 151–159, 225–226

Dematiaceous Fungi

Introduction

Dematiaceous fungi include a large group of organisms that produce dark (olive, brown, gray, or black) colonies because of a melanin pigment in their cell walls.

The diseases produced by some of the dematiaceous fungi are classified according to the clinical presentation and the appearance of the organism in tissue.

• **Chromoblastomycosis:** The fungi are seen in tissue as sclerotic bodies. These structures are round (5–12 μm in diameter), brownish, usually with a single septum or two intersecting septa. The infection is chronic and causes the development of warty nodules, tumorlike masses, or raised, rough, cauliflower-like lesions containing the sclerotic bodies. The lesions usually develop in the subcutaneous tissue of the lower extremities but are sometimes on other exposed areas, such as the hands, head region, or trunk. On rare occasions, the etiologic agents have been known to spread to the central nervous system, lungs, or muscular tissues.

• **Phaeohyphomycosis:** The etiologic agents occur in tissue as dark yeastlike cells, pseudohypha-like elements, variously shaped hyphae, or any combination of these forms. The infection may be cutaneous, subcutaneous, or systemic.

• **Mycetoma:** The infection is chronic and characterized by swollen tumorlike lesions that yield granular pus through draining sinuses. The granules of eumycotic mycetoma may be dark or light (many of the etiologic agents are not dematiaceous) and contain variously shaped fungal elements. The infection occurs most often in the feet or hands but may occur on any exposed parts of the body.

Tinea nigra and black piedra are also caused by dematiaceous fungi.

Many of the infections caused by the dematiaceous fungi are due to traumatic implantation of the organism from the environment into cutaneous or subcutaneous tissue, but pulmonary or disseminated infections have been initiated by inhalation of conidia.

Although the dematiaceous fungi are not highly virulent, some are regularly seen as etiologic agents of disease while others usually are encountered as saprophytes or contaminants and only occasionally act as opportunistic pathogens.

Sporothrix schenckii grows as a dematiaceous fungus when incubated at 25–30°C, but it is yeastlike and nonpigmented at 35–37°C and is therefore placed with the thermally dimorphic fungi (p. 148).

For further information, see
  Murray et al. (ed.), 1999, Manual of Clinical Microbiology, 7th ed., chapters 101 and 102

Fonsecaea pedrosoi

PATHOGENICITY: The most common worldwide cause of chromoblastomycosis (for a description of the disease, see p. 44). The lesions usually develop in the subcutaneous tissue on the lower extremities but sometimes are on other exposed areas. On very rare occasions, the organism has been known to cause internal infections.

RATE OF GROWTH: Slow; mature in 14 days.

COLONY MORPHOLOGY: Surface is dark green, gray, or black, covered with silvery, velvety mycelium; colonies are usually flat and then develop a convex cone-shaped protrusion in the center. Colony becomes slightly imbedded in the medium. Reverse is black. (Color Plates 77 and 78.)

MICROSCOPIC MORPHOLOGY: Hyphae are septate, branched, and brown; conidia are dark, 1.5–3.0 × 2.5–6.0 µm. Conidiation is enhanced on cornmeal agar or potato dextrose agar. Four types of conidial formation may be seen.

1. *Fonsecaea* type: Conidiophores are septate, erect, and compactly sympodial. The distal end of the conidiophore develops swollen denticles that bear primary single-celled ovoid conidia. Denticles on the primary conidia support secondary single-celled conidia that may produce tertiary conidia, but long chains are not formed. Elongate conidia often form in verticils at fertile sites along the conidiophore, producing an asterisk-like appearance.

2. *Rhinocladiella* type: Conidiophores are septate, erect, and sympodial; swollen denticles bear ovoid conidia at the tip and along the side of the conidiophore. Usually only primary conidia develop; secondary conidia are rare.

3. *Cladosporium* type: Conidiophores are erect and give rise to large primary shield-shaped conidia that in turn produce short, branching chains of oval conidia having small dark hila (scars of attachment).

4. *Phialophora* type: Phialides are vase shaped with terminal cuplike collarettes. Round to oval conidia accumulate at the apex of the phialide. This type of conidiation is often scant or lacking.

Note: In tissues, this organism, as well as the other etiologic agents of chromoblastomycosis, appears as large (5–12 µm diameter), round, brownish, thick-walled cells with horizontal and vertical septa. When cultured at 25, 30, or 37°C, the organisms are filamentous.

(continued on following page)

THERMALLY MONOMORPHIC MOULDS: Dematiaceous Fungi

Fonsecaea pedrosoi (continued)

Fonsecaea-type
conidiation

Rhinocladiella-type
conidiation

Phialophora-type
conidiation

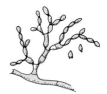

Cladosporium-type
conidiation

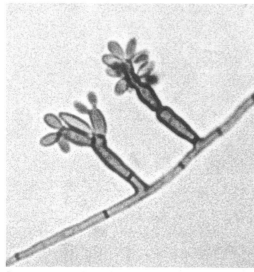

Fonsecaea- and *Rhinocladiella*- type conidiation.

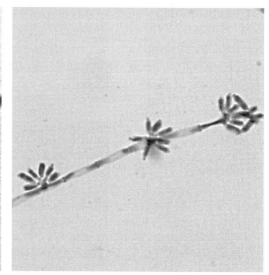

"Asterisk" of *Fonsecaea*-type conidiation.

For further information, see
de Hoog et al., 2000, pp. 676, 679–680
Kwon-Chung and Bennett, 1992, pp. 337–349
McGinnis, 1980, pp. 213–219, 482–484
Rippon, 1988, pp. 276, 287–293
Wentworth, 1988, pp. 117–128

Fonsecaea compacta

PATHOGENICITY: Causes chromoblastomycosis. For a description of the disease, see p. 44. This organism is rarely encountered.

RATE OF GROWTH: Very slow; mature in 28 days.

COLONY MORPHOLOGY: Surface is dark green to black, heaped, and brittle, with irregular indented border. After 3 or 4 weeks, brownish hyphae appear on the surface with typical conidiophores and conidial formations. Reverse is black.

MICROSCOPIC MORPHOLOGY: On Sabouraud dextrose agar, hyphae are septate, brown, and branched and bear predominantly *Fonsecaea*-type conidiophores that produce short chains and masses of almost round conidia (1.5–3 μm in diameter). The outstanding characteristics of this species are (i) the cask-like shape of the conidia with the wide diameter of the septa between conidia and (ii) the compact arrangement of the conidial chains, which are not easily dissociated. *Rhinocladiella*-, *Cladosporium*-, and *Phialophora*-type conidiation (p. 184) may also be seen.

In tissue, the organisms appear as dark, round, septate cells (5–12 μm in diameter).

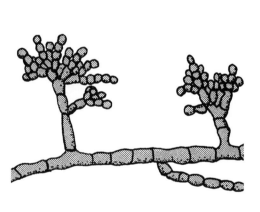
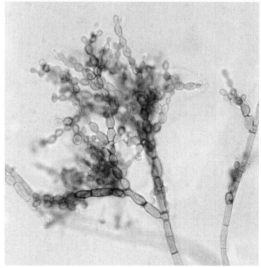

For further information, see
  de Hoog et al., 2000, pp. 677–678
  Kwon-Chung and Bennett, 1992, pp. 349–350
  McGinnis, 1980, pp. 213–218, 221–222, 482–484
  Rippon, 1988, p. 293

TABLE 13 Characteristics of *Phialophora*, *Phaeoacremonium*, *Acremonium*, *Phialemonium*, and *Lecythophora*

Organism	Colony	Basal septum	Phialide		Conidia	Illustration
			Shape	Collarette		
Phialophora (p. 187)	Dark greenish brown to black	Yes, usually	Flask or vase shaped	Flared, distinct (*P. repens* is an exception)	Oval or round; clusters	
Phaeoacremonium (p. 189)	Dark olive gray to dark brown or black	Yes, usually	Cylindrical; rough at base; tapered toward tip	Almost inconspicuous; tubular or slightly funnel shaped	Oblong; some curved; clusters	
Acremonium (p. 279)	White, gray, or rose; cottony	Yes, usually	Erect, cylindrical; unbranched; tapered	Inconspicuous	Oblong; clusters	
Phialemonium (p. 190)	White, then yellow, gray, light brown, or greenish; may become dark	No, usually not	Short, peg-like or long, cylindrical	Inconspicuous	Tear shaped or oblong; curved or straight; clusters	
Lecythophora (p. 282)	Pink or salmon; moist to slimy	No, usually not	Short; volcano shaped along hyphae	Parallel sided	Oval to oblong; straight or slight curve; no clusters	

Phialophora verrucosa

PATHOGENICITY: Causes chromoblastomycosis, of which it is the second common etiologic agent worldwide (*Fonsecaea pedrosoi* is the most co agent). It is also an etiologic agent of phaeohyphomycosis and, on rare occ mycetoma. For descriptions of these diseases, see pp. 44, 43, and 32, respectively.

RATE OF GROWTH: Moderate; mature in 7–12 days.

COLONY MORPHOLOGY: Surface is dark greenish brown to black with a close matlike olive to gray mycelium. Some strains are heaped and granular; others are flat. Colonies become imbedded in the medium. Reverse is black. (Color Plate 79.)

MICROSCOPIC MORPHOLOGY: Hyphae are brown, branched, and septate. Phialides are vase shaped with a flared cuplike collarette; they usually have a distinct septum at the base. Round to oval conidia (1–3 × 2–4 μm) accumulate at the apex of the phialide, giving the appearance of a vase of flowers.

To differentiate *Phialophora* from other similar genera, see Table 13 (p. 186).

Note: In tissue with chromoblastomycosis, the organism appears as dark, round, septate cells, 5–12 μm in diameter.

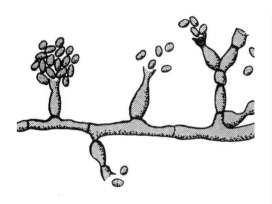
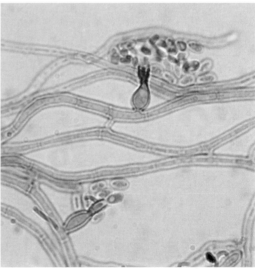

For further information, see
  de Hoog et al., 2000, pp. 864, 878–879
  Kwon-Chung and Bennett, 1992, pp. 346–347
  McGinnis, 1980, pp. 261–265, 482–484
  Rippon, 1988, pp. 293–294

Phialophora richardsiae

PATHOGENICITY: An uncommon agent of cystic subcutaneous phaeohyphomycosis* (see p. 43 for a description of the disease). Most reported cases have been in debilitated or immunocompromised patients.

RATE OF GROWTH: Moderate; mature in 6–10 days.

COLONY MORPHOLOGY: Surface is olive-brown to brownish gray, woolly to velvety or powdery; brown diffusing pigment may develop with age. Reverse is dark.

MICROSCOPIC MORPHOLOGY: Septate hyphae are at first colorless and become brown. The distinguishing phialides usually (but not always) have a distinct septum at the base and are slightly flask shaped with a characteristic flared, saucer-shaped collarette; they produce conidia that are brown and almost round (2–3.5 μm in diameter). Simple, short, unflared phialides may also form along the hyphae and produce conidia that are hyaline and cylindrical or slightly curved (2–3 × 3–6 μm).

To differentiate *Phialophora* from other similar genera, see Table 13 (p. 186).

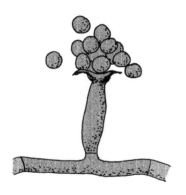
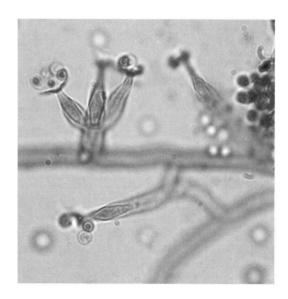

For more information, see
  de Hoog et al., 2000, pp. 864, 876–877
  Kwon-Chung and Bennett, 1992, pp. 658–661
  Rippon, 1988, pp. 307–311

---

*Note that *Phialophora repens* is also an occasional agent of phaeohyphomycosis. The phialides form singly or in penicillately branched groups; the collarettes are typically unflared and inconspicuous. It has been suggested that it be placed in the genus *Cadophora*. The organism formerly known as *Phialophora parasitica* is now *Phaeoacremonium parasiticum* (see p. 189).

THERMALLY MONOMORPHIC MOULDS: Dematiaceous Fungi

Phaeoacremonium parasiticum (formerly *Phialophora parasitica*)

PATHOGENICITY: Has been reported in cases of subcutaneous phaeohyphomycoses, mycetoma, arthritis, endocarditis, and disseminated infection.

RATE OF GROWTH: Moderate; mature within 7 days.

COLONY MORPHOLOGY: Surface initially cream colored and velvety, then becomes olive-gray to black and develops clusters of aerial hyphae. Reverse blackish. (Color Plate 80.)

MICROSCOPIC MORPHOLOGY: Young hyphae appear hyaline, later brown and rough or warty; they may accumulate side by side to form thick bundles (fascicles). Phialides form along the hyphae or on branched or unbranched conidiophores that may be rough walled near the base; phialides are brown, cylindrical (2–3 × 15–35 μm), slightly tapering toward the apex; they usually have a basal septum and a collarette that is small and tubular or vaguely funnel shaped. Conidia are hyaline, oblong (1–2 × 3–6 μm), some curved, gathering in clusters at end of phialide.

To differentiate *Phaeoacremonium* from other similar genera, see Table 13 (p. 186).

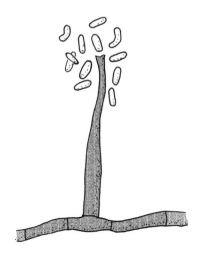

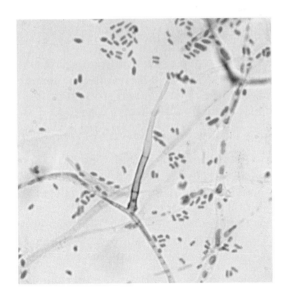

For further information, see
Crous et al., 1996
de Hoog et al., 2000, pp. 846–852

Phialemonium spp.

(Genus is intermediate between *Phialophora* and *Acremonium*.)

PATHOGENICITY: Occasionally isolated from clinical specimens. Has been reported in a subcutaneous phaeohyphomycotic cyst; an endocarditis mixed infection; peritonitis; fungemia due to contaminated venous catheters; infection of cutaneous, subcutaneous, and spleen tissue in a burn patient; and osteomyelitis in a dog. All of the involved patients were immunocompromised.

RATE OF GROWTH: Moderately rapid; mature within 5–7 days.

COLONY MORPHOLOGY: Broadly spreading. Surface is at first white or cream, becoming yellow, grayish, or slightly greenish (the pale yellow or green pigment may diffuse into the agar); with age, light brown or gray areas may develop; some colonies produce chlamydoconidia and develop dark centers. Texture may be smooth or slightly fuzzy or may have superficial radiating hyphal strands. Reverse is light with pale wine-buff or brown areas sometimes developing.

MICROSCOPIC MORPHOLOGY: Hyphae are septate and hyaline or very pale yellow-brown; they may accumulate side by side to form thick bundles (fascicles). Phialides form singly along the hyphae, usually with no septum at the base to delimit it from the hypha; they may be short and peg-like (0.5–1.5 × 1.0–9.0 μm) or longer and cylindrical (up to 30 μm long, 1–2 μm wide), usually lacking a visible collarette when grown on routine mycology media (rarely forms a very inconspicuous cylindrical, parallel-walled collarette). Conidia are single celled (1.0–2.5 × 3.0–6.0 μm), hyaline, and smooth walled and form clusters. Hyaline chlamydoconidia sometimes form in old colonies.

Note: The two major species of *Phialemonium* can be differentiated as follows.

- *P. obovatum* produces conidia that are oval to tear shaped, may appear slightly cut off at the base, consistently straight; old colonies become greenish; pale brown chlamydoconidia may develop in old cultures and result in brown spots or a black center on the colony.
- *P. curvatum* (includes *P. dimorphosporum*) produces conidia that are oval, elongate, and curved (some may remain straight). Chlamydoconidia are not formed. Colonies may develop pale wine-buff zones on reverse side.

Phenotypic characteristics of this genus show significant variation depending on culture medium and temperature. It is therefore recommended to standardize conditions, e.g., use potato dextrose agar and incubate at 24–25°C.

To differentiate *Phialemonium* from other similar genera, see Table 13 (p. 186).

Phialemonium spp. *(continued)*

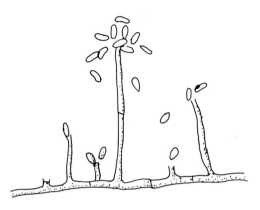

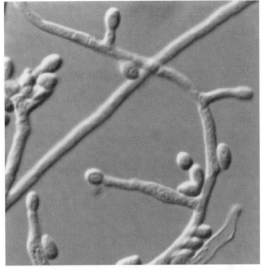

Courtesy of Wiley Schell.

For further information, see
  de Hoog et al., 2000, pp. 859–863
  Gams and McGinnis, 1983
  Guarro et al., 1999

Cladosporium spp.

PATHOGENICITY: Commonly considered saprophytic contaminants. They have only occasionally been implicated in infections.

RATE OF GROWTH: Moderately rapid; mature within 7 days at 25°C. Most strains do not grow at 37°C, but some do.

COLONY MORPHOLOGY: Surface is greenish brown or black with grayish velvety nap, becoming heaped and slightly folded. Reverse is black. (Color Plate 81.)

MICROSCOPIC MORPHOLOGY: Hyphae are septate and dark; conidiophores are dark and branched, vary in length, and usually produce 2 or more conidial chains. Conidia are brown, round to oval (3–6 × 4–12 μm), and usually smooth; they form branching treelike chains and are easily dislodged, showing dark spots (hila) at the point where they were attached to the conidiophore or other conidia. The cells bearing the conidial chains are large and sometimes septate, resemble shields, and may be mistaken for macroconidia when seen alone.

See Table 14 (p. 193) for differentiation from *Cladophialophora* spp.

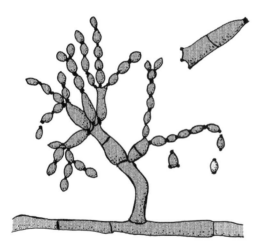 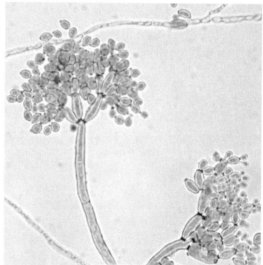

For further information, see
de Hoog et al., 2000, pp. 582–592
Kwon-Chung and Bennett, 1992, pp. 801–802
McGinnis, 1980, pp. 198–201, 203
Rippon, 1988, pp. 771, 773

TABLE 14 Characteristics of *Cladosporium* and *Cladophialophora* spp.[a]

Organism	Distinct conidiophores	"Shield cells"	Shape of conidia	Distinct hila on conidia	Conidial chain length	Conidial chain branching	Maximum growth temp (°C)	Gelatin hydrolysis	Growth with 15% NaCl	Pathogenicity
Cladosporium spp.	+	+	Oval	+	Short	Frequent	<37 (V)[b]	+ (V)[c]	+	Nonpathogenic
Cladophialophora carrionii	±	±	Oval	±	Medium	Moderate	35–37	–	–	Causes chromoblastomycosis
Cladophialophora bantiana	–	–	Oval	–	Long	Sparse	42–43	–	–	Causes cerebral phaeohyphomycosis
Cladophialophora emmonsii	–	–	Bent	–	Medium	Sparse	37	–	–	Rare cause of subcutaneous phaeohyphomycosis

[a]Reprinted (updated) by permission of the publisher from Larone, 1989. Copyright by Elsevier Science Inc. Abbreviations: +, positive; –, negative; ±, sometimes difficult to distinguish; V, variable.

[b]29% grow at 40°C.

[c]86% positive.

Cladophialophora carrionii (formerly *Cladosporium carrionii*)

PATHOGENICITY: Causes chromoblastomycosis, most commonly in Australia, Venezuela, and South Africa (for a description of the disease, see p. 44).

RATE OF GROWTH: Slow; mature within 18 days.

COLONY MORPHOLOGY: Dark surface, flat with slightly raised center, covered with velvety dull gray, gray-green, or purplish-brown short-napped mycelium. Reverse is black. (Color Plate 82.)

MICROSCOPIC MORPHOLOGY: Hyphae are septate and dark with lateral and terminal conidiophores of various sizes. Conidiophores produce long, branching chains of brown, smooth-walled, oval, somewhat pointed conidia (~2.5 × 4.5–7 μm) that are easily dispersed with handling. The conidia typically have relatively pale scars of attachment (i.e., hila that are not as dark and prominent as those of *Cladosporium* spp.). Phialides with wide collarettes occasionally form on nutritionally deficient media.

For differentiation from *Cladosporium* spp. and other species of *Cladophialophora*, see Table 14 (p. 193).

In tissue, the organism appears as large (5–12 μm in diameter), dark, round, septate cells.

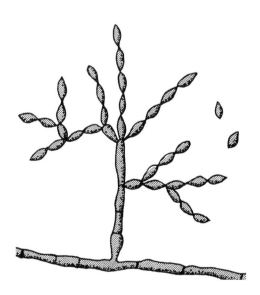
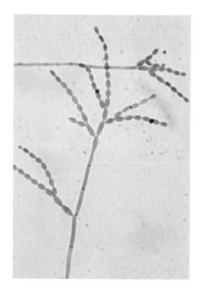

For further information, see
  de Hoog et al., 2000, pp. 570–572
  Kwon-Chung and Bennett, 1992, pp. 350–351
  McGinnis, 1980, pp. 198–203
  Rippon, 1988, pp. 291, 295

Cladophialophora bantiana (previously known as *Xylohypha bantiana, Cladosporium bantianum,* and *Cladosporium trichoides*)

PATHOGENICITY: The organism has a predilection for the central nervous system and consequently causes cerebral phaeohyphomycosis. Infection might be contracted through inhalation; extreme care and a biological safety cabinet must be used when handling this organism. Slide cultures should NOT be made. It is only rarely involved in cutaneous and subcutaneous infections.

RATE OF GROWTH: Slow; mature within 15 days.

COLONY MORPHOLOGY: Surface is olive-gray to brown or black and velvety. Reverse is black.

MICROSCOPIC MORPHOLOGY: Brown septate hyphae with conidiophores that are similar to the vegetative hyphae; long, sparsely branched wavy chains of smooth oval conidia (2.5–5 × 5–9 μm); the conidia do not display conspicuous scars of attachment. For differentiation from similar organisms, see Table 14 (p. 193).

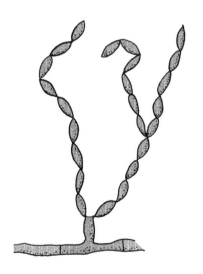

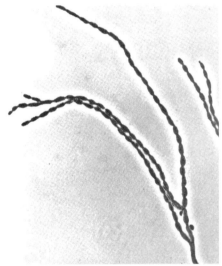

From Michael McGinnis, *Manual of Clinical Microbiology,* 4th ed.

For further information, see
de Hoog et al., 2000, pp. 564–566
Kwon-Chung and Bennett, 1992, pp. 642–645
Rippon, 1988, p. 309

Pseudallescheria boydii (sexual state); *Scedosporium apiospermum* (asexual state)*

PATHOGENICITY: Has been known for many years to cause mycetoma (see p. 32 for a description of the disease). The infection occurs most often in the feet or hands but may occur on any exposed parts of the body. This organism is now also recognized as an agent of phaeohyphomycosis. It can infect the subcutaneous tissue, bones, brain, eyes, lungs, sinuses, meninges, and other body sites. Disseminated infection has been reported in immunocompromised patients.

RATE OF GROWTH: Moderately rapid; mature in 7 days. The sexual stage (*P. boydii)* is inhibited by cycloheximide; the asexual stage (*S. apiospermum*) is not inhibited.

COLONY MORPHOLOGY: Surface has a spreading, white, cottony aerial mycelium which later turns gray or brown. Reverse is at first white but usually becomes gray or black. (Color Plates 83 and 84.)

MICROSCOPIC MORPHOLOGY: Hyphae are septate (2–4 μm in diameter), with simple long or short conidiophores bearing conidia singly or in small groups (may resemble mould phase of *Blastomyces dermatitidis,* p. 152). The conidia (4–7 × 5–12 μm) are unicellular and oval, with the larger end toward the apex, and appear cut off at the base (i.e., truncate); they become dark with age. The *Graphium* type of asexual conidiation (p. 215) is seen occasionally; it is characterized by long, erect, narrow conidiophores that are cemented together, diverge at the apex, and bear clusters of oval, truncate conidia (2–3 × 5–7 μm). In the sexual stage, large brown cleistothecia (50–250 μm in diameter) are formed and release elliptical ascospores when ruptured. The sexual stage may sometimes be induced by culturing on corn-meal agar or potato dextrose agar; the cleistothecia are most likely to form in the center of the colony.

---

*The sexual-stage name has priority over the asexual-stage name. The designation *P. boydii* should therefore be used if the sexual stage is demonstrated; if only the asexual stage is seen, the organism should be called *S. apiospermum.*

Pseudallescheria boydii (sexual state); *Scedosporium apiospermum* (asexual state) *(continued)*

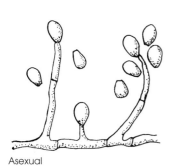

Asexual

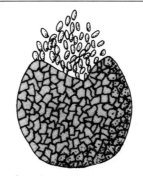

Sexual

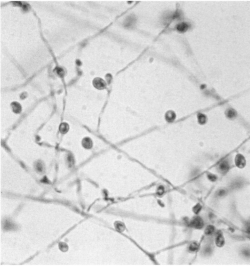

Asexual stage.

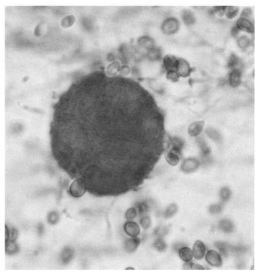

Sexual stage.

For further information, see
  de Hoog et al., 2000, pp. 305–309
  Kwon-Chung and Bennett, 1992, pp. 577, 678–794
  McGinnis, 1980, pp. 172–173, 227–228, 268–271, 505–508
  Rippon, 1988, pp. 105, 651–676
  Wentworth, 1988, pp. 106–113, 117

THERMALLY MONOMORPHIC MOULDS: Dematiaceous Fungi

Scedosporium prolificans (formerly *Scedosporium inflatum*)

PATHOGENICITY: Causes invasive infection which is often characterized by arthritis or osteomyelitis. Localized and disseminated infections occur in a variety of sites. The isolates are often resistant to antifungal agents, and disseminated infections are commonly fatal. Both immunocompromised and immunocompetent patients have presented with infections due to this organism. Asymptomatic colonization has also been reported.

RATE OF GROWTH: Rapid; mature within 5 days. Growth is inhibited by cycloheximide.

COLONY MORPHOLOGY: Young colony is cottony or moist (yeasty) and light gray to black. Mature colony becomes dark gray to black and may develop white mycelial tufts with age. Reverse is gray to black. (Color Plates 85 and 86)

MICROSCOPIC MORPHOLOGY: Hyphae are septate, with conidiogenous cells (annellides) having a swollen base and elongated "neck"; conidia form small clusters at the apex. Conidia (2–5 × 3–12 μm) are olive to brown, one celled, smooth, and ovoid with a slightly narrowed, truncated (cut-off) base. There is no known sexual state.

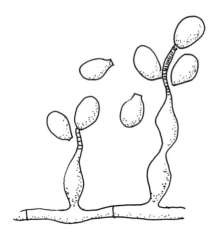
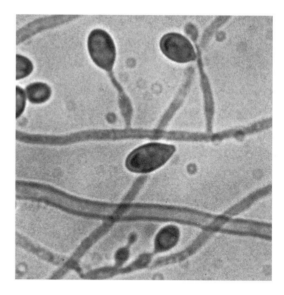

For further information, see
  de Hoog et al., 2000, pp. 899–901
  Kwon-Chung and Bennett, 1992, pp. 678–694
  Rippon, 1988, pp. 675–676

*Dactylaria constricta**

PATHOGENICITY: *D. constricta* var. *gallopava* has caused subcutaneous and disseminated infections in immunocompromised patients with underlying diseases. The organism is known to have a predilection for the central nervous system and to cause encephalitis in turkeys, chickens, and other birds. *D. constricta* var. *constricta* is not known to be pathogenic.

RATE OF GROWTH: Rapid; mature within 5 days.

COLONY MORPHOLOGY: Surface is woolly and dark olive-gray, reddish brown, or gray-black. Reverse is dark; a red to brown pigment usually diffuses into the medium. (Color Plate 87.)

MICROSCOPIC MORPHOLOGY: Hyphae are septate, with conidiophores that are hyaline, erect, and sometimes knobby or bent at the point of conidial formation. Conidia (average, 3.5 × 10 μm) form on threadlike denticles; they are brownish, two celled, oval to tear shaped, and typically have a marked constriction at the central septum. A frill of the denticle often remains on the base of the conidium after detachment from the conidiophore. Young conidia may be round and single celled.

See Table 15 (p. 200) for differentiation of varieties.

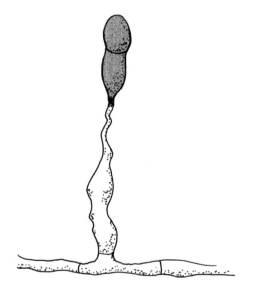

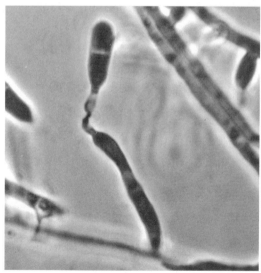

Courtesy of Dennis Dixon.

For more information, see
  de Hoog et al., 2000, pp. 779–783
  Dixon and Salkin, 1986
  Kwon-Chung and Bennett, 1992, pp. 667–668

---

*There is disagreement among mycologists as to whether the varieties of this organism should be considered separate species and into which genus they should be classified, i.e., *Dactylaria*, *Ochroconis*, or *Scolecobasidium*.

TABLE 15 Differentiation of the varieties of *Dactylaria constricta*[a]

Organism	Growth with cycloheximide[b]	Gelatinase at ≤7 days	Growth at 37–45°C	Pathogenic for humans and birds
D. constricta var. gallopava	0	0[c]	+[d]	+
D. constricta var. constricta	+	+	0	0

[a]Some mycologists consider the varieties *gallopava* and *constricta* to be separate species, while others place them in the genera *Ochroconis* and *Scolecobasidium*. Abbreviations: 0, negative; +, positive.
[b]Mycosel agar (BBL, Cockeysville, Md.).
[c]Delayed positive; ≥21 days.
[d]Grows more rapidly at 37–45°C than at 30°C.

TABLE 16 Characteristics of some of the "black yeasts"[a]

Organism	Decomposition of:		Growth in 15% NaCl	KNO₃ assimilation	Maximum growth temp (°C)
	Casein (% positive)	Tyrosine (% positive)			
Exophiala jeanselmei	0	+ (78)	0	+	≤37
Wangiella dermatitidis	0	+ (83)	0	0	42
Phaeoannellomyces werneckii	+ (78)	0 (22)	+	+	Varying reports

[a]Reprinted by permission of the publisher from Larone, 1989. Copyright Elsevier Science Inc. Abbreviations: +, positive; 0, negative.

Exophiala jeanselmei

PATHOGENICITY: Causes mycetoma and phaeohyphomycosis. Chromoblastomycosis-like infections have only rarely been reported. For descriptions of diseases, see pp. 32, 43, and 44, respectively.

RATE OF GROWTH: Slow; mature within 14 days when incubated at 25–30°C. Grows more slowly or not at all at 37°C.

COLONY MORPHOLOGY: Surface is at first brownish black or greenish black and skinlike; it then becomes covered with short, velvety, grayish hyphae. Reverse is black. (Color Plates 88 and 89.)

MICROSCOPIC MORPHOLOGY: Young culture consists of many yeastlike budding cells. Eventually, septate hyphae form with numerous conidiogenous cells (annellides) that are slender, tubular, sometimes branched, and characteristically tapered to a narrow, elongated tip. The conidia (1–3 × 2–5 μm) are oval and gather in clusters at the end and sides of the conidiophore and at points along the hyphae. Conidium formation is often best exhibited on cornmeal agar or potato dextrose agar.

See Table 16 (p. 200) for differentiation from similar organisms.

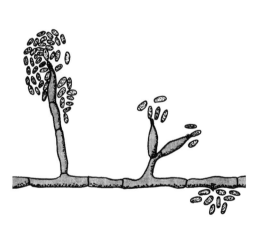 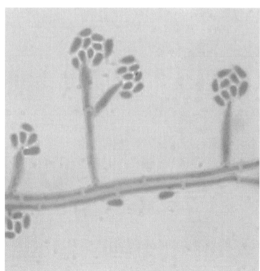

For further information, see
  de Hoog et al., 2000, pp. 655–657
  Kwon-Chung and Bennett, 1992, pp. 575–577, 646–653
  McGinnis, 1980, pp. 211–213, 505–508, 511
  Rippon, 1988, pp. 108–109, 308–309
  Wentworth, 1988, pp. 127–142

Wangiella dermatitidis (Exophiala dermatitidis)

PATHOGENICITY: Causes phaeohyphomycosis (for a description of the disease, see p. 43). The organism appears to have a predilection for the central nervous system; it has been involved in infections of the brain and eye as well as cutaneous and subcutaneous tissue.

RATE OF GROWTH: Slow; mature and filamentous within 25 days (yeastlike in 10 days).

COLONY MORPHOLOGY: At first the colony is black, moist, shiny, and yeastlike. After 3 or 4 weeks or upon repeated subculture, olive-gray aerial hyphae develop at the periphery and sometimes near the center of the colony. Reverse is dark. (Color Plates 90 and 91.)

MICROSCOPIC MORPHOLOGY: Young cultures are composed of dark (may originally be hyaline), oval to round, budding, yeastlike cells. These cells eventually produce dark, septate hyphae and flask-shaped to cylindrical phialides that lack a flared lip. Round to oval, single-celled, pale brown conidia (2–4 × 2.5–6 μm) accumulate at the apex of the phialide and down the sides of the conidiophore. Conidia may also be produced at projections along the hyphae; annellides of the *Exophiala* type have been observed in some isolates. Production of conidia is often sparse.

See Table 16 (p. 200) for differentiation from similar organisms.

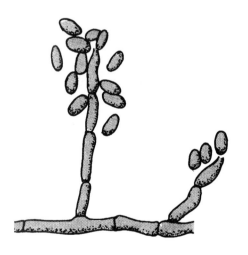

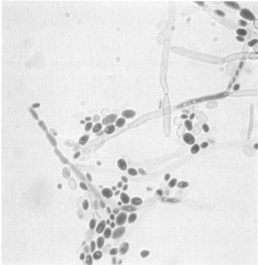

For further information, see
   de Hoog et al., 2000, pp. 652–654
   Kwon-Chung and Bennett, 1992, pp. 647–650
   McGinnis, 1980, pp. 300, 304, 311, 511
   Rippon, 1988, pp. 305–307
   Wentworth, 1988, pp. 141–142, 146–147

Phaeoannellomyces werneckii (Hortaea werneckii, Exophiala werneckii)

PATHOGENICITY: Etiologic agent of tinea nigra, a superficial asymptomatic fungal infection of the skin, usually on the palms of the hands and occasionally on other parts of the body. The lesions are flat, smooth, and not scaly and appear as irregularly shaped brown to black spots resembling silver nitrate stains.

RATE OF GROWTH: Develops slowly; mature within 21 days.

COLONY MORPHOLOGY: Surface is at first light colored, moist, shiny, and yeast-like but soon becomes olive-black. Later, grayish green hyphae may form at the periphery, and the center may lose its shine and become olive colored due to thin layer of mycelium. Reverse is black.

MICROSCOPIC MORPHOLOGY: The very early phase consists mainly of pale or dark brown yeastlike cells, some having a central septum. These cells (2–5 × 5–10 μm) are actually annellides; they are round at one end while tapered and elongated with striations at the other end where conidia are formed. With age, dark, closely septated, thick-walled hyphae may develop. The one- or two-celled annelloconidia may form and accumulate at annellidic points along the hyphae. Each conidium can function as an annellide and produce new conidia.

For characteristics differentiating *Phaeoannellomyces werneckii* from *Wangiella dermatitidis* and *Exophiala jeanselmei*, see Table 16 (p. 200).

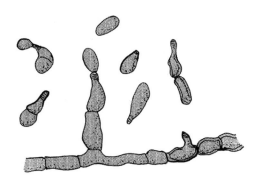
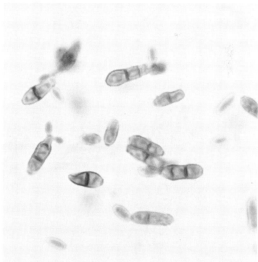

For further information, see
de Hoog et al., 2000, pp. 720–722
Kwon-Chung and Bennett, 1992, pp. 191–197
McGinnis, 1980, pp. 211–213, 215
Rippon, 1988, pp. 159–163
Wentworth, 1988, pp. 34–40

Madurella mycetomatis

PATHOGENICITY: Causes black grain mycetoma (for a description of the disease, see p. 32).

RATE OF GROWTH: Moderate at 37°C; mature in 10 days. Grows much more slowly at 25°C.

COLONY MORPHOLOGY: Varies greatly; may be smooth or folded and glabrous or powdery and ranges in color from white to yellowish brown. There is usually a brown diffusible pigment in the agar. Reverse is dark brown.

MICROSCOPIC MORPHOLOGY: On Sabouraud dextrose agar, forms only septate hyphae (1–6 μm in diameter) with numerous chlamydoconidium-like enlarged cells. On cornmeal agar, some strains produce phialides that bear round or oval conidia at their tips. May form large, black masses of modified hyphae (sclerotia) in old cultures.

M. mycetomatis differs biochemically from *Madurella grisea* in assimilating lactose but not sucrose.

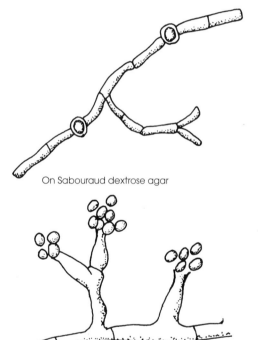

On Sabouraud dextrose agar

On cornmeal agar

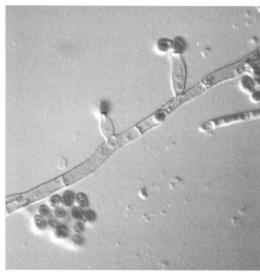

On cornmeal agar. Courtesy of Arvind Padhye.

For further information, see
   Kwon-Chung and Bennett, 1992, pp. 574–579; McGinnis, 1980, pp. 232–234, 236–237, 505–508; Rippon, 1988, pp. 103–107; Wentworth, 1988, pp. 106–114, 117

Madurella grisea

PATHOGENICITY: Causes black grain mycetoma (for a description of the disease, see p. 32).

RATE OF GROWTH: Moderately slow at 25–30°C; mature in 12 days. Does not grow well, if at all, at 37°C.

COLONY MORPHOLOGY: Surface is somewhat folded in the center with radial grooves toward the periphery. Very short, tan or gray aerial hyphae cover a dark gray or olive-brown mycelial mat. Reverse is dark. May form diffusible pigment, but not as commonly as does *Madurella mycetomatis.*

MICROSCOPIC MORPHOLOGY: Hyphae are septate, mostly wide (3–5 μm), branched, and dark. These hyphae sometimes appear to be made up of chains of rounded cells, suggesting a budding process. Thinner (1–3 μm in diameter), cylindrical, branched hyphae are also present. Conidia are not commonly formed. Some strains may produce pycnidia; chlamydoconidia are occasionally produced.

M. grisea differs biochemically from *M. mycetomatis* in assimilating sucrose but not lactose.

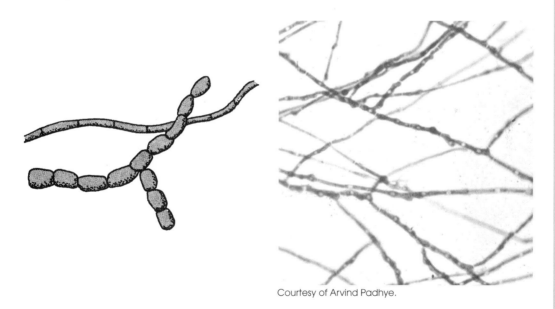

Courtesy of Arvind Padhye.

For further information, see
  Kwon-Chung and Bennett, 1992, pp. 574–575, 579
  Rippon, 1988, pp. 104–107
  Wentworth, 1988, pp. 106–114, 116–117

Piedraia hortae

PATHOGENICITY: Causes black piedra, a fungal infection of the hairs of the scalp seen most commonly in the tropics. It is characterized by the formation of small, stony hard, dark nodules along the hair shafts. White piedra is caused by *Trichosporon ovoides* and *Trichosporon inkin* (p. 140).

RATE OF GROWTH: Slow; mature in 21 days.

COLONY MORPHOLOGY: Colonies are small, adherent, compact, somewhat raised, and dark greenish brown to black and may be glabrous or covered with very short aerial hyphae. Reddish brown diffusible pigment may form. Reverse is black.

MICROSCOPIC MORPHOLOGY: Hyphae are closely septate, dark, and thick walled and vary in diameter, with many intercalary chlamydoconidium-like cells. Asci may be produced in culture. The walls of the asci readily dissolve, releasing single-celled, curved ascospores (5–10 × 30–35 μm) that taper at the ends to form whiplike extensions. The ascospores are more likely to be seen on direct microscopic examination of the specimen than on culture.

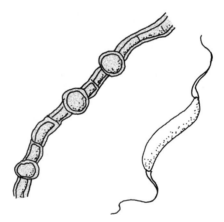

For further information, see
  de Hoog et al., 2000, pp. 303–304
  Kwon-Chung and Bennett, 1992, pp. 183–190
  Rippon, 1988, pp. 163–168
  Wentworth, 1988, pp. 39–43

Aureobasidium pullulans

PATHOGENICITY: Relatively rare agent of phaeohyphomycosis; reported cases include corneal, peritoneal, cutaneous, pulmonary, and systemic infections. May also be encountered as a contaminant in clinical specimens.

RATE OF GROWTH: Rapid; growth appears within 3–5 days, but pigment production and characteristic morphology may require extended incubation.

COLONY MORPHOLOGY: Colony is at first white, very occasionally pale pink; appears moist and creamy. Eventually develops areas of brown or black (when arthroconidia develop) and becomes shiny, with a white to grayish fringe. Reverse is dark when colony is mature. (Color Plate 92.)

MICROSCOPIC MORPHOLOGY: Young colonies consist of unicellular, budding, yeastlike cells. Two types of hyphae develop: (i) hyaline, delicate, and thin walled, producing blastoconidia directly from the walls at certain fertile points, and (ii) thick-walled, dark, and closely septated segments that become arthroconidia. The blastoconidia are hyaline and oval, vary in size (average, 3–6 × 6–12 μm), and may continue to multiply by budding; they form synchronously on the hyaline hyphae. The early yeastlike form may be similar to *Candida* spp. or young cultures of *Phaeoannellomyces werneckii* (p. 203) and *Wangiella dermatitidis* (p. 202), but it can be distinguished by careful examination of growth rate and mature microscopic morphology.

A. pullulans is most likely to be confused with *Hormonema dematioides* (p. 210); for differentiation of these two fungi, see Table 17 (p. 209).

(continued on following page)

THERMALLY MONOMORPHIC MOULDS: Dematiaceous Fungi

Aureobasidium pullulans (continued)

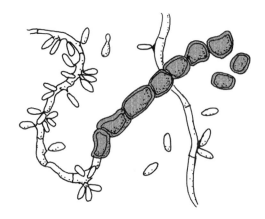

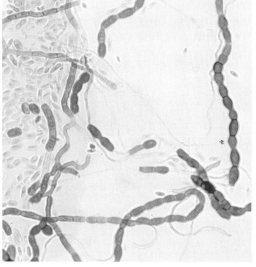

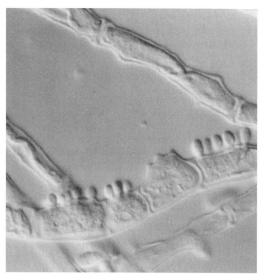

Synchronous production of blastoconidia. Courtesy of Wiley Schell.

For further information, see
  de Hoog et al., 2000, pp. 520–522
  Kwon-Chung and Bennett, 1992, pp. 664–665, 799, 800

TABLE 17 Differential characteristics of *Aureobasidium pullulans* vs *Hormonema dematioides*

Organism	Assimilation of methyl-α-D-glucoside[a]	Formation of hyaline blastic conidia[b]
Aureobasidium pullulans (p. 207)	Positive	Form mostly on hyaline hyphae. Develop in a synchronous fashion (i.e., conidia are formed simultaneously, each **from a separate fertile point**; these points are often very close together, producing clusters of conidia)
Hormonema dematioides (p. 210)	Negative	Form on both hyaline and dematiaceous hyphae. Develop in an asynchronous fashion (i.e., conidia are produced in succession **from the same single fertile point**; the conidia may form short chains or gather in loose clusters)

[a]Methyl-α-D-glucoside (MDG) assimilation can be tested with the API 20C AUX panel (bioMerieux, Hazelwood, Mo.). This one substrate appears to give credible results with these organisms, but the overall identification profile number cannot be accepted.

[b]The microscopic morphology of these organisms is best demonstrated by utilizing the Dalmau method (p. 335) on cornmeal-Tween 80 medium incubated at 25°C for an extended period of time (until dematiaceous hyphae develop).

Hormonema dematioides

PATHOGENICITY: Has been reported to cause peritonitis, fungemia, and cutaneous phaeohyphomycosis. It may also be encountered as a contaminant. There is a high probability that this organism has been misidentified as *Aureobasidium pullulans* in the past.

RATE OF GROWTH: Rapid; growth appears within 3–5 days, but pigment production and characteristic morphology may require extended incubation.

COLONY MORPHOLOGY: Colony is initially white to cream, sometimes pinkish; appears smooth and becomes moister as conidia develop; poorly conidiating strains may have a woolly mycelial mat; color eventually becomes brownish black as arthroconidia develop. Reverse is dark when colony is mature.

MICROSCOPIC MORPHOLOGY: Young colonies consist of unicellular, budding, yeastlike cells. Two types of hyphae develop: (i) hyaline, delicate, and thin walled, producing blastoconidia directly from the walls at certain fertile points, and (ii) thick-walled, dark, and closely septated segments that become arthroconidia. The blastoconidia are hyaline and oval, vary in size (average, 3–6 × 6–12 μm), and may continue to multiply by budding; they are produced asynchronously on both the hyaline and dematiaceous hyphae.

H. dematioides can easily be mistaken for *Aureobasidium pullulans* (p. 207); for differentiation of these two fungi, see Table 17 (p. 209).

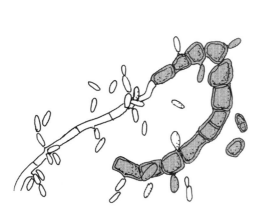

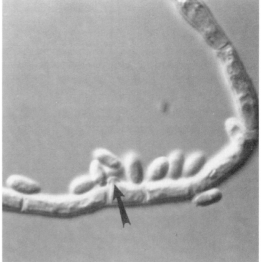

Asynchronous production of blastoconidia. Courtesy of Wiley Schell.

For further information, see
  de Hoog et al., 2000, pp. 717–719
  Shin et al., 1998

Scytalidium spp.

PATHOGENICITY: Known to commonly cause nail and skin infections; there are also rare reports of more deep-seated infections, e.g., subcutaneous abscess, sinusitis, endophthalmitis, lymphadenitis, and fungemia in immunocompromised patients. Infection is predominantly in individuals who live in or have visited tropical or subtropical areas; recently, a few cases have been reported in people who have never left temperate zones.

RATE OF GROWTH: Rapid; mature within 3 days. Growth is inhibited by cycloheximide.

COLONY MORPHOLOGY: Colonies are usually woolly, and growth quickly fills the agar plate or covers the agar slant; some isolates do not spread across the agar as robustly. The surface may be gray to brown with a dark reverse (*S. dimidiatum*) or white to cream or gray with a buff to yellowish reverse (*S. hyalinum*). (Color Plate 93.)

MICROSCOPIC MORPHOLOGY: Hyphae are septate and branched, but no conidiophores are formed. Arthroconidia (3–7 × 3–14 μm) develop that have one or two cells, are flattened on the ends, and may be rectangular, square, oval, or roundish and become barrel shaped; they are consecutive, i.e., there are no empty cells between the arthroconidia. A pycnidial form very occasionally develops in old cultures; it is known as *Nattrassia mangiferae* (formerly *Hendersonula toruloidea*); pycnidial conidia are hyaline when young and with age develop 1–5 septa and a dark brown central area.

The wider hyphae and arthroconidia of *S. dimidiatum* are usually dark, while the narrower side branches of hyphae tend to produce pale arthroconidia.

The hyphae and arthroconidia of *S. hyalinum* are colorless but are identical to those of *S. dimidiatum* in every other way; some mycologists consider it a hyaline mutant of *S. dimidiatum*.

See Table 21 (p. 260) for differential characteristics of fungi in which arthroconidia predominate.

(continued on following page)

Scytalidium spp. *(continued)*

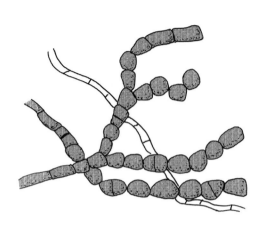 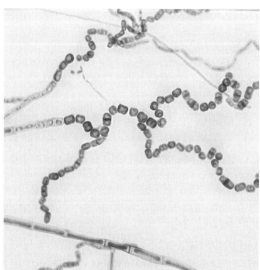

For further information, see
   de Hoog et al., 2000, pp. 329–330
   Kane et al., 1997, pp. 254–257
   Sigler et al., 1997

Botrytis sp.

PATHOGENICITY: Commonly considered a contaminant.

RATE OF GROWTH: Rapid; mature within 5 days.

COLONY MORPHOLOGY: Surface is at first white and then gray or brown, sometimes with blackish spots; woolly. Reverse is usually dark.

MICROSCOPIC MORPHOLOGY: Wide, septate hyphae with dark, septate, long conidiophores that branch only at the apex. The branches have swollen tips that bear round to oval, colorless to pale brown conidia on short denticles. Conidia also form at points along the conidiophore.

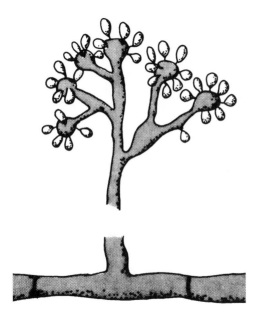

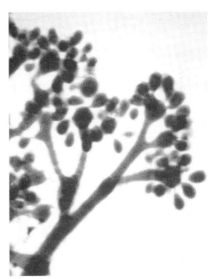

From Rippon, 1988.

For further information, see
Barron, 1977, pp. 105–106
McGinnis, 1980, pp. 192–193, 195
Rippon, 1988, pp. 760, 761

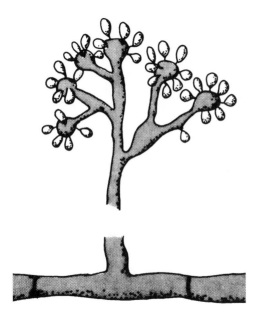

THERMALLY MONOMORPHIC MOULDS: Dematiaceous Fungi

Stachybotrys chartarum (S. alternans, S. atra)*

PATHOGENICITY: Commonly considered a contaminant. It produces several myco-toxins that appear to have the ability to affect humans and animals after ingestion, inhalation, or percutaneous absorption. The fungus has been associated with pul-monary hemorrhage and hemosiderosis in infants. It has also been implicated in ill-nesses (with a variety of symptoms) in occupants (of all ages) of water-damaged homes and other buildings. Additional studies are needed to establish a firm causal relationship.

RATE OF GROWTH: Moderately rapid; usually mature within 7 days but can be rather fastidious on routine laboratory media; prefers medium with high cellulose content.

COLONY MORPHOLOGY: Surface is at first white, becoming dark gray to black with age; powdery to cottony, spreading. Reverse is at first light and then dark.

MICROSCOPIC MORPHOLOGY: Hyphae are septate and colorless to dark. Coni-diophores are simple or branched, may become pigmented and rough with age, and bear clusters of 3–10 phialides. The phialides are colorless or pigmented, non-septate, and cylindrical, with a swollen upper portion. Conidia are dark, oval (aver-age, 4.5×9 μm), single celled, and smooth or rough walled and usually form in clusters on the phialides.

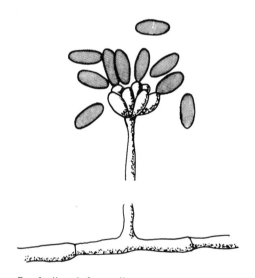

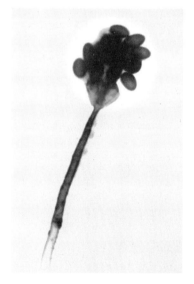

For further information, see
  Etzel et al., 1998
  Fung et al., 1998
  McGinnis, 1980, pp. 282–283

---

*The nomenclature of *Stachybotrys* has been confusing; these three species names have been used interchangeably in the literature.

Graphium sp.

PATHOGENICITY: May be found as a contaminant but is also an asexual form of *Pseudallescheria boydii* (p. 196).

RATE OF GROWTH: Moderately rapid; mature within 7 days.

COLONY MORPHOLOGY: Surface gray, cottony. Reverse is at first light, turning dark.

MICROSCOPIC MORPHOLOGY: Hyphae are septate, with simple, long, dark conidiophores that are cemented together forming synnemata. At the apex of each synnema is a cluster of oval, colorless, single-celled conidia (2–3 × 5–7 μm). Delicate rhizoid-like structures appear at the base of the synnema.

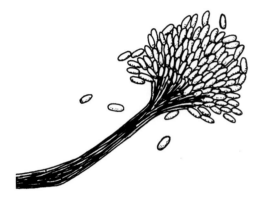 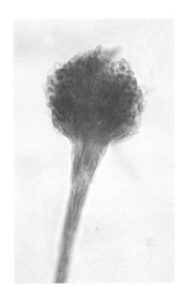

For further information, see
  Barron, 1977, pp. 185–188
  McGinnis, 1980, pp. 227–229

Curvularia spp.

PATHOGENICITY: Etiologic agents of opportunistic infections, most commonly of the cornea and sinuses; also cause mycetoma and phaeohyphomycosis at various sites, including nails, subcutaneous tissue, and systemic organs. Dissemination to the brain is known to occur occasionally. They are also encountered as contaminants.

RATE OF GROWTH: Rapid; mature within 5 days.

COLONY MORPHOLOGY: Colony is dark olive-green to brown or black with a pinkish gray, woolly surface. Reverse is dark. (Color Plate 94.)

MICROSCOPIC MORPHOLOGY: Hyphae are septate and dark. Conidiophores are simple or branched and bent or knobby at points of conidium formation (sympodial geniculate growth). Conidia are large (8–14 × 21–35 μm), usually contain 4 cells, and eventually appear curved due to swelling of a central cell. Conidia differ from those of *Bipolaris* spp. (p. 217) by having a central cell that is darker than the end cells, a thinner cell wall, narrower septations between cells, and a distinct curve that develops with age.

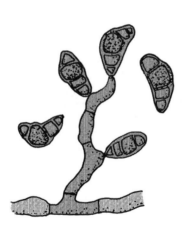 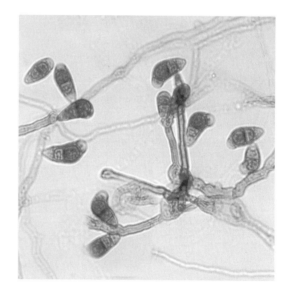

For further information, see
de Hoog et al., 2000, pp. 598–612
Kwon-Chung and Bennett, 1992, pp. 665–666, 802
McGinnis, 1980, pp. 203–204
Rippon, 1988, pp. 311–312, 767

Bipolaris spp.*

PATHOGENICITY: Most commonly cause allergic sinusitis and, in immunocompromised patients, may progress to invade bone and cause lesions in the brain. Occasionally infect a variety of other sites, including the eye, skin, aorta, lung, and central nervous system. Also known to be present as contaminants in clinical specimens.

RATE OF GROWTH: Rapid; mature within 5 days.

COLONY MORPHOLOGY: Surface is at first grayish brown, becoming black with a matted center and raised grayish periphery. Reverse is dark brown to black. (Color Plates 95 and 96.)

MICROSCOPIC MORPHOLOGY: Dark septate hyphae. Conidiophores elongate and bend at the point where each conidium is formed (sympodial geniculate growth); this produces a knobby zigzag appearance. The conidia are brown, oblong to cylindrical (6–12 × 16–35 μm), appear thick walled, and have 3–5 septations and a slightly protruding hilum.

See Table 18 (p. 218) for characteristics that distinguish *Bipolaris* from similar organisms.

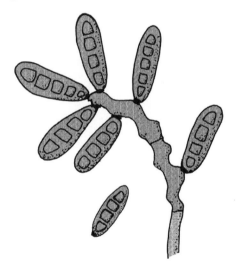
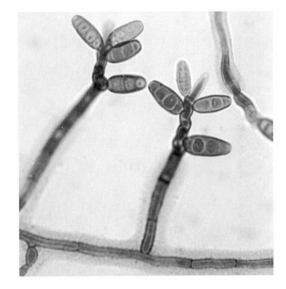

For further information, see
de Hoog et al., 2000, pp. 526–534
Kwon-Chung and Bennett, 1992, pp. 653–657, 799–800
McGinnis et al., 1986
Rippon, 1988, pp. 316–317

*In the past, most isolates of *Bipolaris* spp. were mistakenly called *Drechslera* spp.

TABLE 18 Characteristics of *Bipolaris*, *Drechslera*, and *Exserohilum* spp.[a]

| Genus | Reported as pathogen | Conidia | | | | Germ tubes[b] | | Illustration |
		Conidiation	Avg. size (μm)	No. of septa	Hilum	Origin	Orientation from basal cell	
Bipolaris	+	Profuse	8 × 26	3–5	Protrudes slightly	One or both end cells; adjacent to hilum	Along axis of conidium	
Drechslera	0	Poor	16 × 65	3–5	Does not protrude	Intermediate and end cells; not adjacent to hilum	Perpendicular to conidial axis	
Exserohilum	+	Profuse	14 × 90 or greater	5–12	Protrudes strongly	One or both end cells; adjacent to hilum; often other cells	Along axis of conidium	

[a]Reprinted by permission of the publisher from Larone, 1989. Copyright by Elsevier Science Inc.

[b]See p. 311 for instructions on performance of the germ tube test for these organisms.

Exserohilum spp.

PATHOGENICITY: Cause phaeohyphomycosis (see p. 43 for a description of the disease), most commonly in nasal sinuses, skin, subcutaneous tissue, and cornea. Fatal disseminated infections have been reported to occur on rare occasions.

RATE OF GROWTH: Rapid; mature within 5 days.

COLONY MORPHOLOGY: Surface is dark gray to black, cottony. Reverse is black. (Color Plate 97.)

MICROSCOPIC MORPHOLOGY: Dark septate hyphae. Conidiophores elongate and bend (sympodial geniculate growth) at the point where each conidium is formed; this produces a knobby, zigzag appearance. The conidia are brown, long (average, 14×80 μm or greater), fusiform, appear thick walled, and usually have 7–11 septa. The hilum (scar of attachment) on each conidium is seen as a dark, conspicuous, square protrusion. The most commonly encountered species, *E. rostratum,* displays a distinctive dark septum at each end cell of the mature conidium.

See Table 18 (p. 218) for differentiation from similar organisms.

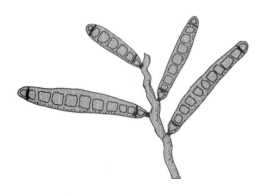
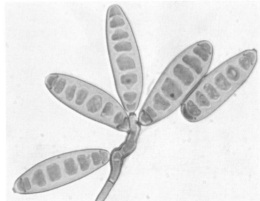

For further information, see
  de Hoog et al., 2000, pp. 669–675
  Kwon-Chung and Bennett, 1992, p. 657
  McGinnis et al., 1986

Helminthosporium sp.

PATHOGENICITY: Commonly considered a contaminant. Not known to cause infection.

RATE OF GROWTH: Rapid; mature within 5 days.

COLONY MORPHOLOGY: Surface is dark gray to black, cottony. Reverse is black.

MICROSCOPIC MORPHOLOGY: Hyphae are septate. Conidiophores are brown, determinate (i.e., not elongating at the point of conidium formation), slightly curved, unbranched, and often in clusters. Conidia form along the sides of the conidiophores, frequently in whorls. Conidia are large (approximately 9×40 μm), dark, thick walled, and club shaped with the broader end toward the conidiophore, and usually contain 6 or more cells.

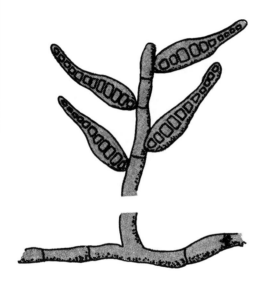

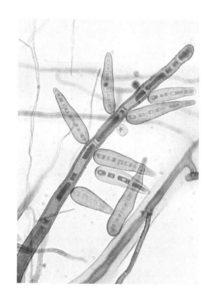

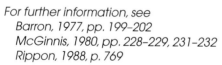

For further information, see
  Barron, 1977, pp. 199–202
  McGinnis, 1980, pp. 228–229, 231–232
  Rippon, 1988, p. 769

Alternaria sp.

PATHOGENICITY: Commonly considered a saprophytic contaminant but occasionally causes phaeohyphomycosis, most commonly in subcutaneous tissue. There have also been a few reports of infection of nails, eye, and nasal sinuses.

RATE OF GROWTH: Rapid; mature within 5 days.

COLONY MORPHOLOGY: Surface is at first grayish white and woolly and later becomes greenish black or brown with a light border. May eventually become covered by short, grayish, aerial hyphae. Reverse is black. (Color Plates 98 and 99.)

MICROSCOPIC MORPHOLOGY: Hyphae are septate and dark. Conidiophores are septate and of variable length and sometimes have a zigzag appearance. Conidia are large (usually $8–16 \times 23–50$ μm) and brown, have both transverse and longitudinal septations, sometimes produce germ tubes, and are found singly or in chains; they are usually rather round at the end nearest the conidiophore while narrowing at the apex, producing a clublike shape.

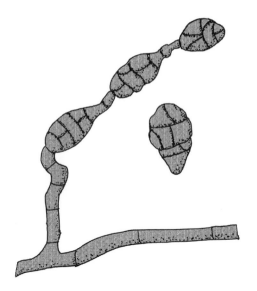
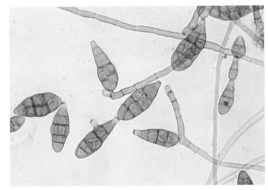

For further information, see
de Hoog et al., 2000, pp. 422–435
Kwon-Chung and Bennett, 1992, pp. 630–631, 662–663
McGinnis, 1980, pp. 181–182
Rippon, 1988, pp. 312–313, 769–770

Ulocladium sp.

PATHOGENICITY: Commonly considered a contaminant; very rarely involved in phaeohyphomycosis.

RATE OF GROWTH: Rapid; mature within 5 days.

COLONY MORPHOLOGY: Surface is dark brown to black, cottony. Reverse is black.

MICROSCOPIC MORPHOLOGY: Septate hyphae, light to dark brown. Conidiophores are simple or branched and bent at points of conidial production, giving a zigzag appearance. Conidia are brown to black, smooth or rough, and round to oval or slightly egg shaped (7–12 × 18–24 μm), with transverse and longitudinal septations.

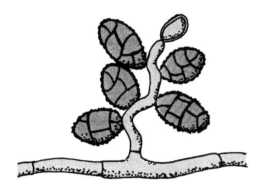
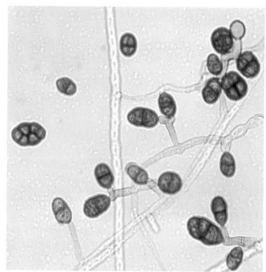

For further information, see
de Hoog et al., 2000, pp. 997–1001
Kwon-Chung and Bennett, 1992, pp. 807–809
McGinnis, 1980, pp. 296, 309
Rippon, 1988, pp. 769, 771

Stemphylium sp.

PATHOGENICITY: Commonly considered a contaminant.

RATE OF GROWTH: Rapid; mature within 5 days.

COLONY MORPHOLOGY: Surface is brown to black, cottony. Reverse is black.

MICROSCOPIC MORPHOLOGY: Septate hyphae, light to dark brown. Conidiophores are simple or occasionally branched, with a dark, swollen terminus bearing individual conidia; the conidiophore develops a nodular or knobby appearance as it ages and produces more conidia. Conidia (12–20 × 15–30 μm) are dark, smooth or rough, and round or oval and have transverse and longitudinal septations, often with marked constriction at the central septum.

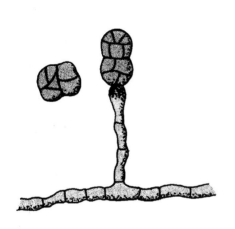

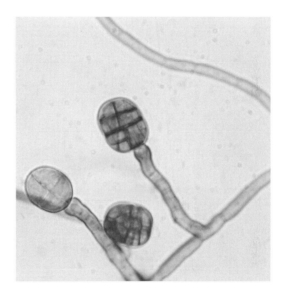

For further information, see
  Barron, 1977, pp. 291–292
  Kwon-Chung and Bennett, 1992, pp. 811–813
  McGinnis, 1980, pp. 283–284
  Rippon, 1988, pp. 769, 770

THERMALLY MONOMORPHIC MOULDS: Dematiaceous Fungi

Pithomyces sp.

PATHOGENICITY: Commonly considered a contaminant, but very occasionally has been implicated as an etiologic agent in immunocompromised hosts. Causes facial eczema in sheep.

RATE OF GROWTH: Rapid; mature within 5 days.

COLONY MORPHOLOGY: Surface is light to dark brownish black, cottony. Reverse is dark.

MICROSCOPIC MORPHOLOGY: Septate hyphae, pale or light brown. Conidiophores are short, simple, and peg-like. Conidia are single, oval (10–20 × 20–30 μm), yellow to dark brown, and usually rough, with transverse and longitudinal septations.

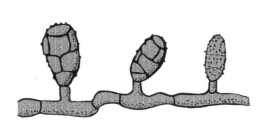
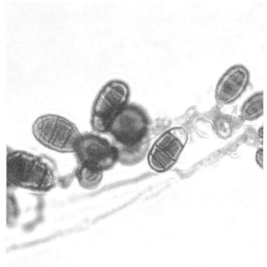

For further information, see
  Barron, 1977, pp. 259–260
  Kwon-Chung and Bennett, 1992, pp. 811, 813
  Rippon, 1988, pp. 771–772

Epicoccum sp.

PATHOGENICITY: Commonly known as a contaminant; not known to cause disease.

RATE OF GROWTH: Moderately rapid; mature within 7 days.

COLONY MORPHOLOGY: Colonies are irregularly cottony and usually yellow to orange at first, becoming brown to black where the dark mature conidia eventually form. Reverse is sometimes red or may be dark brown or grayish. A diffusible pigment may color the medium yellow, orange, red, or brown. (Color Plates 100 and 101.)

MICROSCOPIC MORPHOLOGY: Clusters of short conidiophores form on hyphae by repeated branching to form a dense mass from which conidia arise. Young conidia are round to pear shaped, pale, smooth, and nonseptate. Mature conidia (15–30 μm in diameter) are almost round, multiseptate both longitudinally and transversely, dark brown or black, and often rough and warty. Characteristically, all stages of conidia will be present simultaneously in the clusters.

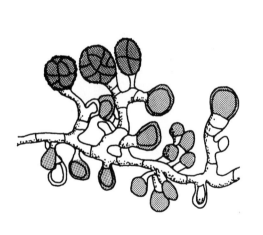
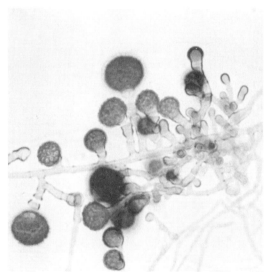

For further information, see
Barron, 1977, pp. 163–164
Kwon-Chung and Bennett, 1992, pp. 809, 810
McGinnis, 1980, p. 209
Rippon, 1988, pp. 761, 764

Nigrospora sp.

PATHOGENICITY: Commonly considered a contaminant; possible involvement in disease has very rarely been reported.

RATE OF GROWTH: Rapid; mature within 4 days.

COLONY MORPHOLOGY: Compact, woolly; at first white, then gray. With age, black areas of conidiation appear. Reverse is black. (Color Plate 102.)

MICROSCOPIC MORPHOLOGY: Hyphae are septate with short conidiophores that swell and then taper at point of conidium formation. The conidia are large, black, and almost round, slightly flattened (approximately 14–20 μm in diameter).

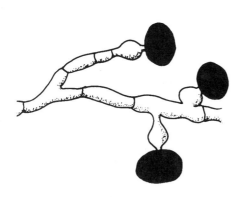

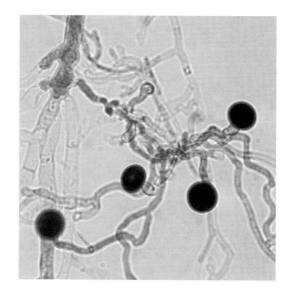

For further information, see
  de Hoog et al., 2000, pp. 777–778
  McGinnis, 1980, pp. 241–242, 251
  Rippon, 1988, pp. 771, 774

Chaetomium sp.

PATHOGENICITY: Commonly considered a contaminant; occasionally implicated in systemic and cutaneous phaeohyphomycosis.

RATE OF GROWTH: Rapid; mature within 5 days.

COLONY MORPHOLOGY: Surface is cottony, spreading, usually white, becoming tannish gray or grayish olive with age. Reverse is usually orange-tan tinted with red but may be brown to black. (Color Plates 103 and 104.)

MICROSCOPIC MORPHOLOGY: Hyphae are septate with large (90–170 × 110–250 μm), round, oval, or flask-shaped perithecia (best seen on potato dextrose agar) that are olive to brown and fragile and have wavy and/or straight filamentous appendages. Asci are stalked and club shaped, contain 4–8 spores, and usually dissolve soon after release from the ostiole (opening) of the perithecium. Ascospores, readily observed, are oval or lemon shaped, single celled, and usually olive-brown but may occur in a variety of sizes, shapes, and colors.

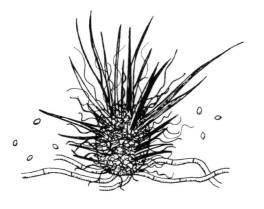 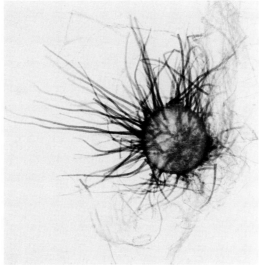

For further information, see
de Hoog et al., 2000, pp. 262–270
Kwon-Chung and Bennett, 1992, pp. 666–667, 800–801
McGinnis, 1980, pp. 165–166
Rippon, 1988, pp. 764–765

Phoma sp.

PATHOGENICITY: Commonly considered a contaminant. Occasional agent of phaeohyphomycosis.

RATE OF GROWTH: Rapid; mature within 5 days.

COLONY MORPHOLOGY: Colony is powdery or velvety, spreading, and grayish brown. Reverse is black. There is a reddish to brown diffusible pigment in some species. (Color Plate 105.)

MICROSCOPIC MORPHOLOGY: Septate hyphae; large (~70–200 μm in diameter) asexual fruiting bodies (pycnidia). The pycnidia are dark and round or flask shaped and have openings (ostioles) through which the conidia are dispersed. The conidia, formed on conidiophores inside the pycnidia, are rather oval, one celled, and hyaline. Chlamydoconidia resembling the conidia of *Alternaria* sp. (p. 221) are produced in some species.

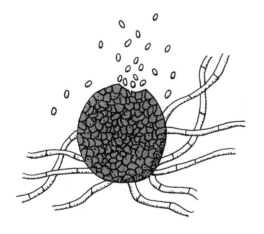

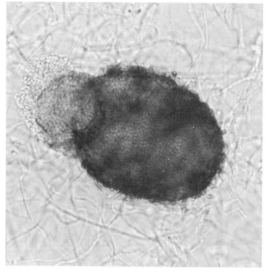

For further information, see
  de Hoog et al., 2000, pp. 332–348
  Kwon-Chung and Bennett, 1992, p. 805
  McGinnis, 1980, pp. 178–179
  Rippon, 1988, pp. 764, 766

Dermatophytes

Introduction

Dermatophytes are filamentous fungi that are able to digest and obtain nutrients from keratin (a relatively insoluble protein; the primary component of skin, hair, and nails). When the organism grows on the host, living tissue is not usually invaded; the organism simply colonizes the keratinized outermost layer of the skin. The "disease" known as tinea or ringworm is the result of the host reaction to the enzymes released by the fungus during its digestive process. Dermatophytes are the only fungi that have evolved a dependency on human or animal infection for the survival of the species. It is therefore not surprising that these fungi are among the most common infectious agents of humans.

The group comprises three genera that can generally be differentiated by their conidium formation.

Microsporum: —Macroconidia numerous, thick walled, rough.
—Microconidia usually present.
(*M. audouinii* is an exception; it seldom forms conidia.)

Trichophyton: —Macroconidia rare, thin walled, smooth.
—Microconidia numerous.
(Some species do not produce conidia.)

Epidermophyton: —Macroconidia numerous, thin and thick walled, smooth.
—Microconidia are not formed.

For further information, see
Kane et al., 1997, Laboratory Handbook of Dermatophytes
Murray et al. (ed.), 1999, Manual of Clinical Microbiology, 7th ed., chapter 100

Microsporum audouinii

PATHOGENICITY: Formerly caused epidemics of ringworm of the scalp in children. Also known to infect skin on other parts of the body. Very rarely infects adults.

RATE OF GROWTH: Moderate; mature in 7–10 days.

COLONY MORPHOLOGY: Surface is flat, downy to silky, with a radiating edge; it is grayish or tannish white. Reverse is light salmon with reddish brown center (pigment is best seen on potato dextrose agar). (Color Plates 106 and 107.)

MICROSCOPIC MORPHOLOGY: Hyphae are septate with terminal chlamydoconidia that are often pointed on the end. Pectinate (comblike) hyphae are commonly seen. This species is usually almost devoid of conidia but sometimes forms poorly shaped, abortive macroconidia or occasionally microconidia that are identical to those occurring in other species of the genus *Microsporum*.

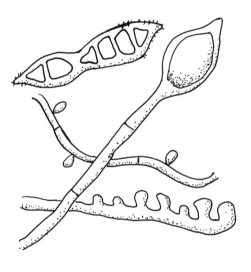 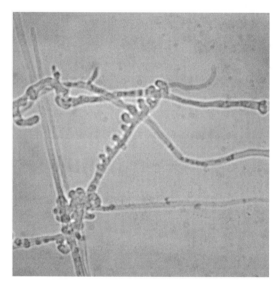

For further information, see
  Kane et al., 1997, pp. 194, 195, 199–200
  Kwon-Chung and Bennett, 1992, pp. 135–136
  Rebell and Taplin, 1970, pp. 16–18
  Rippon, 1988, p. 241

Microsporum canis var. canis

PATHOGENICITY: Causes infections of scalp and skin; it is most prevalent in children. Has occasionally been reported as a cause of nail infections. Most infections in humans are acquired from infected dogs or cats.

RATE OF GROWTH: Moderate; mature within 6–10 days.

COLONY MORPHOLOGY: Surface is whitish, coarsely fluffy, hairy to silky or fur-like, with yellow pigment at periphery and closely spaced radial grooves. Reverse is deep yellow and turns brownish yellow with age. (Color Plates 108 and 109.)

MICROSCOPIC MORPHOLOGY: Hyphae are septate with numerous macroconidia, which are long (10–25 × 35–110 μm), spindle shaped, rough, and thick walled and characteristically taper to knob-like ends. The rough surface of the macroconidia is seen especially at the knob. Usually more than 6 compartments are seen in the macroconidia. A few microconidia are sometimes observed; they are club shaped and smooth walled and form along the hyphae.

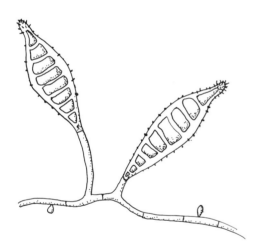
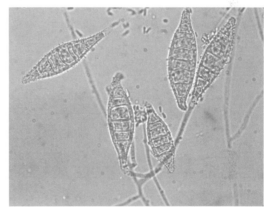

For further information, see
  Kane et al., 1997, pp. 194, 195, 200–201
  Kwon-Chung and Bennett, 1992, pp. 136–137
  Rebell and Taplin, 1970, pp. 13–14
  Rippon, 1988, pp. 47–51, 53

Microsporum canis var. *distortum*

PATHOGENICITY: Occasionally causes ringworm of the scalp and other parts of the body.

RATE OF GROWTH: Moderate; mature within 6–10 days.

COLONY MORPHOLOGY: Surface is fuzzy and flat with raised center; white to buff. Reverse is usually yellow.

MICROSCOPIC MORPHOLOGY: Septate hyphae. Macroconidia resemble those of *M. canis* var. *canis* (p. 233) but are very bent and distorted and have fewer compartments; macroconidia are produced best on potato dextrose agar. Club-shaped microconidia are often abundant (an uncommon finding in *M. canis* var. *canis*).

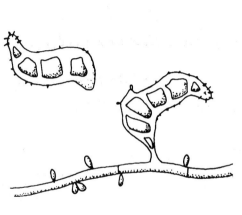
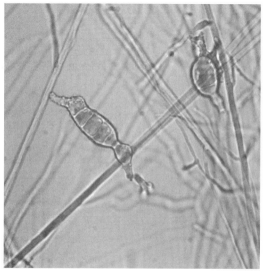

For further information, see
   Kane et al., 1997, pp. 194, 201
   Kwon-Chung and Bennett, 1992, pp. 136–137
   Rebell and Taplin, 1970, p. 15
   Rippon, 1988, pp. 241–245

Microsporum cookei

PATHOGENICITY: Occasionally involved in infections in humans; it is not known to infect hair in vivo.

RATE OF GROWTH: Moderate; mature within 7 days.

COLONY MORPHOLOGY: Surface is coarse, powdery; yellowish or dark tannish central area surrounded by thin, downy, white peripheral zone. Under the aerial mycelium is a characteristic deep grape-red pigment. Reverse is deep purplish red.

MICROSCOPIC MORPHOLOGY: Hyphae are septate and branched. Macroconidia are oval (10–15 × 30–50 μm), thick walled, and rough, with approximately 5 to 8 cells. Thick walls serve to distinguish this species from reddish isolates of *Microsporum gypseum*. Club-shaped microconidia are usually abundant.

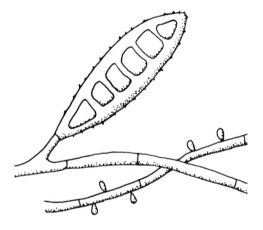 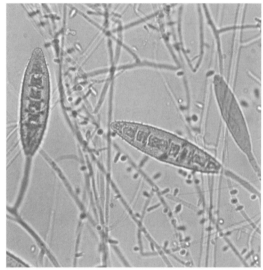

For further information, see
Kane et al., 1997, p. 206
Kwon-Chung and Bennett, 1992, pp. 142–143
Rebell and Taplin, 1970, p. 29
Rippon, 1988, p. 249

Microsporum gypseum complex

PATHOGENICITY: Occasionally infects the scalp and skin on various parts of the body; infections are more common in lower animals than in humans.

RATE OF GROWTH: Moderately rapid; mature within 6 days.

COLONY MORPHOLOGY: Surface is flat and spreading and powdery to granular, developing an irregularly fringed border; it is buff at first, then tan to cinnamon brown. Colony often develops a sterile white hyphal border or cottony white center. Reverse may be yellow, orange-tan, brownish red, or purplish red in spots. (Color Plates 110 and 111.)

MICROSCOPIC MORPHOLOGY: Septate hyphae. Macroconidia (8–16 × 22–60 μm) appear in enormous numbers and are symmetric, rough, and relatively thin walled, with no more than 6 compartments. The ends are rounded, not pointed as in *M. canis*. Microconidia, club shaped, are usually present along the hyphae.

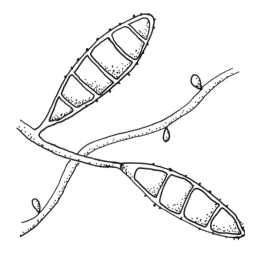 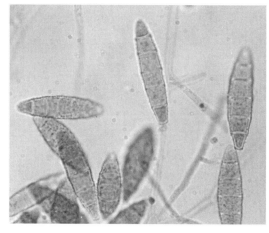

For further information, see
  Kane et al., 1997, pp. 194–196, 202–203
  Kwon-Chung and Bennett, 1992, pp. 138–139
  Rebell and Taplin, 1970, pp. 23–25
  Rippon, 1988, pp. 244–246

Microsporum gallinae

PATHOGENICITY: Rare cause of ringworm of the scalp and other parts of the human body; more often seen as cause of ringworm in chickens or other fowl.

RATE OF GROWTH: Moderate; mature in 6–10 days.

COLONY MORPHOLOGY: Surface is slightly fluffy or satiny and white, becoming pinkish with age. Reverse is yellow at first and later has a red pigment that diffuses into the medium.

MICROSCOPIC MORPHOLOGY: Hyphae are septate. Macroconidia (6–8 × 15–50 μm) have walls that are relatively thin and usually smooth but sometimes slightly rough at the tip; they contain 4–10 cells, are blunt tipped, and are often distinctively curved with a tapering base. Microconidia are usually abundant.

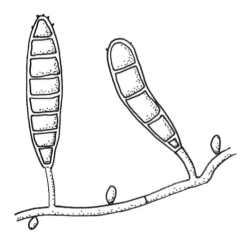 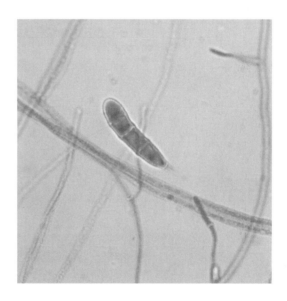

For further information, see
  Kane et al., 1997, p. 204
  Kwon-Chung and Bennett, 1992, p. 138
  Rebell and Taplin, 1970, p. 21
  Rippon, 1988, p. 247

Microsporum nanum

PATHOGENICITY: A rare cause of ringworm in humans; more common in pigs.

RATE OF GROWTH: Moderate; mature within 7 days.

COLONY MORPHOLOGY: Surface is at first white and then yellowish, peachy, or beige; spread thin, downy or powdery, with fringed edges. Reverse is initially orange and later reddish brown. (Color Plates 112 and 113.)

MICROSCOPIC MORPHOLOGY: Septate hyphae; macroconidia (4–8 × 12–18 μm) are rough, fairly thin walled (as in *M. gypseum*), and egg shaped with truncate base, having 1 to 3 cells (usually 2). Microconidia, club shaped and smooth walled, may also be present.

The short conidiophores, singly formed macroconidia with rough walls and no foot-like attachment points, and presence of microconidia serve to distinguish this organism from *Trichothecium roseum* (p. 283).

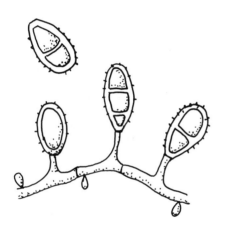
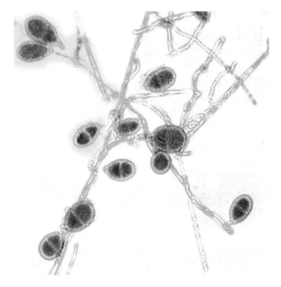

For further information, see
Kane et al., 1997, pp. 194, 196, 203–204
Kwon-Chung and Bennett, 1992, p. 140
Rebell and Taplin, 1970, p. 26
Rippon, 1988, pp. 246–247

Microsporum vanbreuseghemii

PATHOGENICITY: Rare cause of ringworm in humans and lower animals.

RATE OF GROWTH: Moderate; mature within 7 days.

COLONY MORPHOLOGY: Surface is powdery or fluffy; cream, pink, or tan in color. Reverse is colorless or yellow to orange-tan.

MICROSCOPIC MORPHOLOGY: Hyphae are septate; macroconidia are long (10–12 × 58–62 μm), tapered, thick walled, and usually rough and spiny surfaced, with 7 or more cells. The macroconidia are in abundance singly, laterally, or terminally. Microconidia are also present. Care must be taken not to confuse *M. vanbreuseghemii* with *Trichophyton ajelloi* (p. 252).

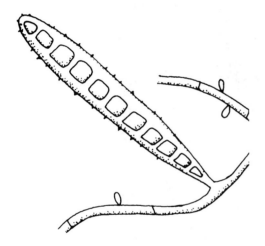 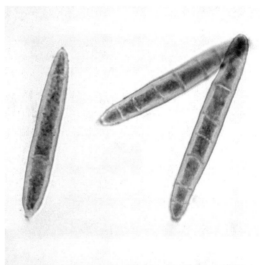

Courtesy of Glenn Roberts.

For further information, see
  Kane et al., 1997, pp. 194, 204
  Kwon-Chung and Bennett, 1992, p. 141
  Rebell and Taplin, 1970, p. 30
  Rippon, 1988, p. 249

THERMALLY MONOMORPHIC MOULDS: Dermatophytes

Microsporum ferrugineum

PATHOGENICITY: Primarily causes ringworm of the scalp (tinea capitis) in children. Also known to infect the skin and nails.

RATE OF GROWTH: Slow; mature in 12–20 days.

COLONY MORPHOLOGY: Isolates from the Far East have a surface that is usually yellow to rusty orange, smooth, waxy, and heaped; on repeated subculture, the pigment is often lost. Another colony type (typical in the Balkans) is also waxy, but white to pale yellow and flatter. Either form may develop a fine velvety overgrowth. Reverse is cream to brownish.

MICROSCOPIC MORPHOLOGY: Hyphae are septate; some are characteristically long and straight with prominent cross walls; these are called "bamboo" hyphae. Other hyphae are irregularly branched, clubbed, and fragmented and may have intercalary chlamydoconidium-like cells. Macroconidia, rarely produced, resemble those of *M. canis* (pp. 233, 234) and *M. cookei* (p. 235).

Note: The orange form of this organism may be differentiated from *Trichophyton soudanense* (p. 247), which it somewhat resembles, by the formation of light yellowish colonies on Lowenstein-Jensen medium; *T. soudanense* will form dark reddish-brown-to-blackish colonies.

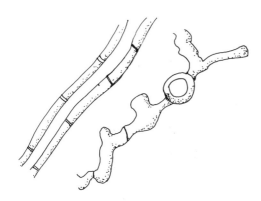 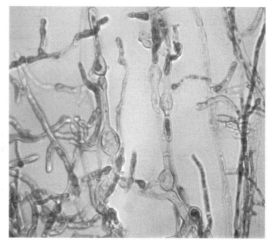

Courtesy of Michael Rinaldi.

For further information, see
  Kane et al., 1997, pp. 194, 201–202
  Kwon-Chung and Bennett, 1992, pp. 137–138
  Rebell and Taplin, 1970, p. 19
  Rippon, 1988, p. 245

Trichophyton mentagrophytes

PATHOGENICITY: Invades all parts of the body surface, including hair and nails. It is a common cause of athlete's foot.

RATE OF GROWTH: Moderate; mature in 7–10 days.

COLONY MORPHOLOGY: Varies greatly; surface may be buff and powdery or white and downy. May become pinkish or yellowish. Powdery form exhibits concentric and radial folds. Colonies rapidly develop a dense fluff with little or no conidiation. Reverse is usually brownish tan but may be colorless, yellow, or red. (Color Plates 114 and 115.)

MICROSCOPIC MORPHOLOGY: Septate hyphae. Microconidia in powdery cultures are very round (4–6 μm in diameter) and clustered on branched conidiophores or, in fluffy strains, are smaller, fewer in number, tear shaped, and more easily confused with those of *Trichophyton rubrum* (p. 243). Macroconidia (4–8 × 20–50 μm) are sometimes, but not always, present; they are cigar shaped and thin walled, have narrow attachments to hyphae, contain 1 to 6 cells, and are more readily found in young primary cultures 5–10 days old. Coiled spiral hyphae are often seen. Nodular bodies are seen in some strains.

See Table 19 (p. 242) to differentiate *T. mentagrophytes* from similar species of *Trichophyton*.

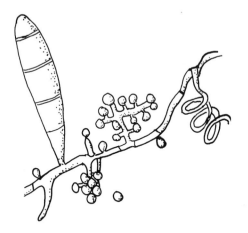
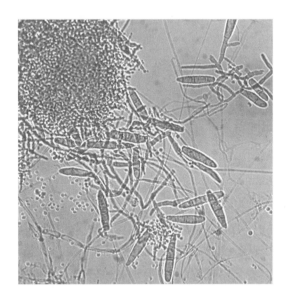

For further information, see
Kane et al., 1997, pp. 149–155
Kwon-Chung and Bennett, 1992, pp. 143–145
Rebell and Taplin, 1970, pp. 40–43
Rippon, 1988, pp. 252–256

TABLE 19 Differentiation of similar conidia-producing *Trichophyton* spp.[a]

| Organism | Growth on *Trichophyton* agars | | | In vitro hair perforation | Red pigment on cornmeal with 1% dextrose | Growth at 37°C | Growth on *Trichophyton* agars[b] | |
	No. 1 (casein base)	No. 4 (casein + thiamine)	Urease (7 days)				No. 6 (NH_4NO_3 base)	No. 7 (NH_4NO_3 + histidine)
T. mentagrophytes	4+	4+	+	+	0	+	4+	2+
T. rubrum	4+	4+	0 or W	0	+	+	3+	4+
T. tonsurans	± or +	4+	+	0[v]	0	+	±	±
T. terrestre	4+	4+	+	+	v	0	2+	2+
T. megninii	4+	2+	+[v, c]	0	v	+	0	4+

[a]Abbreviations: +, positive; 0, negative; W, weak; ±, trace; 4+, maximum growth; v, variable.

[b]As *T. megninii* is the only dermatophyte that requires histidine, *Trichophyton* agar no. 6 and 7 are used only when it is suspected; the organism is very rare in the Americas and in northern Europe.

[c]Use urea broth, not agar, to ensure positive result in 7 days with *T. megninii*.

Trichophyton rubrum

PATHOGENICITY: Infects the skin and nails and only rarely the beard, hair, or scalp. It is presently the most common dermatophyte infecting humans.

RATE OF GROWTH: Moderately slow; mature within 14 days.

COLONY MORPHOLOGY: Surface is granular or fluffy, white to buff. Reverse is deep red or purplish; occasionally it is brown, yellow-orange, or even colorless. The pigment production is best seen on potato dextrose agar (p. 341) or cornmeal dextrose agar (p. 335). (Color Plates 116 and 117.)

MICROSCOPIC MORPHOLOGY: Septate hyphae. Tear-shaped microconidia (2–3.5 × 3–5.5 μm) usually form singly all along the sides of the hyphae (not clustered like *T. mentagrophytes*, p. 241). Macroconidia (4–8 × 40–60 μm) may be abundant, rare, or absent; when present, they are long, narrow, and thin walled, with parallel sides (pencil-like), and have 4–10 cells. Macroconidia may form directly on ends of thick hyphae singly or in groups. Microconidia characteristically form directly on macroconidia. Arthroconidia tend to form from both hyphae and macroconidia. Granular cultures have more macroconidia formation and larger, rounder microconidia than the fluffy form.

See Table 19 (p. 242) for differentiation from similar species of *Trichophyton*.

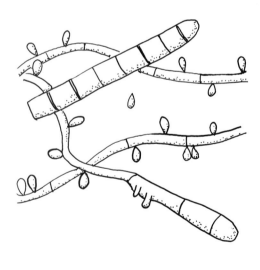
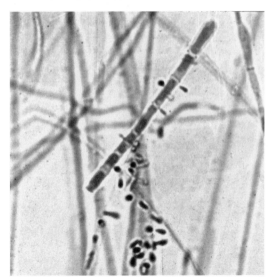

For further information, see
  Kane et al., 1997, pp. 158–164
  Kwon-Chung and Bennett, 1992, pp. 145–148
  Rebell and Taplin, 1970, pp. 50–51
  Rippon, 1988, pp. 255–257

Trichophyton tonsurans

PATHOGENICITY: The principal etiologic agent of scalp ringworm in the United States; also infects the skin and nails.

RATE OF GROWTH: Moderately slow; mature in 12 days.

COLONY MORPHOLOGY: Highly variable. Surface may be white, grayish, yellow, rose, or brownish. Surface is usually suede-like, with many radial or concentric folds. Reverse is usually reddish brown (pigment may diffuse into the medium); sometimes it is yellow or colorless. (Color Plates 118, 119, and 120.)

MICROSCOPIC MORPHOLOGY: Hyphae are septate, with many variably shaped microconidia all along the hyphae or on short conidiophores that are perpendicular to the parent hyphae. Microconidia are usually teardrop or club shaped but may be elongate or enlarge to round "balloon" forms. Intercalary and terminal chlamydo-conidia are common in older cultures. Macroconidia are rare, irregular in form, and a bit thick walled. May have spiral coils and arthroconidia. This species has a partial requirement for thiamine.

See Table 19 (p. 242) for differentiation from similar species of *Trichophyton*.

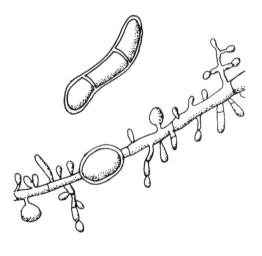 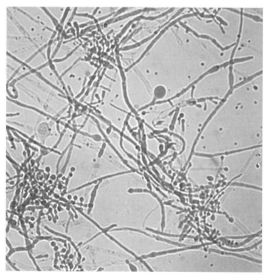

For further information, see
Kane et al., 1997, pp. 174–177
Kwon-Chung and Bennett, 1992, pp. 148–149
Rebell and Taplin, 1970, pp. 52–53
Rippon, 1988, pp. 257–259

Trichophyton terrestre

PATHOGENICITY: Not known to cause infection in humans but may be confused with other *Trichophyton* spp.

RATE OF GROWTH: Moderate; mature within 8 days. It does not grow at 35–37°C.

COLONY MORPHOLOGY: Surface is white to yellow and velvety or granular. Reverse is colorless, yellow, reddish, or brown. (Color Plates 121 and 122.)

MICROSCOPIC MORPHOLOGY: Hyphae are septate, with club-shaped microconidia (often on short stalks) or characteristic larger peg-shaped microconidia that usually exhibit transition forms to rather numerous smooth, thin-walled macroconidia (4–5 × 8–50 μm). The conidia often stain more intensely with lactophenol cotton blue than do the hyphae and are cut off on a relatively broad base.

See Table 19 (p. 242) for differentiation from similar species of *Trichophyton*.

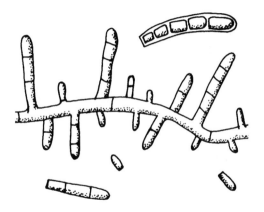 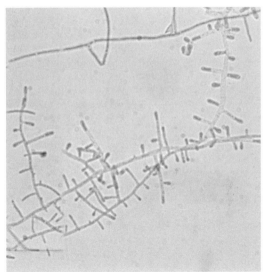

For further information, see
Kane et al., 1997, pp. 172–174
Rebell and Taplin, 1970, pp. 33–34

Trichophyton megninii

PATHOGENICITY: Primarily infects the scalp and beard and the skin on other parts of the body. Very rarely encountered in the Americas; it is endemic in parts of southern Europe and in north and east central Africa.

RATE OF GROWTH: Moderate; mature within 6–10 days.

COLONY MORPHOLOGY: Surface is suede-like, at first white and then pink to violet with widely spaced radial grooves. Reverse is red.

MICROSCOPIC MORPHOLOGY: Hyphae are septate, with teardrop-shaped microconidia along the sides. Macroconidia, infrequently produced, are long, narrow, and pencil shaped. There is a close resemblance to *T. rubrum* (p. 243), but *T. megninii* differs by requiring histidine (in *Trichophyton* agar no. 7) and often giving a positive test for urease within 7 days.

See Table 19 (p. 242) for differentiation from similar species of *Trichophyton*.

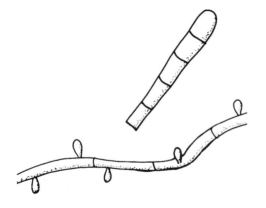

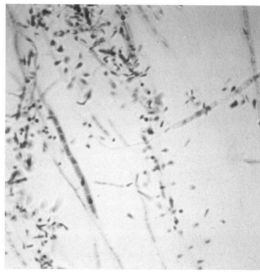

Courtesy of Michael Rinaldi.

For further information, see
Kane et al., 1997, pp. 145–149
Kwon-Chung and Bennett, 1992, p. 151
Rebell and Taplin, 1970, p. 49
Rippon, 1988, p. 263

Trichophyton soudanense

PATHOGENICITY: Primarily infects the scalp and hair and may spread to other parts of the body. It is endemic in central and west Africa and has occasionally been reported in Europe, the United States, and South America.

RATE OF GROWTH: Slow; mature within 15 days. Growth factor requirements are variable.

COLONY MORPHOLOGY: Surface is yellow to orange, suede-like, and flat to folded, with a radiating fringe. Purplish red variants exist. Reverse is similar in color to the surface.

MICROSCOPIC MORPHOLOGY: Septate hyphae that often break up to form arthroconidia. Characteristically, branches form at both forward and backward angles to the parent hypha (i.e., in directions that are both the same and opposite to that of the elongating hypha). This is known as "reflexive" branching; when adjacent branches point in opposite directions, they often give the appearance of barbed wire. The unique characteristic microscopic formations are most likely to be found in the radiating fringe of the colony. Teardrop-shaped microconidia may also form along the hyphae; no macroconidia are seen.

Note: The orange form of this organism may be differentiated from *Microsporum ferrugineum* (p. 240), which it somewhat resembles, by the formation of dark reddish-brown-to-blackish colonies on Lowenstein-Jensen medium; *T. soudanense* will form pale yellow colonies.

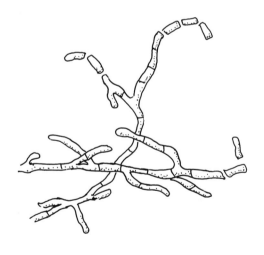 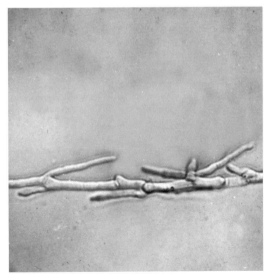

Courtesy of Stanley Rosenthal.

For further information, see
 Kane et al., 1997, pp. 168–172; Kwon-Chung and Bennett, 1992, p. 152;
 Rebell and Taplin, 1970, pp. 56–57; Rippon, 1988, pp. 263–264

TABLE 20 Growth patterns of *Trichophyton* species on nutritional test media[a] (p. 346)

Organism	Percent	Growth on *Trichophyton* agar no.						
		1	2	3	4	5	6	7

USUALLY NO CONIDIA ON SABOURAUD AGAR; INCUBATE *TRICHOPHYTON* AGARS AT 37°C

Organism	Percent	1	2	3	4	5	6	7
T. verrucosum	84	0	±	4+	0			
	16	0	0	4+	4+			
T. schoenleinii		4+	4+	4+	4+			
T. concentricum[b]	50	4+	4+	4+	4+			
	50	2+	2+	4+	4+			
T. violaceum[c]		± or 1+			4+ (in 3 weeks)			

USUALLY PRODUCES MICROCONIDIA AND SOMETIMES MACROCONIDIA ON SABOURAUD AGAR; INCUBATE *TRICHOPHYTON* AGARS AT ROOM TEMPERATURE

Organism	Percent	1	2	3	4	5	6	7
T. tonsurans		± or 1+			4+			
T. rubrum[d]		4+			4+			
T. mentagrophytes[d]		4+			4+	4+		
T. equinum[e]		0				4+		
T. megninii[f]		4+			2+		0	4+
T. terrestre[g]		4+			4+			

[a]Abbreviations: 1, casein agar base (vitamin free);
2, casein + inositol;
3, casein + inositol and thiamine;
4, casein + thiamine;
5, casein + nicotinic acid;
6, ammonium nitrate agar base;
7, ammonium nitrate + histidine;
0, no growth;
+, growth;
1+, ¼ as much growth as 4+.
2+, ½ as much growth as 4+.
3+, ¾ as much growth as 4+.
4+, maximum growth.

[b]For more information, see Rebell and Taplin, 1970 (p. 61) or Kane et al., 1997 (pp. 135–136).
[c]Usually has distinct pigment on primary isolation.
[d]Differentiation of *T. rubrum* and *T. mentagrophytes* is by morphology, urease test, in vitro hair perforation test, and pigment production on cornmeal dextrose agar. See Table 19 (p. 242).
[e]Commonly found in horses; has been confused with *T. mentagrophytes*, but *T. equinum* usually requires nicotinic acid. For more information, see Rebell and Taplin, 1970 (p. 45) or Kane et al., 1997 (pp. 136–138).
[f]No other dermatophyte shows this regular requirement for histidine.
[g]Not known to cause infections, but may be confused with some pathogenic species. See Table 19 (p. 242).

Trichophyton schoenleinii

PATHOGENICITY: Causes favus, a severe, chronic, scarring scalp infection that results in permanent hair loss; sometimes infects the nails and skin.

RATE OF GROWTH: Slow; mature within 15 days.

COLONY MORPHOLOGY: Colony is whitish, waxy, or slightly downy; heaped or folded; primary isolates are sometimes yeastlike. Growth is often submerged and splits the agar medium. Reverse is colorless or pale yellowish orange to tan.

MICROSCOPIC MORPHOLOGY: Hyphae are septate, highly irregular, and knobby. The subsurface hyphae usually form characteristic antler-like branching structures commonly called favic chandeliers; they have swollen tips that resemble nail heads. Chlamydoconidia are numerous. Microconidia and macroconidia are absent. Initial growth from clinical specimen may resemble yeast both macroscopically and microscopically.

See Table 20 (p.248) for growth pattern on *Trichophyton* agars.

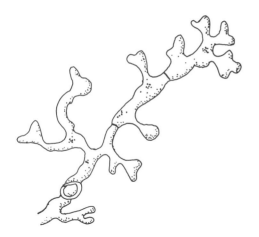 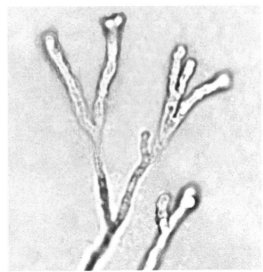

For further information, see
   Kane et al., 1997, pp. 164–166
   Kwon-Chung and Bennett, 1992, pp. 149–150
   Rebell and Taplin, 1970, pp. 59–60
   Rippon, 1988, pp. 260–262

THERMALLY MONOMORPHIC MOULDS: Dermatophytes

Trichophyton verrucosum

PATHOGENICITY: Infects scalp, beard, nails, and skin on various parts of the body. Usually contracted from cattle.

RATE OF GROWTH: Slow; mature in 14–21 days. Unlike other dermatophytes, this fungus grows best at 37°C.

COLONY MORPHOLOGY: Usually small, heaped, and button-like but sometimes flat. Texture skinlike, waxy, or slightly downy. Usually white, but can be gray or yellow. Reverse varies from nonpigmented to yellow.

MICROSCOPIC MORPHOLOGY: On Sabouraud dextrose agar (SDA) at 37°C, forms hyphae with many chlamydoconidia (often in chains) and some antler-like branches. On enriched media with thiamine, produces many small, delicate, single microconidia and occasional long, thin, irregular macroconidia shaped like string beans or "rats' tails."

See Table 20 (p. 248) for growth patterns on *Trichophyton* agars. This species requires thiamine and usually inositol as well.

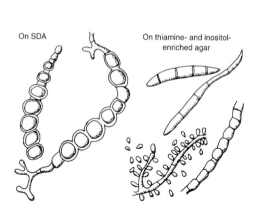

On SDA

On thiamine- and inositol-enriched agar

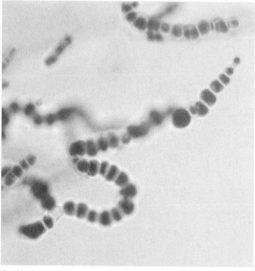

On SDA.

For further information, see
  Kane et al., 1997, pp. 177–181
  Kwon-Chung and Bennett, 1992, pp. 148–149
  Rebell and Taplin, 1970, pp. 47–48
  Rippon, 1988, pp. 259–260

Trichophyton violaceum

PATHOGENICITY: Most commonly infects the scalp and hair but also causes infection in skin and nails.

RATE OF GROWTH: Slow; mature in 14–21 days.

COLONY MORPHOLOGY: Original cultures are waxy, wrinkled, heaped, and deep purplish red. Subcultures are more downy, and they decrease in color. Reverse is lavender to purple.

MICROSCOPIC MORPHOLOGY: Hyphae are tangled, branched, irregular, and granular, with intercalary chlamydoconidia. Microconidia and macroconidia are not usually seen on Sabouraud dextrose agar, but a few may form on thiamine-enriched media.

See Table 20 (p. 248) for growth pattern on *Trichophyton* agars. This species has a partial requirement for thiamine.

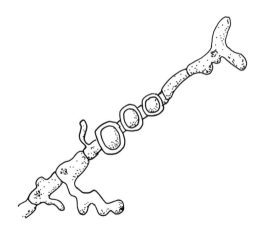
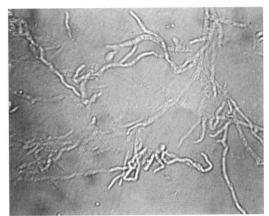

Courtesy of Michael Rinaldi.

For further information, see
Kane et al., 1997, pp. 181–185
Kwon-Chung and Bennett, 1992, pp. 150–151
Rebell and Taplin, 1970, p. 54
Rippon, 1988, p. 259

Trichophyton ajelloi

PATHOGENICITY: Has only rarely been reported as a possible cause of infections in humans.

RATE OF GROWTH: Moderate; mature within 7 days.

COLONY MORPHOLOGY: Surface is cream to orange-tan, rather powdery, and flat or folded. Reverse may be colorless or have a reddish purple or bluish black pigment that diffuses into the medium.

MICROSCOPIC MORPHOLOGY: Hyphae are septate with many macroconidia that are long (5–10 × 20–65 μm), cigar shaped, or cylindric with tapering ends, smooth surfaced, and moderately thick walled and that contain 5–12 cells. Microconidia are sparse in most isolates but may be absent in others. Care must be taken not to confuse this organism with *Microsporum vanbreuseghemii* (p. 239) or *Epidermophyton floccosum* (p. 253).

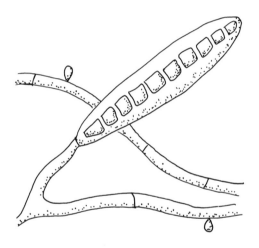 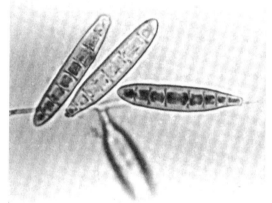

From Murray et al. (ed.), 1999, *Manual of Clinical Microbiology*, 7th ed., chapter 100.

For further information, see
  Kane et al., 1997, pp. 133–135
  Rebell and Taplin, 1970, p. 31
  Rippon, 1988, pp. 263–265

Epidermophyton floccosum

PATHOGENICITY: Produces infection in skin and nails (not hair).

RATE OF GROWTH: Moderate; mature within 10 days.

COLONY MORPHOLOGY: Surface is brownish yellow to olive-gray or khaki; it is at first lumpy and sparse and then folded in the center and grooved radially, becoming velvety. After several weeks, fluffy white sterile mycelium covers the colony. Reverse is orange to brownish, sometimes with a thin yellow border. (Color Plates 123 and 124.)

MICROSCOPIC MORPHOLOGY: Septate hyphae; no microconidia. Macroconidia (7–12 × 20–40 μm), seen best in young cultures, are smooth, both thin and slightly thick walled, and club shaped with rounded ends; they contain 2 to 6 cells and are found singly or in characteristic clusters. With age, macroconidia often transform into chlamydoconidia. Microconidia are not formed. Older cultures commonly develop white sterile hyphae; stock cultures are best maintained on Sabouraud dextrose agar containing 3–5% sodium chloride.

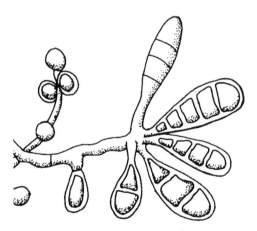 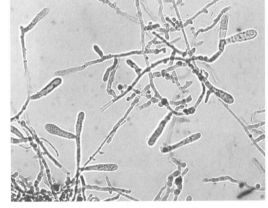

For further information, see
   Kane et al., 1997, pp. 186–189
   Kwon-Chung and Bennett, 1992, p. 154
   Rebell and Taplin, 1970, p. 62
   Rippon, 1988, pp. 266–269

Hyaline Hyphomycetes

Introduction

This section contains the fungi that have not been discussed earlier in this guide. These moulds have colorless, septate hyphae and produce conidia that may be colorless or pigmented. Their colony surfaces are white, gray, tan, yellow, pink, or green; the reverse is white or lightly pigmented. Some of these organisms are known pathogens (e.g., *Coccidioides immitis*), but most of them are opportunistic and cause disease only in the immunocompromised patient.

In the past, all fungi were categorized as pathogens or saprophytes—those days are gone forever. Almost any fungus isolated from a clinical specimen might be an etiologic agent of infection in a predisposed individual. All fungal isolates should be identified; most of those commonly considered saprophytes are identified in most laboratories only to genus level, as it often requires an expert to differentiate the species.

In the medical laboratory, the saprophytic fungi are frequently encountered as contaminants. The source of the organism may be the transport container, the medium, or the laboratory environment, but most often it is the site from which the specimen was taken. Every effort should be made to instruct clinicians on proper techniques for specimen collection.

Other fungi that are commonly considered saprophytes, contaminants, and/or possible opportunists are described in previous sections of this guide.

For further information, see
  Murray et al. (ed.), 1999, Manual of Clinical Microbiology, 7th ed.,
    chapter 97

THERMALLY MONOMORPHIC MOULDS: Hyaline Hyphomycetes

PATHOGENICITY: Causes coccidioidomycosis, which is a highly infectious disease that may be an acute but benign, self-limiting respiratory disease or a chronic, malignant, sometimes fatal infection involving the skin, bone, joints, lymph nodes, adrenals, and central nervous system. It is endemic in the arid southwestern United States and in dry regions of Mexico, Central America, and South America.

RATE OF GROWTH: Moderate; mature within 10 days. Growth occurs in 3–5 days, but production of arthroconidia may take 1–2 weeks.

COLONY MORPHOLOGY: There may be great variation in colony morphology. On Sabouraud dextrose agar (SDA) at 25 or 37°C the colony often is at first moist, grayish, and membranous and soon develops a white, cottony aerial mycelium, which becomes gray or tan to brown with age; may also be pinkish or yellow. Reverse is white to gray; sometimes yellow or brownish. Only when grown on special Converse medium with increased CO_2 at 37–40°C is the spherule, or tissue phase, formed in vitro (this is not routinely performed in clinical laboratories).

MICROSCOPIC MORPHOLOGY: Cultures exhibit coarse, septate, branched hyphae that produce thick-walled, barrel-shaped arthroconidia (3–4 × 3–6 μm) that alternate with empty cells. The walls of the empty cells break and are characteristically present on either end of the freed conidia. Racquet hyphae are present in young colonies. Careful microscopic examination should prevent confusion with *Geotrichum candidum* (p. 143). *C. immitis* is more likely to be confused with *Malbranchea* (p. 261), which also forms alternating arthroconidia along the hyphae but has a more delicate appearance.

See Table 21 (p. 260) for differential characteristics of fungi in which arthroconidia predominate.

To confirm the identity of *C. immitis* and definitively differentiate it from organisms that it may closely resemble, it is necessary to perform one of the following tests: (i) specific DNA probe (commercially available; be aware that isolates killed by suspension in formaldehyde will yield false-negative reactions with the AccuProbe (Gen-Probe Inc., San Diego, Calif.) system, while heat-killed isolates remain positive), (ii) immunodiffusion test for exoantigen (may be performed by a few reference laboratories), (iii) cultivation of spherules in special synthetic Converse medium in increased CO_2 at 37–40°C, or (iv) animal inoculation for in vivo production of spherules.

In tissues or body fluids, *C. immitis* exists as large, round, thick-walled spherules (10–80 μm in diameter), which contain endospores (2–5 μm in diameter). When cultured on routine media, whether incubated at 25, 30, or 37°C, the organism is filamentous (for that reason, it is not placed with the thermally dimorphic fungi in this guide).

Coccidioides immitis *(continued)*

Note: Because the arthroconidia are highly infectious, the cultures must be handled with great care and grown in tubes only, not petri plates. The tubed growth should be wet down with sterile water before being handled. A biological safety cabinet must be used. Slide cultures should NOT be made.

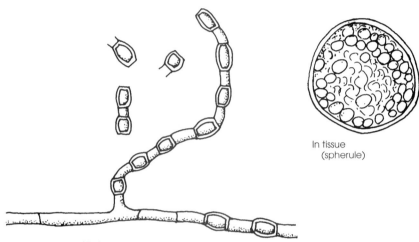

Cultured at 25° or 37°C

In tissue
(spherule)

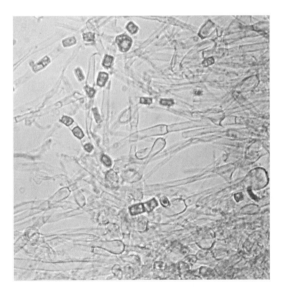

For further information, see
de Hoog et al., 2000, pp. 593–595; Kwon-Chung and Bennett, 1992, pp. 356–396;
McGinnis, 1980, pp. 201–203, 484–486; Rippon, 1988, pp. 433–473;
Saubolle and Sutton, 1994

TABLE 21 Differentiating characteristics of fungi in which arthroconidia predominate[a]

Genus	Dark pigment	Pseudohyphae	Conidiophores	Alternating arthroconidia[b]	Arthroconidia barrel shaped	Blastoconidia	Illustration of microscopic morphology
Geotrichum (p. 143)	0	0	0	0	0	0	
Trichosporon (p. 140)	0	+	0	0	0	+	
Arthrographis (p. 263)	0	0	+	0	0	+^{v}	
Geomyces (p. 262)	0	0	+	+	+	0	
Coccidioides (p. 259)	0	0	0	+	+	0	
Malbranchea (p. 261)	0	0	0	+	0	0	
Scytalidium (p. 211)	+^{v}	0	0	0	+^{v}	0	

[a] Abbreviations: +, positive; 0, negative; V, variable.
[b] Empty cells appear between the arthroconidia.

Malbranchea spp.

PATHOGENICITY: Not known to cause infection. Commonly considered a contaminant.

RATE OF GROWTH: Moderately rapid; mature within 7 days.

COLONY MORPHOLOGY: Surface may be white, beige, orange, pinkish, or brownish; texture is granular, powdery, or woolly. Reverse is light. (Color Plates 127 and 128).

MICROSCOPIC MORPHOLOGY: Hyphae are septate, hyaline; no conidiophores are formed. Arthroconidia alternating with empty cells develop in the hyphae. The arthroconidia may be of various lengths but are the same width as the fairly narrow hypha (usually less than 4 μm). Arthroconidia are released by breakage of the empty cells, and a portion of the adjacent empty cell often remains attached to separated arthroconidia. The arthroconidia are not swollen and not thick walled, differentiating them from those of *Coccidioides immitis*. In its sexual state (which is rarely seen in routine culture), large round asci-producing fruiting bodies (gymnothecia) are formed; they have no opening and are surrounded by loosely organized hyphae. One species of *Malbranchea* forms large, round, dark masses of cells (sclerotia).

If the identification is questionable, and there is suspicion that the isolate could be *C. immitis*, safety precautions must be diligently observed, wet preps should be made rather than slide cultures, and an exoantigen test or nucleic acid probe test specific for *C. immitis* should be performed.

See Table 21 (p. 260) for differential characteristics of fungi in which arthroconidia predominate.

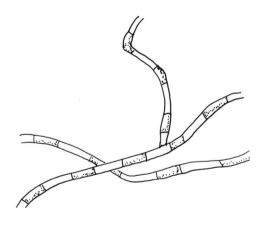

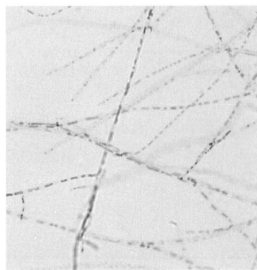

For further information, see
Kane et al., 1997, pp. 306–309
Sigler and Carmichael, 1976

Geomyces pannorum

PATHOGENICITY: Commonly considered a contaminant; encountered in specimens of skin and nails. There are rare reports of it causing skin infection in dogs.

RATE OF GROWTH: Moderate to slow; mature in 10–21 days. Grows well at 5–25°C; no growth at 37°C. Grows on media with cycloheximide.

COLONY MORPHOLOGY: Surface is white, pale yellow, gray, or tan; usually cottony or powdery. May be flat or elevated in the center; radial grooves sometimes form. Reverse can be colorless, but yellow is more typical, and a yellow or tan pigment may diffuse into the agar.

MICROSCOPIC MORPHOLOGY: Hyphae are septate. Conidiophores are erect, narrow, and measure 10–100 μm long; branches form in whorls around the central structure. Conidia (2–4 × 2–6 μm) are smooth or rough, form at the tips of the branches and also in intercalary positions separated by short empty spaces to create chains of 2 to 4 alternating, barrel-shaped arthroconidia. Conidia may also form along the sides of the conidiophore. Terminal and lateral conidia are somewhat clavate, having a rounded apex and truncate (cut-off, flattened) base.

See Table 21 (p. 260) for differential characteristics of fungi in which arthroconidia predominate.

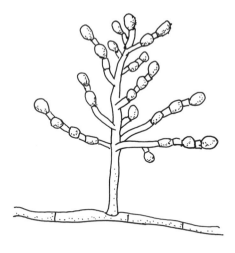

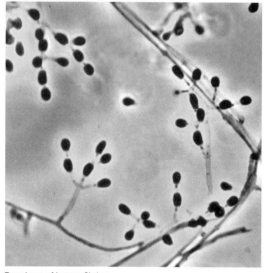

Courtesy of Lynne Sigler.

For further information, see
de Hoog et al., 2000, pp. 706–707
Kane et al., 1997, pp. 300–301

Arthrographis kalrae

PATHOGENICITY: Reported rarely as a cause of mycetoma and corneal infection. It has been isolated from various sites with questionable etiologic significance. Most commonly considered a contaminant, mainly in skin and nails.

RATE OF GROWTH: Slow at 25–30°C; mature in 10–21 days. Growth is enhanced at 37°C; also grows at 45°C. Grows on media containing cycloheximide. *Arthrographis cuboidea* is a rapid grower, reaching maturity in 3–5 days.

COLONY MORPHOLOGY: Surface at first smooth and yeastlike, later velvety; cream to pale yellow or tan. Reverse pale yellow, may become tan. (Color Plate 129.)

MICROSCOPIC MORPHOLOGY: Yeastlike cells seen on early growth; later hyphae are septate and colorless. Conidiophores are simple or branched in a treelike fashion; they produce chains of consecutive arthroconidia that are mostly rectangular, some oval (2–3.5 × 3–7 μm). Intercalary arthroconidia also form. Round blastoconidia (3.5–5.5 μm in diameter) may develop directly on the hyphae (most commonly on submerged hyphae).

See Table 21 (p. 260) for differential characteristics of fungi in which arthroconidia predominate.

Note: A. cuboidea differs from *A. kalrae* by growing rapidly (3–5 days) at 25–30°C but not growing at 45°C and by producing a pink-to-lavender pigment at 35–37°C that may form slowly and diffuse into the medium. It is not known to cause infection.

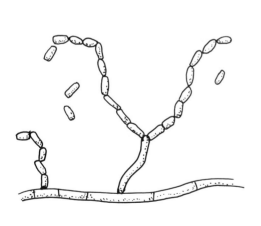
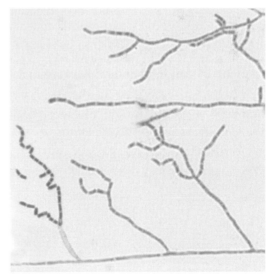

For further information, see
de Hoog et al., 2000, pp. 440–441
Sigler and Carmichael, 1983

Emmonsia spp.*

PATHOGENICITY: Cause adiaspiromycosis, a pulmonary disease seen mainly in rodents and small animals living in soil; only occasionally in humans. This mycosis is characterized by the in vivo enlargement, without multiplication, of inhaled conidia. The mycosis is usually self-limited, benign, localized, and relatively asymptomatic but may be more severe; disseminated infection has been reported in patients with AIDS. Lung biopsy is usually required for diagnosis; sputum or bronchoalveolar lavage will not suffice. *E. crescens* is the main etiologic agent in animals and the only agent of the disease in humans. *E. parva* is very rarely reported.

RATE OF GROWTH: Moderate; mature in 7–14 days. For primary isolation, minced lung tissue should be cultured on routine mycology agar at 25°C; both species grow best at 20–25°C. *E. parva* grows well in the presence of cycloheximide; *E. crescens* is somewhat inhibited.

COLONY MORPHOLOGY: Surface is white, occasionally buff to pale brown in the center; some areas may be glabrous, while others will have tufts of matted mycelia; slight radial grooves may form. Reverse is cream to pale brown.

MICROSCOPIC MORPHOLOGY: Hyphae are septate (1–2.5 μm wide); conidiophores are at right angles to the vegetative hyphae and produce conidia that are round or almost so (2–4.5 μm in diameter) and may become finely roughened with age. The conidiophores may swell at the apex and produce 2 or 3 conidia on short, narrow denticles. The conidia also form directly on short stalks along the sides of the hyphae.

When the hyphae and conidia are incubated at their maximum temperatures on enriched medium, the hyphae become distorted and usually disintegrate while the conidia swell to become round, thick-walled adiaconidia (formerly called adiaspores). The adiaconidia of *E. crescens* are produced at 37°C and measure 20–140 μm in diameter. The adiaconidia of *E. parva* are best produced at 40°C and range from 10–25 μm in diameter. Adiaconidia in vivo are larger and have thicker walls.

At various temperatures and stages of development, *Emmonsia* may resemble a number of other fungi, including *Blastomyces dermatitidis*, *Paracoccidioides brasiliensis*, *Histoplasma capsulatum*, and *Chrysosporium* spp.

Note: Isolates may give false-positive results with the *B. dermatitidis* DNA probe, exoantigen, and direct immunofluorescent-antigen tests.

---

*In the older literature, these organisms are referred to as *Emmonsia parva* var. *crescens* and *Emmonsia parva* var. *parva* or *Chrysosporium parvum* and *Chrysosporium parvum* var. *crescens*.

Emmonsia spp. *(continued)*

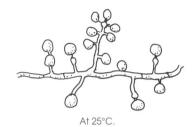

At 25°C.

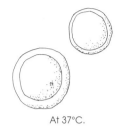

At 37°C.

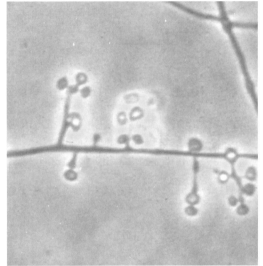

At 25°C. Courtesy of Lynne Sigler.

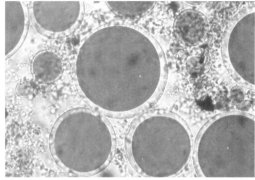

At 37°C. Courtesy of Lynne Sigler.

For further information, see
  de Hoog et al., 2000, pp. 633–637
  Kane et al., 1997, pp. 293–294
  Kwon-Chung and Bennett, 1992, pp. 733–739
  Rippon, 1988, pp. 718–721

TABLE 22 Identification of the most common species of *Aspergillus* (see description of genus on p. 268)

A. fumigatus[a]	A. niger	A. flavus	A. versicolor
PATHOGENICITY			
Most common cause of invasive disseminated aspergillosis; frequent agent of sinusitis	Most common in ear infections; frequently in aspergilloma; rarely disseminated	Involved in pulmonary, systemic, sinus, ear, and other infections; produces aflatoxins	Only occasionally involved in nail or invasive infection
MACROSCOPIC MORPHOLOGY[b]			
Velvety or powdery, at first white, then turning dark greenish to gray. Reverse white to tan	Woolly, at first white to yellow, then turning black. Reverse white to yellow	Velvety, yellow to green or brown. Reverse goldish to red-brown	Velvety; at first white, then yellow, orangey, tan, green, or occasionally pinkish. Reverse white; may be yellow, orange, or red
MICROSCOPIC MORPHOLOGY OF CONIDIOPHORES			
Short (<300 μm) Smooth	Long Smooth	Variable length Rough; pitted; spiny	Long Smooth
MICROSCOPIC MORPHOLOGY OF PHIALIDES			
Uniseriate, usually only on upper two-thirds of vesicle, parallel to axis of conidiophore	Biseriate; cover entire vesicle; form "radiate" head	Uniseriate and biseriate; cover entire vesicle; point out in all directions	Biseriate; loosely radiate; cover most of vesicle (Hülle cells may be present)

[a]*A. fumigatus* grows well at 45°C or higher.
[b]Classically studied on Czapek-Dox agar; on Sabouraud dextrose agar, most species of *Aspergillus* grow luxuriantly but not always characteristically.

A. nidulans	A. glaucus group	A. terreus	A. clavatus
PATHOGENICITY			
Can cause infection at various sites; seen in patients with chronic granulomatous disease	Rarely involved in nail, ear, and systemic disease	Involved in nail, skin, eye, ear, and systemic infections	An agent of allergic aspergillosis; rarely in nail and lung infections
MACROSCOPIC MORPHOLOGY[b]			
Velvety, usually green, but buff to yellow where cleistothecia form. Reverse purplish red becoming dark	Feltlike, green with yellow areas. Reverse yellow (osmophilic, growth enhanced by 20% sucrose in medium)	Usually velvety, cinnamon-brown. Reverse white to brown	Feltlike, blue-green. Reverse white, may become brown with age
MICROSCOPIC MORPHOLOGY OF CONIDIOPHORES			
Short (<250 μm) Smooth; brown	Variable length Smooth	Short (<250 μm) Smooth	Long Smooth
MICROSCOPIC MORPHOLOGY OF PHIALIDES			
Biseriate; short; columnar; cleistothecia usually present with reddish ascospores; Hülle cells often abundant	Uniseriate; radiate to very loosely columnar; cover entire vesicle (cleistothecia generally present)	Biseriate; compactly columnar (round hyaline cells produced on mycelium submerged in agar)	Uniseriate; closely crowded on huge clavate vesicle (approximately 200 × 40 μm)

⟩GENICITY: Members of the genus *Aspergillus* cause a group of diseases ι as aspergillosis; the disease may be in the form of invasive infection, colo-n, toxicoses, or allergy. The organisms are opportunistic invaders, the most common moulds to infect various sites in individuals with lowered resistance due to neutropenia and/or treatment with high-dose corticosteroids or cytotoxic drugs. *Aspergillus* spp. are widespread in the environment and are commonly found as contaminants in cultures. Approximately 175 species of *Aspergillus* are known, but only about 20 have been found to cause disease.

RATE OF GROWTH: Usually rapid; mature within 3 days; some species are slower growing.

COLONY MORPHOLOGY: Surface is at first white and then any shade of green, yellow, orange, brown, or black, depending on species. Texture is velvety or cottony. Reverse is usually white, goldish, or brown. (Color Plates 130–142.)

MICROSCOPIC MORPHOLOGY: Hyphae are septate (2.5–8.0 μm in diameter); an unbranched conidiophore arises from a specialized foot cell. The conidiophore is enlarged at the tip, forming a swollen vesicle. Vesicles are completely or partially covered with flask-shaped phialides (formerly referred to as sterigmata), which may develop directly on the vesicle (uniseriate form) or be supported by a cell known as a metula (biseriate form). The phialides produce chains of mostly round, sometimes rough conidia (2–5 μm in diameter).

See Table 22 (p. 266) for differentiation of species most commonly encountered in the clinical laboratory.

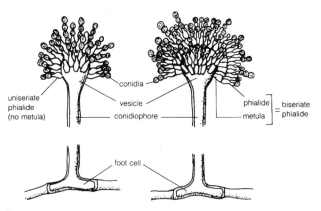

For further information, see
   de Hoog et al., 2000, pp. 442–519; Kwon-Chung and Bennett, 1992, pp. 201–247; McGinnis,
   1980, pp. 182–190, 475–477; Rippon, 1988, pp. 618–650; Wentworth, 1988, pp. 174–183

For detailed descriptions and keys to all species of Aspergillus, see
   Raper and Fennell, 1973

Penicillium spp.

PATHOGENICITY: Commonly considered contaminants, but found in a variety of diseases in which their etiologic significance is uncertain. They have been known to cause corneal, cutaneous, external ear, respiratory, and urinary tract infections, as well as endocarditis after insertion of valve prostheses. Disseminated disease has been reported in severely immunocompromised patients. Many strains produce toxins.

See also *Penicillium marneffei* (p. 156).

RATE OF GROWTH: Rapid; mature within 4 days. Usually no or poor growth at 37°C.

COLONY MORPHOLOGY: Surface at first is white, then becomes very powdery and bluish green with a white border. Some less common species differ in color and texture. Reverse is usually white, but may be red or brown. (Color Plate 143.)

If the isolate produces a red reverse and diffuse pigment in the agar, *P. marneffei* (p. 156) must be considered, and the organism should be tested for thermal dimorphism; this is especially relevant if the patient has recently visited Southeast Asia.

MICROSCOPIC MORPHOLOGY: Hyphae are septate (1.5–5 μm in diameter) with branched or unbranched conidiophores that have secondary branches known as metulae. On the metulae, arranged in whorls, are flask-shaped phialides that bear unbranched chains of smooth or rough, round conidia (2.5–5 μm in diameter). The entire structure forms the characteristic "penicillus" or "brush" appearance.

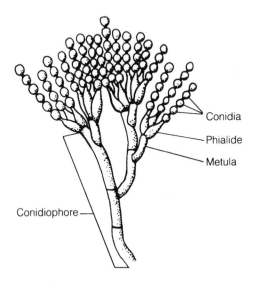

Conidia
Phialide
Metula
Conidiophore

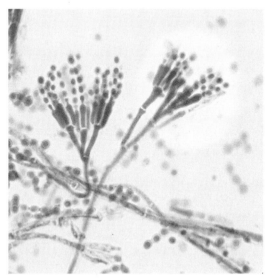

For further information, see
Barron, 1977, pp. 247–248; de Hoog et al., 2000, pp. 814–845; Kwon-Chung and Bennett, 1992, pp. 750–752, 804–805; McGinnis, 1980, pp. 251–261; Rippon, 1988, pp. 728–730, 754–755

Paecilomyces spp.

PATHOGENICITY: Usually considered contaminants, but are increasingly associated with disease, especially sinusitis and eye infections. They have also been reported to occasionally cause endocarditis; nephritis; nail, cutaneous, and subcutaneous infections; pulmonary infection; catheter-related fungemia; and infection at various other sites. Most deep infections have been in immunocompromised individuals.

RATE OF GROWTH: Rapid; mature within 3 days.

COLONY MORPHOLOGY: Surface is flat and powdery or velvety; may be yellowish brown, pinkish mauve, or another color, but it is never bright green or blue-green; often has whitish border. Reverse is off-white, pinkish, yellow, or pale brown. (Color Plate 144.)

MICROSCOPIC MORPHOLOGY: Resembles *Penicillium* spp. (p. 269), but the phialides of *Paecilomyces* spp. are more elongated and taper to a long, slender tube, giving them the shape of tenpins; they bend away from the axis of the conidiophore and may appear singly along the hyphae. The conidia (approximately 2–4 × 2.5–5 μm) are elliptical or oblong and occur in long, unbranched chains.

For differentiation of the two species most commonly involved in disease, *P. lilacinus* and *P. variotii*, see Table 23 (p. 274).

Paecilomyces **spp.** *(continued)*

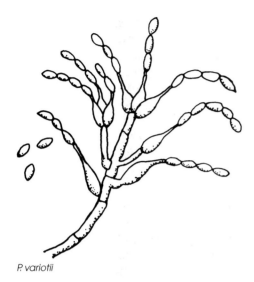

P. variotii

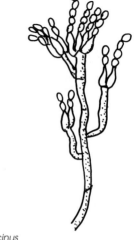

P. lilacinus

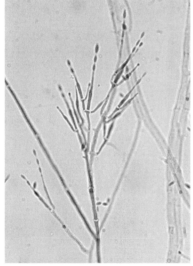

P. variotii

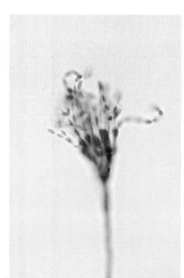

P. lilacinus

For further information, see
  de Hoog et al., 2000, pp. 794–809
  Kwon-Chung and Bennett, 1992, pp. 747–750, 753, 803–804
  McGinnis, 1980, pp. 244, 247–248
  Rippon, 1988, pp. 735–736, 756

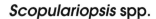
THERMALLY MONOMORPHIC MOULDS: Hyaline Hyphomycetes

PATHOGENICITY: Known to infect the nails (usually toenail) and are rarely associated with subcutaneous and invasive infection at various sites, primarily in immunocompromised patients. They have also commonly encountered as a contaminant.

RATE OF GROWTH: Rapid; mature within 5 days.

COLONY MORPHOLOGY: Surface is at first white and glabrous and then usually becomes powdery light brown with a light tan periphery. Some less frequently encountered species may be dark grayish, brown, or black. Reverse is usually tan with brownish center; occasionally darker. (Color Plates 145 and 146.)

MICROSCOPIC MORPHOLOGY: Septate hyphae with short, often branched conidiophores bearing annellides that may be cylindrical or tenpin shaped (swollen at the base and narrowing to an extended apex). The annellides form in brush-like groups or singly. The conidia, in chains, are roundish (4–9 μm in diameter), thick walled, rough and spiny when mature, sometimes slightly pointed at the apex, and are cut off at the base, forming a short neck. *Scopulariopsis* spp. somewhat resemble *Penicillium* spp. (p. 269) but have shorter and sometimes simpler conidiophores; the conidium-bearing cells are annellides (rather than phialides) and may be more cylindrical; the conidia are larger, rough, and uniquely shaped by being cut off at one end and sometimes slightly pointed at the other.

The two species that are most commonly encountered in the clinical laboratory and have been reported to cause invasive disease are *S. brevicaulis* and *S. brumptii*. For differentiation of these species, see Table 24 (p. 274).

Scopulariopsis **spp.** *(continued)*

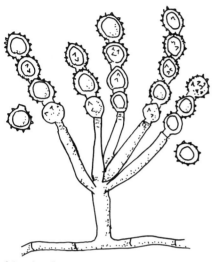

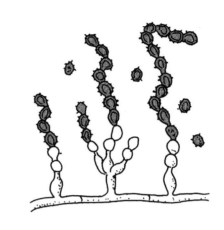

S. brevicaulis

S. brumptii

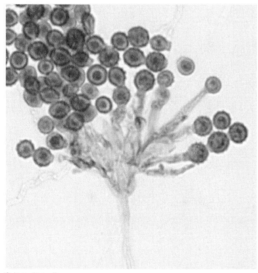

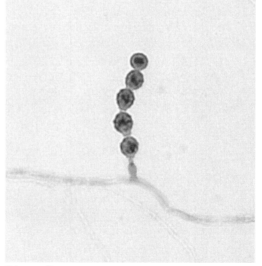

S. brevicaulis

S. brumptii

For further information, see
  de Hoog et al., 2000, pp. 902–916
  Kane et al., 1997, pp. 252–254
  Kwon-Chung and Bennett, 1992, pp. 752–753, 806–807
  McGinnis, 1980, pp. 272–275
  Rippon, 1988, pp. 736, 756, 758

TABLE 23 Differential characteristics of *Paecilomyces variotii* vs *P. lilacinus*

Organism	Colony color	Conidiophores	Phialides	Conidia	Temp
P. variotii	Tan to yellowish brown	Smooth walled	More broadly spaced; 2–7 form on each metula	Smooth; 2–4 × 3–5 μm (or longer)	Reported to grow well at 50°C, but many do not grow at >40°C
P. lilacinus	Pinkish, violet, or reddish gray	Rough walled	Densely clustered; 2–4 form on each metula	Smooth or rough; 2.0–2.2 × 2.5–3.0 μm	Restricted at 37°C

TABLE 24 Differential characteristics of *Scopulariopsis brevicaulis* vs *S. brumptii*

Organism	Pathogenicity	Colony	Annellides		Conidia		
			Shape	Size (μm)	Arrangement	Diameter (μm)	Color
S. brevicaulis	Frequently involved in nail infections; occasional reports of invasive disease	Light brown	Fairly cylindrical	2.5–3.5 × 9.0–25.0	Most in brush-like groups, some single	5.0–8.0	Hyaline or pale brown
S. brumptii	Occasionally found in pulmonary disease	Dark gray or grayish brown	Like tenpins; swollen at base, narrowing at apex	2.5–3.5 (at base) × 5.0–10.0	Most single, some in groups	3.5–5.5	Dark brown to blackish

Gliocladium sp.

PATHOGENICITY: Commonly considered a contaminant; not known to cause disease.

RATE OF GROWTH: Rapid; mature within 4 days.

COLONY MORPHOLOGY: Surface is at first white. The center then becomes dark green; some strains may be pinkish. Fluffy growth spreads over plate in 1 week. Reverse is white. (Color Plates 147 and 148.)

MICROSCOPIC MORPHOLOGY: The hyphae, conidiophores, and phialides are similar to those of *Penicillium* spp. (p. 269); however, the conidia of *Gliocladium* do not remain in chains but clump together with the conidia of adjacent phialides to form large clusters or balls.

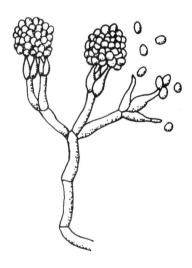 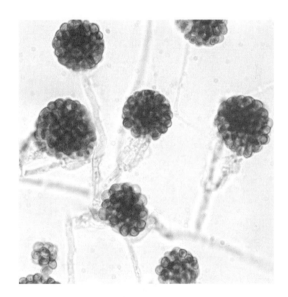

For further information, see
  Barron, 1977, pp. 177–179
  Kwon-Chung and Bennett, 1992, pp. 809–810
  McGinnis, 1980, pp. 224, 226
  Rippon, 1988, pp. 756–757

Trichoderma sp.

PATHOGENICITY: Commonly considered a contaminant, but there have been occasional reports of infection in immunocompromised patients and several cases of peritonitis in patients undergoing peritoneal dialysis.

RATE OF GROWTH: Rapid; mature within 5 days.

COLONY MORPHOLOGY: White fluff covers agar in a few days and then becomes more compact and woolly. Green patches are eventually produced due to formation of conidia (initially at the center of the colony and spread to the margin). Reverse is colorless or light orangey tan to yellow. (Color Plates 149 and 150.)

MICROSCOPIC MORPHOLOGY: Hyphae are septate. Conidiophores are short and often branched at wide angles; phialides are flask shaped and form at wide angles to the conidiophore. Conidia are round (3–4 μm in diameter) or slightly oval (2–3 × 2.5–5.0 μm), single celled, and clustered together at the end of each phialide. Clusters are easily disrupted unless microscopic preparations are handled with exceptional care.

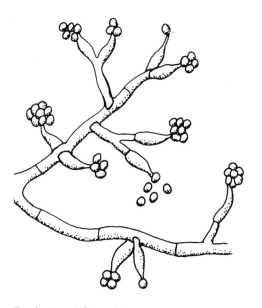 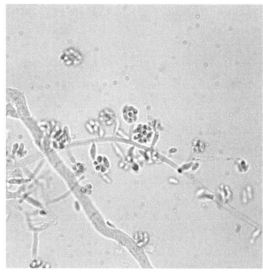

For further information, see
de Hoog et al., 2000, pp. 943–953
Kwon-Chung and Bennett, 1992, pp. 754–755, 812–814
McGinnis, 1980, pp. 288–289
Rippon, 1988, pp. 756, 758

Beauveria bassiana

PATHOGENICITY: Commonly considered a contaminant. Known to be pathogenic in insects and especially silkworms; very rarely involved in infection of humans.

RATE OF GROWTH: Rapid; mature within 4 days.

COLONY MORPHOLOGY: Surface is white to cream, occasionally pinkish; fluffy to powdery. Reverse is white. (Color Plate 151.)

MICROSCOPIC MORPHOLOGY: Hyphae are septate, narrow, and delicate. Conidia-producing structures are rather flask shaped with a narrow zigzag terminal extension bearing a conidium at each bent point (sympodial geniculate growth). Conidia are small (2–4 μm in diameter), one celled, and round to oval, each forming singly on a tiny denticle. It is best to examine young cultures before dense clusters of conidiogenous cells form, making it difficult to observe the characteristic arrangement of conidia.

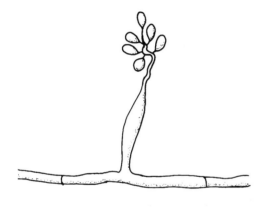
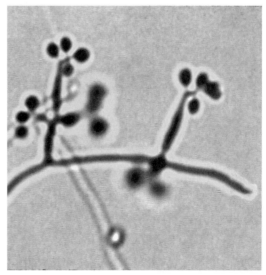

For further information, see
  de Hoog et al., 2000, pp. 523–524
  Kwon-Chung and Bennett, 1992, pp. 745, 799–800
  McGinnis, 1980, pp. 186–187, 192–193
  Rippon, 1988, pp. 730–731, 760

Verticillium sp.

PATHOGENICITY: Commonly known as a contaminant. Reported as rare agent of keratitis (inflammation of the cornea).

RATE OF GROWTH: Rapid; mature within 4 days.

COLONY MORPHOLOGY: Surface is at first white and then may become pinkish brown, red, green, or yellow; powdery or velvety in texture; spreading. Reverse is white or rust in color. (Color Plate 152.)

MICROSCOPIC MORPHOLOGY: Septate hyphae. Conidiophores are simple or branched at several levels and in whorls (i.e., verticillate); phialides are very elongate, having pointed apex, also arranged in whorls. Conidia are oval and single celled, appear singly or in clusters at ends of phialides, and remain in place only if slide preparations are handled with great care.

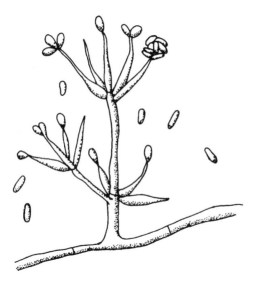

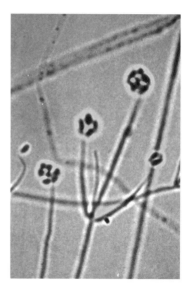

For further information, see
  Barron, 1977, pp. 321–323
  McGinnis, 1980, pp. 296, 300, 310
  Rippon, 1988, pp. 757, 759

Acremonium spp. (formerly *Cephalosporium* spp.)

PATHOGENICITY: *Acremonium* is most commonly known as an etiologic agent of white grain mycetoma but has also been involved in localized disease, such as nail infections and corneal or endophthalmic infections. Disseminated infection has been reported on rare occasions, mostly in immunosuppressed patients. The organism may also be encountered as a contaminant.

RATE OF GROWTH: Moderately rapid; mature within 5–7 days.

COLONY MORPHOLOGY: At first compact, glabrous; later becomes feltlike, powdery, or cottony. May be white, yellowish, light gray, or pale rose in color. Colony does not spread. Reverse is colorless, pale yellow, or pinkish. (Color Plates 153 and 154.)

MICROSCOPIC MORPHOLOGY: Extremely delicate. Hyphae are septate. Phialides are erect, unbranched, tapering, have no conspicuous collarette, and form directly on the fine, narrow hyphae; most (but not all) have a septum at the base delimiting them from the hyphae. Conidia are oblong (2–3 × 4–8 μm) and usually one celled but occasionally two celled. The conidia form easily disrupted clusters at the tips of the phialides.

To differentiate *Acremonium* from similar genera, see Table 13 (p. 186).

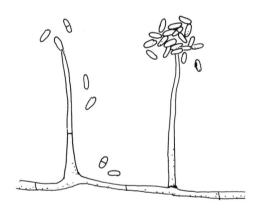

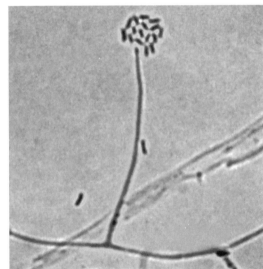

For further information, see
  de Hoog et al., 2000, pp. 395–419
  Guarro et al., 1997
  Kwon-Chung and Bennett, 1992, pp. 573–575, 577, 744–745, 797–798
  McGinnis, 1980, pp. 179–181
  Rippon, 1988, pp. 109–110, 731–732, 761, 763

THERMALLY MONOMORPHIC MOULDS: Hyaline Hyphomycetes

PATHOGENICITY: Frequent agents of mycotic eye infections, most commonly affecting the cornea. They are also occasionally involved in a variety of infections, including mycetoma, sinusitis, septic arthritis, and nail infections. *Fusarium* spp. are increasingly the cause of disseminated systemic infections in severely neutropenic hosts; in these cases, the organism can often be cultured from skin lesions and blood specimens. Additionally, disease has been reported in individuals who ingested food prepared from grain that had been overgrown by toxin-producing species. *Fusarium* is also encountered as a contaminant.

RATE OF GROWTH: Rapid; mature within 4 days.

COLONY MORPHOLOGY: At first white and cottony, but often quickly develops a pink or violet center with a lighter periphery. Some species remain white or become tan or orangey. *F. solani* is unique in becoming blue-green or bluish brown where clusters of conidiogenous cells develop. Reverse is usually light, but may be deeply colored. (Color Plate 155.)

MICROSCOPIC MORPHOLOGY: Septate hyphae. There are two types of conidiation: (i) unbranched or branched conidiophores with phialides that produce large (2–6 $\times$ 14–80 μm) sickle- or canoe-shaped macroconidia (with 3–5 septa) and (ii) long or short simple conidiophores bearing small (2–4 $\times$ 4–8 μm), oval, 1- or 2-celled conidia singly or in clusters resembling those of *Acremonium* spp. (p. 279).

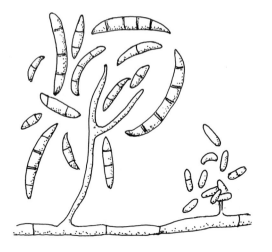

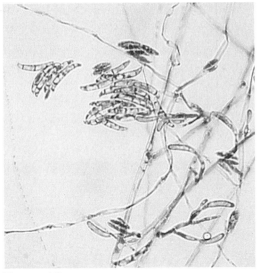

Macroconidia.

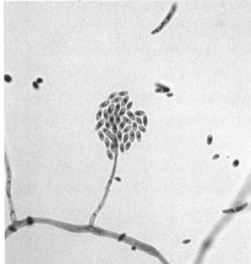

Microconidia.

For further information, see
   de Hoog et al., 2000, pp. 681–705
   Kwon-Chung and Bennett, 1992, pp. 574–575, 745–752, 802–803
   McGinnis, 1980, pp. 218–220, 223
   Rippon, 1988, pp. 732–735, 757, 759

Lecythophora spp.

PATHOGENICITY: Have occasionally been involved in subcutaneous abscess, corneal infection, endophthalmitis, sinusitis, peritonitis, and endocarditis.

RATE OF GROWTH: Moderate; mature within 7 days.

COLONY MORPHOLOGY: At first flat, smooth, moist to slimy, somewhat yeastlike, pink to salmon or orange; may develop clumps of erect hyphal fuzz. If isolate produces chlamydospores, the center of the colony will become blackish brown. Reverse is pink or tan.

MICROSCOPIC MORPHOLOGY: Hyphae septate, hyaline, or very lightly pigmented. Phialides usually do not have a septum at the base; most are extremely short volcano-shaped structures along the sides of the hyphae, but they may be larger and flask shaped or nearly cylindrical. Phialides have parallel-sided collarettes that may require oil immersion microscopy to be seen. Conidia are hyaline or almost so, single celled (1.5–2.5 × 3.0–6.0 μm), oval to cylindrical, sometimes slightly curved, and do not regularly unite in clusters. May form chlamydoconidia that are brown, approximately 4.5 × 7.0 μm, thick walled, broadly club shaped, and cut off at the base.

Note: The two clinically encountered species of *Lecythophora* differ in that *L. mutabilis* produces brown chlamydoconidia that eventually turn the colony brown, whereas *L. hoffmannii* does not produce chlamydoconidia and the colony therefore remains pink or salmon.

To differentiate *Lecythophora* from similar genera, see Table 13 (p. 186).

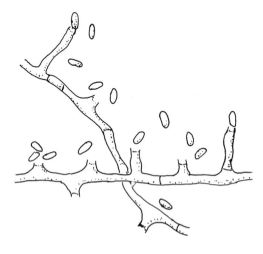

*For further information, see
de Hoog et al., 2000, pp. 725–729;
Gams and McGinnis, 1983, p. 985*

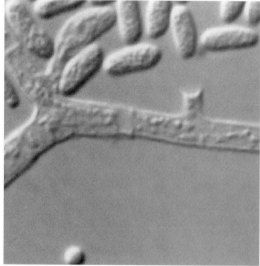

Courtesy of Wiley Schell.

Trichothecium roseum

PATHOGENICITY: Commonly considered a contaminant. Not known to cause infection.

RATE OF GROWTH: Rapid; mature within 4 days.

COLONY MORPHOLOGY: At first white and woolly and then becomes pink or peach colored. Reverse is light. (Color Plate 156.)

MICROSCOPIC MORPHOLOGY: Septate hyphae. Conidiophores are long, slender, and mostly unbranched. Conidia (8–10 × 12–18 µm) are smooth, slightly thick walled, two celled, and pear or club shaped, with a well-marked truncate attachment point frequently off to one side, forming a "foot." The conidia are produced in alternating directions and remain side by side in an elongated group.

The long conidiophores and the smooth walls, attachment points, and arrangement of the conidia serve to distinguish this organism from *Microsporum nanum* (p. 238).

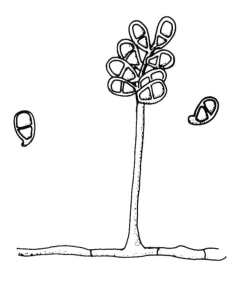

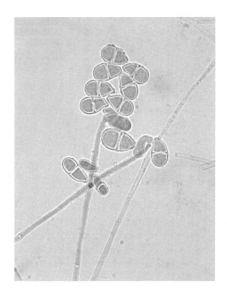

For further information, see
  Barron, 1977, pp. 309–310
  Kwon-Chung and Bennett, 1992, pp. 812, 814
  McGinnis, 1980, pp. 293–294, 303, 304

Chrysosporium spp.

PATHOGENICITY: Commonly considered a contaminant. Isolated from specimens of skin and nails, but its significance is often uncertain. There has been a recent report of systemic infection in a patient with chronic granulomatous disease (Roilides et al., 1999).

RATE OF GROWTH: Moderately rapid; mature within 6 days.

COLONY MORPHOLOGY: Varies greatly among the many species. May be spreading or compact; surface cottony or powdery; flat or raised; usually white, yellow, or tan but may be pink or slightly orange. Reverse is usually white, yellow, tan, or brown but may be another color. (Color Plates 157 and 158.)

MICROSCOPIC MORPHOLOGY: Septate hyphae. Conidia may form directly on the hyphae or at the ends of simple or branched, stalk-like, short or long conidiophores. Conidia are usually one celled (2–9 × 3–13 μm), clavate, with a rounded apex and broad flattened base; the walls may be thin or a bit thick and are most often smooth, occasionally rough. A fringe or remnant of supporting cell wall may stay on the base of the conidium after it matures and detaches. Intercalary conidia (referred to as alternating arthroconidia by some mycologists) are sometimes formed; they are cylindrical or barrel shaped or may bulge on only one side. *Chrysosporium* is the asexual form of several sexual genera; thus, large sexual fruiting bodies (ascocarps) may occasionally be seen in culture.

- The morphology of *Chrysosporium* may resemble that of *Emmonsia parva* (p. 264), but adiaconidia do not develop at 37°C; some species will not grow at 37°C.

- Young conidial formation may mimic that of *Blastomyces dermatitidis* (p. 152), but it will not display thermal dimorphism and will be negative with specific nucleic acid probe.

- Morphology may also resemble that of microconidium-producing *Trichophyton* spp., and some species of *Chrysosporium* will grow on dermatophyte test medium (p. 336) and turn it red.

- For differentiation of *Chrysosporium* from *Sporotrichum*, see Table 25 (p. 286).

Chrysosporium spp. *(continued)*

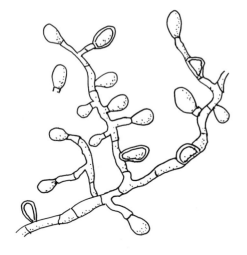

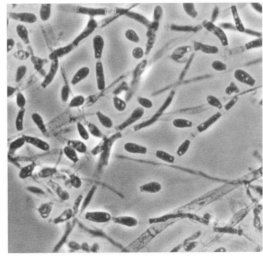

Courtesy of Lynne Sigler.

For further information, see
de Hoog, 2000, pp. 545–559
Kane et al., 1997, pp. 261–311 (extremely informative)

TABLE 25 Differential characteristics of *Chrysosporium* vs *Sporotrichum*[a]

Organism	Colony	Media with cycloheximide[b]	Alternating arthroconidia	Urease[c]	Temp tolerance	Large[d] chlamydospores at 37°C
Chrysosporium (p. 284)	Usually discrete; may spread to cover entire plate	Growth	Remain in chains; may be rare or absent	+	Grows slowly or not at all at 37°C	0
Sporotrichum (p. 287)	Spreads; rapidly covers entire plate	No growth	Usually abundant; often break from hyphae and form clusters	0	Grows well at 37–40°C; some grow at 45°C	+

[a]Abbreviations: +, positive; 0, negative.

[b]Cycloheximide at 0.04%, as in Mycosel agar.

[c]Christensen's urea with 10 days of incubation.

[d]Chlamydospores up to 65 μm in diameter when isolate is subcultured.

Sporotrichum pruinosum

PATHOGENICITY: Commonly considered a contaminant. Has been found in sputa from patients with chronic respiratory disorders, but its significance is unclear.

RATE OF GROWTH: Rapid; mature within 3–5 days. Thermotolerant, grows well at 40°C; many strains can grow at 45°C. It is inhibited by cycloheximide.

COLONY MORPHOLOGY: Spreads rapidly to cover entire surface of plate. Colony is initially cottony, then powdery; at first white, may become cream, yellowish, tan, pinkish, or slightly orange. Reverse is colorless or light tan. (Color Plate 159.)

MICROSCOPIC MORPHOLOGY: Hyphae are broad, lightly pigmented, and septate with bridges known as clamp connections at the septa. Conidiophores form at acute angles to the hyphae and then branch at acute angles; each branch ends with a conidium, giving a tree- or candelabrum-like appearance. The conidia are single celled, ovoid (3–6 × 5–10 µm), typically somewhat pointed at the apex and abruptly flattened at the base. The conidia often retain a portion of attached conidiophore after separation. The conidial walls are fairly thick and are usually smooth. Alternating arthroconidia are often abundant; they may be cylindrical or barrel shaped.

Large (up to 65 µm in diameter), round to oval, thick-walled chlamydospores form when incubated at 37°C, and may also develop at 25°C.

To distinguish *Sporotrichum* from *Chrysosporium*, see Table 25 (p. 286).

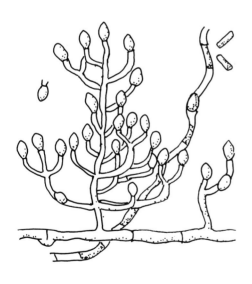

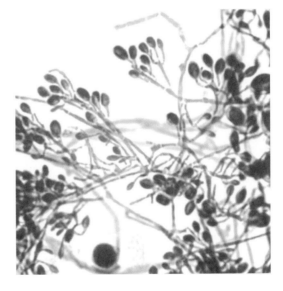

For further information, see
  de Hoog et al., 2000, pp. 928–929
  Kane et al., 1997, pp. 302–303

Sepedonium sp.

PATHOGENICITY: Commonly considered a contaminant; not known to cause disease.

RATE OF GROWTH: Moderately rapid; mature within 7 days.

COLONY MORPHOLOGY: At 25–30°C, colonies are at first white and waxy, then become fluffy, and with age often turn yellow. At 37°C, there is little or no growth. Reverse is white. (Color Plate 160.)

MICROSCOPIC MORPHOLOGY: Hyphae are septate with simple or branched conidiophores. Conidia are large (7–17 μm), round, thick walled, and usually rough and knobby. Differs from *Histoplasma capsulatum* (p. 150) in not forming microconidia, not converting to a yeast at 35–37°C, and not reacting with the DNA probe specific for *H. capsulatum*.

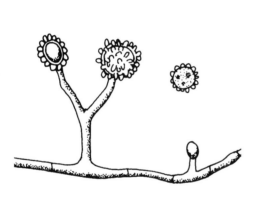 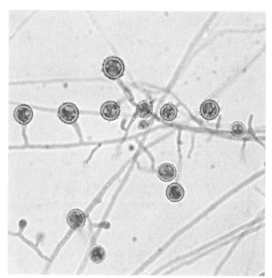

For further information, see
  Barron, 1977, pp. 278–279
  Kwon-Chung and Bennett, 1992, p. 493
  McGinnis, 1980, pp. 276–278
  Rippon, 1988, pp. 760, 762

Monilia sitophila

PATHOGENICITY: Commonly considered a contaminant; rarely involved in infections of the cornea.

RATE OF GROWTH: Rapid; mature within 3 days.

COLONY MORPHOLOGY: White at first and then salmon colored. Thin fluff rapidly spreads over surface of agar.

MICROSCOPIC MORPHOLOGY: Hyphae are septate; simple conidiophores produce branching chains of oval conidia by continuous budding. The older hyphae break up, forming thick-walled arthroconidia.

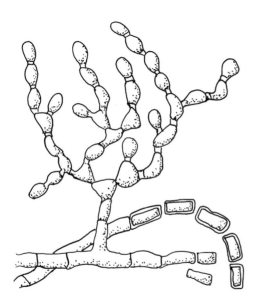

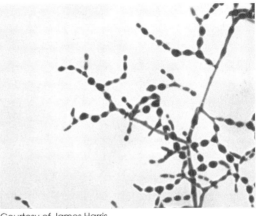

Courtesy of James Harris.

For further information, see
Barron, 1977, p. 227
McGinnis, 1980, pp. 238–239, 247

Laboratory
PART III Technique

Laboratory Procedures

Collection and Preparation of Specimens

No matter how experienced the mycologist, isolation and identification of fungi from clinical specimens are not likely to be accomplished unless the specimen is properly collected and sent immediately to the laboratory. All specimens should be transported in sterile containers and processed as soon as possible. If a specific fungus is suspected by the physician, the laboratory should be notified, as special media and culture procedures may be needed, and the information will be helpful for the safety of laboratory personnel.

Consult references (p. 389) if more information on specimen handling is required.

BLOOD. Blood for fungal cultures must be collected aseptically and inoculated into broth or tubes containing sodium polyanethol sulfonate in a final concentration of 0.03–0.05%; the incorporation of saponin to lyse the blood cells is also desirable. Since recovery of fungi increases with the volume of blood tested and since fungal sepsis may be intermittent, at least two blood samples should be separately collected and cultured.

Special methods and media for fungal blood cultures are now available from a variety of manufacturers. The lysis-centrifugation system (ISOLATOR; Wampole Laboratories, Cranbury, N.J.) has been shown to detect more fungi in less time than the more conventional methods. It is definitely the method of choice for the detection and isolation of *Histoplasma capsulatum*. The automated, continuous-monitoring blood culture systems (BacT/Alert [Organon Teknika, Durham, N.C.], BACTEC [Becton Dickinson, Sparks, Md.], and ESP [Difco Laboratories, Detroit, Mich.]) are now used in the majority of clinical microbiology laboratories. Studies have shown their acceptable ability to detect fungemia caused by yeasts; extending incubation to 10 days provides increased recovery of *Candida glabrata* and *Cryptococcus neoformans*.

While the continuous-monitoring broth systems do sometimes yield positive cultures of moulds, lysis-centrifugation is recommended in general and is still considered essential for the recovery of *H. capsulatum* in most instances. If only an automated broth culture is performed, it has been found that *H. capsulatum* can be recovered after the routine 5-day incubation of the bottle by removing a 5-ml aliquot, centrifuging it, streaking the sediment onto a supportive agar medium, and incubating it for up to 4 weeks (James Snyder, University of Louisville, personal communication).

If a manual method is to be used, biphasic blood culture medium consisting of broth with an agar slant (e.g., Septi-Chek; Becton Dickinson, Cockeysville, Md.) is significantly better than broth alone. Conventional broth blood cultures may require 20–30 days before becoming positive and should be subcultured at regular intervals regardless of gross appearance.

For the recovery of *Malassezia furfur* from broth blood cultures, it is advisable to add palmitic acid or olive oil to make final concentrations of 3 and 5%, respectively.

The membrane filter technique has long been a very successful means of recovering yeasts from blood, but it is impractical for most clinical laboratories.

For membrane filtration, 8 ml of blood is collected in sodium polyanethol sulfonate (yellow-stoppered Vacutainer tube; Becton Dickinson), and a 0.45-μm-pore-size filter is used. The specimen should be kept no longer than 1 h at 35–37°C before being filtered.

BONE MARROW.   Samples of bone marrow should consist of at least 0.5 ml of aspirated marrow. The pediatric ISOLATOR (Wampole Laboratories) is well designed for this small-volume culture. Alternatively, the specimen can be collected in a heparinized syringe and inoculated onto appropriate fungal media at the bedside. Many laboratories use the same bottled broth methods used for fungal blood cultures (see above). The specimen should also be smeared and stained with Giemsa or Wright stain if the presence of *Histoplasma capsulatum* is a possibility.

CEREBROSPINAL FLUID (CSF).   CSF should be centrifuged at 2,000 × *g* for 10 min. The supernatant fluid should not be decanted unless a portion is needed for cryptococcal antigen testing. With a sterile pipette, the sediment is removed and used to inoculate the medium and prepare smears for microscopic examination. Any remaining sediment is resuspended, and the medium is reinoculated with fairly large amounts of the whole specimen. If less than 2 ml of specimen is received, it should be inoculated directly onto the media. Filtration of CSF through a 0.45-μm-pore-size membrane filter, followed by culture of the filter, is sometimes the preferred method.

CUTANEOUS SPECIMENS
Skin.   Specimens of skin are taken from an area previously cleansed with 70% alcohol. The active, peripheral edge of a lesion is scraped with a scalpel or the end of a microscope slide, and the scales are placed in a sterile petri plate.

Nails.   When nails are suspected to have fungal infection, they should be cleansed with an alcohol wipe and then scraped deeply enough to obtain recently invaded nail tissue. The initial scrapings should be discarded, as they are usually contaminated.

Scalp and Hair.   Invaders of the scalp and hair are best isolated by culturing the basal portion of the infected hair. Infected hairs may be selected by placing the patient under a UV light (Wood's lamp); hairs infected with some dermatophytes fluoresce under UV light. Hairs that are fluorescent, distorted, or fractured should be cultured.

EXUDATES, PUS, AND DRAINAGE.   Specimens of exudates, pus, and drainage should be examined for granules by using a dissecting microscope. If granules are present, the color is noted, and then a portion of the specimen is teased apart gently, crushed between two glass slides, and examined microscopically; the remainder is washed several times in sterile distilled water, crushed with a sterile glass rod, and inoculated onto appropriate media (granules may be bacterial and should be plated accordingly). If no granules are present, the specimen is examined microscopically for hyphae and other fungal elements and directly inoculated onto isolation medium.

EYE. Eye cultures for fungi are most successful when the medium is directly inoculated by the ophthalmologist. Corneal scrapings are transferred from a platinum spatula to an agar plate (blood agar plates are the most commonly used) by making a series of C-shaped cuts on the medium. Scraped material should also be smeared on alcohol-cleaned, flamed slides.

FLUIDS. Fluids (e.g., pleural, peritoneal, or joint fluids) must sometimes be collected with heparin to prevent clotting. The fluid is centrifuged at 2,000 $\times$ g for 10 min; any clotted material should be minced with a sterile scalpel and combined with the concentrated fluid. At least 0.3 ml of inoculum is placed onto each medium. The use of lysis-centrifugation (ISOLATOR; Wampole Laboratories) is a recommended alternative.

SPUTUM. Sputum should be collected as a first early-morning sample after the patient's teeth are brushed and the mouth is well rinsed; 24-h specimens are not satisfactory, as they easily become overgrown with bacteria and saprophytic fungi. Flecks containing pus, blood, or caseous material should be sought and used in culture and smears. Sputum decontaminated for culturing acid-fast bacilli is not acceptable, because the sodium hydroxide in the procedure destroys a large number of fungi; a mucolytic agent without sodium hydroxide may be used with very viscous specimens.

STOOL. Specimens of stool are rarely worth culturing for fungi, as their presence in such a contaminated material is usually without meaning. Growth of a large amount (predominance) of yeast has possible significance, but only in indicating a lack of normal fecal flora. Colonization by yeasts is very common in both healthy individuals and compromised patients. If fungal infection of the gastrointestinal tract is suspected, biopsy specimens of tissue are usually required for diagnosis.

TISSUES. Tissues should be minced with a scalpel or ground with a mortar and pestle or tissue grinder. If necessary, a small amount of sterile saline or broth may be added to facilitate grinding. If infection with a zygomycete is suspected, the tissue should be minced, not ground or homogenized, as these procedures destroy the hyphae and decrease the viability of the organisms. Direct microscopic examination is best accomplished with thin paraffin sections stained with Gomori methenamine silver. Subcutaneous tissue should be carefully examined for granules; if granules are present, they should be handled as described above (see "Exudates, Pus, and Drainage").

URINE. Urine should be collected in a sterile container as a first morning "midstream" specimen. Upon reaching the laboratory, the urine is centrifuged at 2,000 $\times$ g for 10 min, the supernatant is decanted, and approximately 0.5 ml of the sediment is placed on each medium to be used. If quantitation is required, a calibrated loop is used to streak uncentrifuged urine onto a plate of appropriate medium. The interpretation of the colony count is still in dispute. The clinical presentation of the patient must be given prime consideration in the determination of the significance of *Candida* spp. in urine. It should be kept in mind that yeast in urine may be a sign of dissemination in severely immunocompromised patients.

For further information on collection and preparation of specimens, see
Isenberg, 1992, pp. 6.1.1–6.1.5, 6.6.1–6.6.5
McGinnis, 1980, pp. 88–99
Miller, 1999
Murray et al. (ed.), 1999, Manual of Clinical Microbiology, 7th ed., chapters 4 and 5
Wentworth, 1988, pp. 11–32

Methods for Direct Microscopic Examination of Specimens

Any specimen submitted for fungus culture can be examined microscopically for fungal elements. This examination is made in addition to, not instead of, a culture. As well as providing the physician with early information regarding the possible need for treatment, it may be helpful in determining the significance of the organism that will later be identified on culture. For a guide to interpreting direct microscopic examinations of clinical specimens, see Part I (pp. 9–64).

POTASSIUM HYDROXIDE (KOH) PREPARATION

Most organic substances that might be confused with fungi when seen through the microscope are converted to an almost clear background in the presence of moderately strong alkaline solutions. The fungi remain unaffected and are therefore rather easily demonstrated. Ink, added to the KOH, stains fungal elements and helps them stand out against the background.

Reagent (Clearing and Staining Agent)
1. Make a 10% KOH solution in Parker Super Quink Ink, permanent blue-black (50 ml of ink + 5 g of KOH pellets).
2. Centrifuge KOH-ink solution at 2,000 × *g* for 10 min.
3. Pour supernatant into plastic (not glass) sterile tube. Store at room temperature.

Slide Preparation
1. Place a portion of the specimen on a labeled slide.
2. Add 1 drop of KOH-ink solution to the slide; mix.
3. Put a coverslip over the preparation.
4. Heat gently over flame. Do not boil. Portions of nails may demand repeated and prolonged heating for the necessary degree of chemical softening so that the material can be pressed out to afford good visibility; alternatively, submerge the nail in the KOH overnight for complete softening and clearing.
5. The slide must be carefully examined microscopically to detect hyphal segments, spores or conidia, budding yeasts, spherules, or sclerotic bodies. Cotton swabs should not be used in preparing these slides, as the cotton strands may resemble hyphae.

KOH preparations are not permanent; the reagent will eventually destroy the fungi. The addition of a small amount of glycerol to the preparation will preserve it for several days.

INDIA INK PREPARATION

1. Place a small drop of India ink on a glass slide

2. Mix with an equal amount of centrifuged (2,000 × g for 10 min) spinal fluid sediment or a suspension of isolated yeast. Sputum or pus can be cleared with KOH and heat and then mixed with India ink.

3. Coverslip, and examine the slide for yeast cells with capsules.

If the India ink is too dark, dilute it by placing a drop of sterile distilled water on the slide next to the edge of the coverslip and allowing the water to slowly diffuse into the ink.

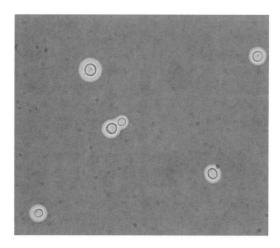

Capsular material is exhibited by the appearance of a clear, well-demarcated halo around a yeast cell. When seen in CSF, it is suggestive of *Cryptococcus neoformans*, but identification must be confirmed by culture and biochemical testing of the isolate. Other species and genera also produce capsules. The capsules of cryptococci vary from 2–10 μm or more in width; they tend to be small in specimens from immunodeficient patients. Leukocytes may also appear haloed, but the halo has a fuzzy, irregular appearance at the periphery, and the cell within the halo has a much paler cell wall than does *C. neoformans*.

Cryptococci often lose their ability to produce capsules when grown on artificial media.

The cryptococcal latex antigen test has been proven to be significantly more sensitive than the India ink preparation and is therefore recommended for the initial diagnosis of cryptococcal disease.

STAINED PREPARATIONS

Calcofluor White (p. 316) is an excellent fluorescent stain for detection of fungi in specimens. It can be combined with KOH (discussed above) if clearing is required. It is a valuable tool and is highly recommended.

Gram stain (p. 320) is most useful in the mycology laboratory for examining specimens for the presence of aerobic actinomycetes. It is commonly used in bacteriology laboratories and may demonstrate mycelial elements and yeast cells, but it does not allow for the best observation of morphologic features.

A modified Kinyoun acid-fast stain (p. 315) is used to detect the partially acid-fast filaments of *Nocardia* spp. The routine Kinyoun method is used to stain ascospores.

Wright's stain (commonly performed in hematology laboratories) or Giemsa stain (p. 317) is used for detecting intracellular yeast forms of *Histoplasma capsulatum* in blood and bone marrow.

The periodic acid-Schiff (PAS; customarily performed in histology laboratories) and Gomori methenamine silver (GMS, p. 318) stains are considered the best for demonstrating fungi in tissue.

Primary Isolation

Specimens to be cultured for fungus must be inoculated onto media that in combination will ensure the growth of all fungi that may be clinically significant. A variety of possible batteries of media can be used, and the ultimate choice often depends on factors such as patient population, fungi endemic in the area, cost, availability, and personal preference. In any case, the battery should include media that have different factors and that complement each other.

There are a few major points to be considered when selecting a battery of fungal media.

- Chloramphenicol and/or gentamicin or other antibiotics are commonly employed to inhibit bacterial contamination. The antibiotics are likely to also prevent the growth of aerobic actinomycetes; therefore, if *Nocardia* or any other filamentous bacteria are suspected, it is necessary to inoculate media lacking the antibiotics commonly used in fungal media.

- Cycloheximide is incorporated in media to inhibit the rapidly growing saprophytic fungi which could overgrow slow-growing primary pathogens. It is necessary to simultaneously use media lacking cycloheximide to grow the organisms that are commonly considered saprophytes or contaminants but can act as opportunistic pathogens; in addition, cycloheximide is known to inhibit the growth of some significant pathogens, e.g., *Cryptococcus neoformans, Penicillium marneffei, Aspergillus fumigatus, Pseudallescheria boydii,* some *Candida* species, and most zygomycetes.

- It is also generally recommended that an enriched medium be used to ensure the growth of very fastidious thermally dimorphic fungi. An enriched medium containing an antibacterial agent(s) can serve a double purpose by eliminating contaminant bacteria while supporting fastidious fungal pathogens. Blood enrichment may promote the growth of fastidious dimorphic fungi, but it inhibits conidiation in the mould form.

Media that are commonly used for primary isolation of fungi from specimens are separated into five groups in Table 26. One medium each can be selected from as many groups as necessary, but cost containment dictates the use of as few media as possible while still guaranteeing recovery of possibly significant fungi. In days gone by, it was common practice to use one battery of media for all fungal cultures. Generally speaking, that usually increased the number of media used. A more efficient system is to establish batteries according to the source of the specimen or the specific organism suspected. It may also be beneficial to use media that have different bases; for example, if using Sabouraud dextrose agar (SDA) without antibiotics,

TABLE 26 Media for primary isolation of fungi

Type of medium[a]	Properties/purpose
A. *Without antimicrobial agents* SDA (p. 344) PDA or PFA (p. 341) BHI agar (p. 333) SABHI agar (p. 343)	SDA provides classic pigment and morphology but not necessarily the best growth or sporulation; it is poor for the recovery of dermatophytes PDA and PFA enhance production of reproductive structures BHI enhances the growth of the fastidious dimorphic fungi SABHI has some of the ingredients of both SDA and BHI
B. *With antibacterial agent(s)* SDA, BHI, or SABHI (usually with chloramphenicol, but may be gentamicin or penicillin with streptomycin) IMA (p. 339) (usually contains chloramphenicol; some formulations also include gentamicin)	Inhibit bacteria while allowing fungi to grow IMA, BHI, and SABHI are enriched media and provide better recovery of fastidious fungi than does SDA
C. *With antibacterial and antifungal agents* Mycosel agar (p. 340) (contains chloramphenicol and cycloheximide) SDA, BHI, or SABHI (with any antibacterial agent in above plus cycloheximide)	Chloramphenicol (or other antibacterial agent) inhibits bacterial growth Cycloheximide inhibits saprobic fungi that could otherwise overgrow pathogens Opportunists and true pathogens may also be inhibited by cycloheximide
D. *For dermatophytes* DTM (p. 336) RSM (p. 343)	Partially selective and differential for dermatophytes Contain antibiotics to inhibit bacteria and cycloheximide to inhibit many nondermatophytes Contain indicator to demonstrate rise in pH, consistent with growth of dermatophytes
E. *Selective and differential for yeasts* CHROMagar (p. 334) Candida ID (p. 333)	Chloramphenicol inhibits bacteria Differentiation of yeast species is possible due to chromogenic substrates in the agar CHROMagar is better able to yield reliable presumptive identification of certain species of *Candida* Both are useful in detecting mixed cultures of yeasts

[a]Abbreviations: SDA, Sabouraud dextrose agar; PDA, potato dextrose agar; PFA, potato flake agar; BHI, brain heart infusion; IMA, Inhibitory Mold Agar; DTM, dermatophyte test medium; RSM, rapid sporulation medium; SABHI, combination of Sabouraud and BHI.

use a different base medium containing antibiotics (e.g., Inhibitory Mold Agar [IMA]).

The following are suggested batteries consisting of a minimum number of media:

- Sterile body sites: one choice from group A and one from group B (or two from group A)
- Respiratory tract: one from group A, one from group B, one from group C
- Throats, vaginals, and most urines: one from group E
- Skin, hair, and nails: one from group B and one from group C or D

Some special situations require specific media.

- If *Histoplasma capsulatum* or *Blastomyces dermatitidis* is suspected, an enriched medium must be one of the choices (and remember, the yeast phase of these organisms is inhibited by cycloheximide).
- If *Histoplasma capsulatum, Blastomyces dermatitidis,* or *Coccidioides immitis* is suspected in a heavily contaminated specimen, yeast extract phosphate medium with ammonia (p. 348) should also be inoculated.
- If an aerobic actinomycete (e.g., *Nocardia*) is suspected, a medium without the antibacterials used in fungal media must be included.

Whenever possible, and unless otherwise indicated, at least 0.5 ml of specimen should be inoculated onto each agar surface. If tubes are used, the media should be slanted in wide tubes (at least 20 mm in diameter) and optimally left in a horizontal position (e.g., on a culture rack commonly used for acid-fast bacilli) for 24 h after inoculation in order for the inoculum to remain dispersed rather than accumulating at the bottom of the slant. The tubes can then be stood vertically for subsequent incubation. The screw caps must be kept partially loosened to ensure proper atmospheric conditions.

Petri plates provide a larger surface area for isolation of fungi but are more hazardous to handle. If plates are used, they should contain 40 ml of medium and be surrounded by a shrink seal to prevent dehydration; the shrink seal also prevents unintentional opening. Plates should NOT be used if *Coccidioides immitis* is suspected.

The optimal temperature for growth of most clinically encountered fungi is 30°C. If a 30°C incubator is not available, cultures should be incubated at room temperature (approximately 25°C). There is no advantage to simultaneously incubating routine primary cultures at 35–37°C; this should be reserved for when there is reason to suspect the presence of thermally dimorphic organisms or one of the few fungi that prefer the higher temperature. If the incubator is not well humidified, it is essential to place pans of water near the cultures.

Most cultures should be incubated for 4 weeks before being considered negative for fungus. Cultures for yeasts in oral thrush, vaginitis, or urine need to be held only 7 days; cultures suspected of containing thermally dimorphic systemic fungi should be incubated for 8 weeks before being reported as negative.

Macroscopic Examination of Cultures

After initial inoculation and incubation, cultures should be examined for growth every 2–3 days during the first week and at least weekly thereafter. Rapid growers will appear by the first or second time the culture tubes are checked, whereas slow-growing fungi may not be evident for 2–3 weeks or longer. It is imperative that any yeast, mould, or actinomycete that grows on a primary medium be subcultured immediately to ensure the viability and isolation of the organism. When mature growth has developed on Sabouraud dextrose agar (SDA), the texture and surface color of the colony should be carefully noted. The color of the reverse (underside) of the colony must also be recorded, along with any pigment that diffuses into the medium. If growth is enhanced on enriched medium, that fact should be noted and a thermally dimorphic fungus should be suspected. It is also helpful to observe whether the fungus grows on medium containing cycloheximide.

To ensure the cultivation of all fungi in a specimen (especially the slower-growing pathogens), it is advisable in many cases to hold the cultures for at least a month, even though some fungi may have been isolated. When more than one fungus is seen on the slant, a carefully streaked plate is usually necessary for isolation. The lid may be taped closed in several places for safety and prevention of dehydration, but care must be taken not to create anaerobic conditions. Shrink seals are perfect for this situation. As previously mentioned, to prevent dehydration of the plates, they should contain 40 ml of agar and a pan of water should be placed in the incubator. If *Coccidioides immitis* is suspected, plates should NOT be used.

Microscopic Examination of Growth

It is best to examine a fungus microscopically when the culture first begins to grow and form conidia or spores and again a few days later. In many instances the manner of conidiation or sporulation, which is so important to identification, is obscured in old cultures. Potato flake or potato dextrose agar often promotes conidiation or sporulation better than does Sabouraud dextrose agar (SDA).

There are several methods for microscopically examining a fungus culture.

A. *Tease mount.* Place a drop of lactophenol cotton blue (LPCB) on a clean glass slide. With a bent dissecting needle, remove a small portion of the colony from the agar surface and place it in the drop of LPCB. With two dissecting needles, gently tease apart the mycelial mass of the colony on the slide, cover with a coverslip, and observe under the microscope with low-power (100×) and high-dry (430×) magnifications. Unfortunately, this method does not always preserve the original position and structure of the conidia, spores, and other characterizing elements, but it is a very rapid method and is always worth a try. All moulds should be examined with this type of wet mount before setting up a slide culture.

B. *Cellophane tape mount.* Another rapid method of studying the microscopic morphology of a mould is with the aid of clear cellophane tape. Loop back on itself a 1.5-in. (~4-cm) strip of clear tape, sticky side out, and hold the tip of the loop securely with a forceps. Press the lower, sticky side very firmly to the surface of the fungal colony, and then pull the tape gently away; aerial hyphae will adhere to the tape. Then, with the tape strip opened up, place it on a small drop of LPCB on a glass slide so that the entire sticky side adheres to the slide, and examine it under the microscope. This method is usually successful in retaining the original positions of the characteristic fungal structures but has the drawback of requiring the organism to be grown on plated medium.

An alternative method has recently been described. It utilizes frosted tape on an applicator stick. The frosted tape is generally more readily available, more pliable, and easier to tear than is clear tape; the use of an applicator stick better permits sampling of fungi in tubed cultures (see Harris, 2000).

C. Slide culture. The best method for preserving and observing the actual structure of a fungus is the slide culture. It is not a rapid technique, but it is unsurpassed as a routine means of studying the fine points of the microscopic morphology of fungi. (Always do a tease mount before a slide culture; organisms suspected of being *Histoplasma, Blastomyces,* or *Coccidioides* spp. or *Cladophialophora bantiana* should NOT be set up on slide culture.)

The procedure is carried out as follows.

1. Cover the inside bottom of a 100-mm-diameter sterile petri plate with a piece of filter paper.
2. Place a bent glass rod, two pieces of plastic tubing (about 6 cm long, 5 cm apart), or the bending end of a flexible drinking straw in the petri plate.
3. Place a clean, flamed glass microscope slide on the glass rod, plastic tubing, or bent straw.
4. From a plate of PDA (or other agar when desired) poured 4 mm deep, cut a 1- × 1-cm block with a sterile scalpel. Transfer the block to the center of the glass slide.

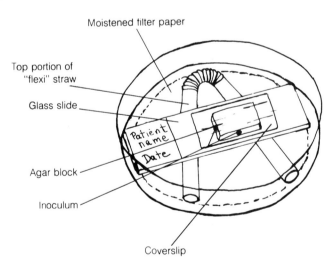

5. With a heavy nichrome wire needle (22 gauge) or sterile applicator stick, inoculate the fungus onto the centers of the four sides of the agar block.

6. Place a flamed coverslip over the block, and apply slight pressure to ensure adherence.

7. Place approximately 1.5 ml of sterile water in the bottom of the petri plate, replace the cover, and incubate the plate at room temperature.

8. Examine periodically for growth, and add water if the plate begins to dry out. The fungus will ordinarily grow on the surface of the slide and also on the undersurface of the coverslip. The closed petri plate can be placed on the microscope stage, and the slide culture can be examined with the low-power (10×) objective.

9. When reproductive structures are well developed, use forceps to carefully remove the coverslip and place it on a drop of LPCB on a second slide.

10. With a heavy needle or applicator stick, gently flip the agar block off the original slide into a container of antifungal disinfectant. Place a drop of LPCB on the slide, and place a new coverslip over it.

11. Both microscopic preparations from steps 9 and 10 can be sealed around the edges with nail polish or mounting fluid and kept for further study or as teaching aids. These slide preparations have been found to last longer if they are stored in a flat position rather than standing on their sides. Huber's modified LPCB with polyvinyl alcohol (p. 322) is now widely used and is definitely the best method available for preserving slide preparations for long periods or for shipping.

Procedure for Identification of Yeasts

The extent to which a yeast needs to be identified depends primarily on the body site from which it is isolated. The particular needs of the patient population and economic issues in the laboratory also play major roles. The following is a scenario that meets minimum requirements while being cost-effective.

Traditionally *Candida albicans*, at least, is differentiated from the other species of *Candida*, but even that level of identification is not usually necessary for isolates from the lower respiratory tract; *Cryptococcus neoformans* is typically the only yeast of concern in such specimens (aside from the yeast forms of the thermally dimorphic fungi). *C. neoformans* can be ruled out, and the result can be reported as "yeast, not *Cryptococcus neoformans*."

For throat cultures requested for fungus, it may be sufficient to identify only *C. albicans* (the need for differentiation from *C. dubliniensis* is at the discretion of each laboratory). Other species can be reported as "yeasts, not *Candida albicans*."

In genital tract specimens, identification of *C. albicans* and *Candida glabrata* to species level is usually adequate. Other species can be reported as "yeasts, not *Candida albicans* or *Candida glabrata*."

Whenever complete identification to species level is not performed, it is advisable to hold the isolate for at least a week after reporting and to add a note to the report that says, "If further identification is required, please call Microbiology, extension *xxxx*."

For blood and other body sites, complete identification of yeasts is the norm.

The decision on how far to go with species identification lies with each laboratory, the primary factors being the patients' needs and the clinical relevancy of the results.

With the above in mind, proceed.

A. *If the colony is mucoid.* Determination should immediately be made as to whether it may be *Cryptococcus neoformans;* this can be accomplished by

- a simple wet prep in sterile water or saline (*C. neoformans* appears as round, dark-walled cells of various sizes)
- addition of India ink (p. 299; will exhibit capsules, if present)
- a urease slant (p. 348) inoculated to the top end of the slant (that area may turn positive more rapidly than the rest of the agar)

If any of the tests listed above suggests *Cryptococcus*, the isolate should be

- inoculated to cornmeal-Tween 80 (or analogous agar that shows microscopic morphology and is glucose free)
- from the cornmeal agar, tested for phenoloxidase with the caffeic acid disk test (p. 308)

The first isolate of *Cryptococcus* from a patient should be confirmed with one of the commercial yeast identification kits. If the isolate is shown to be *C. neoformans*, it is reasonable to do only the caffeic acid disk test on subsequent isolates.

B. *If the colony is not mucoid*

1. Perform a germ tube test (p. 307). Only *Candida albicans* (and *Candida dubliniensis*) will produce germ tubes in serum within 3 h, and they can be differentiated (if desired) by the characteristics in Table 5 (p. 118).

2. If the germ tube test is negative and the colony is small and relatively slow growing, and the wet prep shows small, oval cells, perform the rapid assimilation of trehalose (RAT) test (p. 341) for the identification of *C. glabrata.*

3. If the isolate is not *C. albicans* or *C. glabrata* and further identification is desired, use a pure culture to perform biochemical tests for yeast identification; this is most commonly done with the use of a commercially prepared system, such as one of the following:

> API 20C AUX (bioMerieux, Hazelwood, Mo.)
> ID 32 C (bioMerieux, Marcy l'Etoile, France)
> Minitek (BBL, Cockeysville, Md.)
> RapID Yeast Plus (Remel, Lenexa, Kans.)
> Uni-Yeast-Tek (Remel, Lenexa, Kans.)
> Vitek YBC (bioMerieux, Hazelwood, Mo.)
> Vitek 2 ID-YST (bioMerieux, Hazelwood, Mo.)
> Yeast Identification Panel (MicroScan, Sacramento, Calif.)

4. Using the Dalmau method (p. 335), inoculate a plate of cornmeal-Tween 80 agar or another yeast morphology agar; this should accompany all biochemical identification systems.

C. *If an acceptable identification is not obtained.* After the purity of the isolate is rechecked, subsequent tests may be required for

- fermentation (p. 336)
- assimilation of potassium nitrate or additional carbohydrates (p. 328)
- appearance of isolate in Sabouraud broth (p. 345)
- inhibition of isolate by cycloheximide (p. 340)
- urease activity, if not included in the commercial system (p. 348)
- phenoloxidase (caffeic acid disk test [p. 308])

Consult Tables 3–10 (pp. 114, 116, 118, 123, 130, 131, and 141, respectively) for identification of genus and species.

Isolation of Yeast When Mixed with Bacteria

Yeasts often grow mixed with bacteria on primary culture. It is absolutely essential that only pure cultures be used in assimilation, fermentation, and other biochemical tests for identification.

Careful streaking of the organisms onto plated medium with or without antibiotics often yields isolated colonies. If the yeast is sensitive to cycloheximide, Inhibitory Mold Agar (p. 339) with chloramphenicol should be used. Persistent bacterial contamination may be eliminated with the following acidification method.

1. Place 10 ml of Sabouraud dextrose broth in each of four tubes.
2. To tube no. 1, add 1 drop of 1 N HCl.
3. To tube no. 2, add 2 drops of 1 N HCl.
4. To tube no. 3, add 3 drops of 1 N HCl.
5. To tube no. 4, add 4 drops of 1 N HCl.
6. Make a suspension of the yeast-bacterium mixture in sterile water. Add a drop of the suspension to each of the four Sabouraud dextrose broth-HCl tubes. Incubate at 25–30°C for 24 h.
7. Subculture a loopful of broth from each tube to plated media and incubate for 48 h.

In most instances, there will be an acid concentration at which the bacteria are inhibited and the yeast is allowed to grow.

Germ Tube Test for the Presumptive Identification of *Candida albicans*

1. Make a very light suspension of a yeastlike organism in 0.5–1.0 ml of sterile serum. The optimum inoculum is 10^5–10^6 cells per ml; an increased concentration of inoculum causes a significant decrease in the percentage of cells forming germ tubes. Pooled human sera (negative for hepatitis and human immunodeficiency virus [HIV]) can be used, as well as animal sera or a variety of media. A clean Pasteur pipette tip can be used to inoculate the serum and can be left in the tube during incubation.

2. Incubate at 35–37°C for no longer than 3 h.

3. Place 1 drop of the yeast-serum mixture on a slide with a coverslip. Examine microscopically for germ tube production.

A known strain of *C. albicans* should be tested with each new batch of serum.

Germ tubes are the beginnings of true hyphae and appear as filaments that are NOT constricted at their points of origin on the parent cell. If the filaments are constricted and septate at their points of origin, they are pseudohyphae, not germ tubes.

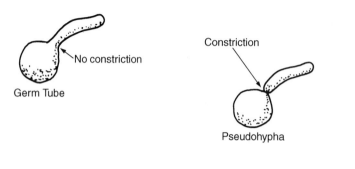

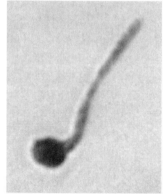

Positive germ tube test.

Rapid Enzyme Tests for the Presumptive Identification of *Candida albicans*

Several systems are now commercially available for the rapid (5–30 min) presumptive identification of *C. albicans* in culture. Each system utilizes two substrates, one for the detection of β-galactosamidase and the other for the detection of L-proline aminopeptidase. Of the clinically encountered yeasts, only *C. albicans* produces both of these enzymes. These tests cannot be used to reliably differentiate *C. albicans* from *C. dubliniensis*. Evaluations of the systems show them to be rapid, acceptable alternatives to the germ tube test. Manufacturers' instructions must be followed.

Caffeic Acid Disk Test

Caffeic acid is one of several good substrates for the detection of phenoloxidase enzyme activity. When phenoloxidase is present, the caffeic acid is broken down to melanin, resulting in a dark brown to black color. As *Cryptococcus neoformans* is the only clinically encountered yeast that produces phenoloxidase, the test is extremely useful for identification and/or confirmation of this organism. Although birdseed agar may also be used, the advantages of the disk test are speed and improved reliability.

1. Culture the isolated yeast on cornmeal-Tween 80 agar. Because phenoloxidase is inhibited by glucose, it is essential that the growth medium be glucose free; cornmeal-Tween 80 agar is usually the most readily available medium to meet this requirement.

2. Place a caffeic acid disk (available from Remel) on a glass slide. Moisten the disk with 30–40 µl of water.

3. Inoculate the disk with several colonies of the isolated yeast.

4. Incubate the disk at 22–35°C in a moist chamber.

5. Read for development of brown to black pigment. Most positive reactions are seen within 30 min, but the test should be held at least 4 h before being considered negative. On rare occasions, an organism may require several generations of growth on cornmeal agar before the enzyme can be detected. (Color Plate 54.)

Olive Oil Disks for Culturing *Malassezia furfur* (K. McGowan, Children's Hospital of Philadelphia, personal communication)

M. furfur (p. 136) requires long-chain fatty acids for growth. This need is usually met in the laboratory by overlaying an agar plate surface with sterile olive oil. As an alternative method, olive oil-saturated paper disks can be used.

1. Place large (½-in. [~13-mm]-diameter) disks (catalog no. 231122; BBL, Sparks, Md.) in a screw-cap sterile flask or jar (a urine specimen container is suitable).

2. Pour in enough olive oil to reach a depth of 10–20 mm.

3. Allow disks (no more than can be easily covered by the oil) to soak in the olive oil; add oil and disks as needed. They can be kept for many months without deterioration.

4. When screening for *M. furfur*, streak specimen or aliquot of blood culture broth (after ~48 h of incubation) onto mycology agar without cycloheximide.

5. Remove a saturated disk from the olive oil, using a swab or forceps (allow excess oil to drip down the side of the container).

6. Place the disk on the area of initial inoculation of the plate.

7. Incubate at 35–37°C.

   M. furfur, if present, will grow well in the area surrounding the disk.

Conversion of Thermally Dimorphic Fungi in Culture

A mycelial colony that is morphologically suggestive of a thermally dimorphic fungus at room temperature is classically grown in its yeastlike form at 35–37°C to confirm its identification. This, or another confirmation method, is essential, as there are several monomorphic moulds that resemble the filamentous phase of thermally dimorphic fungi. In addition, the mould forms of some dimorphic fungi may not be definitive microscopically, and the yeast phase can serve to identify them.

   These organisms MUST be handled in a biological safety cabinet. To test for the ability of a mycelial form to convert to a yeast phase, proceed as follows.

1. Inoculate mycelial growth onto a fresh moist slant of brain heart infusion agar in a screw-cap tube. A small amount of brain heart infusion broth added to the tube ensures sufficient moisture. After the fragment of mould inoculum has been emulsified in the moisture, pull it up and place it on the agar slant.

2. Incubate the slant at 35–37°C, preferably in CO_2. Keep the screw cap closed tightly to retain the moisture, but loosen it daily to allow the colony to "breathe."

3. Periodically examine the slant, and make a wet preparation of any yeastlike area.
4. If only a mycelial form grows, transfer it to another moistened brain heart infusion slant and incubate it again at 35–37°C. It may be necessary to make several serial transfers to attain complete conversion to the yeast phase.

In some instances, in vitro conversion is exceedingly difficult or slow, and exoantigen tests or DNA probes may be preferred or required to confirm identification. The manufacturer's instructions (GenProbe, San Diego, Calif.) should be followed for performing DNA probe tests. For complete instructions on performing the exoantigen test, see Isenberg, 1992, pp. 6.11.10–6.11.12.

Method of Inducing Sporulation of *Apophysomyces elegans* and *Saksenaea vasiformis* (Padhye and Ajello, 1988)

This procedure is recommended for use in identifying all nonsporulating zygomycetes isolated from clinical specimens. The growth on Sabouraud dextrose agar (SDA) at 25°C should consist of broad, nonseptate to sparsely septate, branched, hyaline hyphae without sporangial formation.

1. Grow the isolate on an SDA plate at 25°C for 1 week.
2. Aseptically cut out a 1-cm² agar block permeated with the hyphal growth.
3. Transfer the block to a petri plate containing 20 ml of sterile distilled water and 0.2 ml of filter-sterilized 10% yeast extract. Shrink-seal the plates to prevent spillage.
4. Incubate the blocks in the water solution at 35–37°C (lower temperature will yield fewer or no sporangia). After 5 days of incubation, a thin film of growth should appear over the surface of the water.
5. Make wet preparations (with lactophenol cotton blue) of portions of the film on days 5, 10, and 15 of incubation. Examine microscopically for sporangia. See pp. 170 and 172 for descriptions of *A. elegans* and *S. vasiformis*, respectively.

In Vitro Hair Perforation Test (for differentiation of *Trichophyton mentagrophytes* and *Trichophyton rubrum*)

1. Place 1-cm-long fragments of healthy human hair in a petri plate or tube. Sterilize by autoclaving at 15 lb/in² for 15 min. The clearest and fastest results are obtained with light-colored hair from a child (less than 12 years old). Adult hair will give correct results if the hair has not been exposed to hair spray or a combination of bleach and permanent wave (Salkin et al., 1985b).
2. In a sterile 50-ml screw-cap tube, place 8–10 of the sterile hair fragments; add 20–25 ml of sterile distilled water and 0.1 ml of 10% filter-sterilized yeast extract. (Plastic conical tubes used for concentrating specimens for acid-fast bacilli work well; tubes have proven safer to handle than petri plates when doing this test.)
3. Place several fragments of the fungal culture in the tube.
4. Incubate at room temperature for 4 weeks or until a positive reaction is seen (average, 8–10 days). Examine at weekly intervals by placing one or two hairs from the culture onto a slide with a drop of lactophenol cotton blue and a coverslip.

Look for wedge-shaped perforations caused by hyphae that penetrate the hairs perpendicularly. (Color Plate 126.)

The hair is perforated by *T. mentagrophytes* but not by *T. rubrum* (see Table 19, p. 242).

Positive in vitro hair perforation test

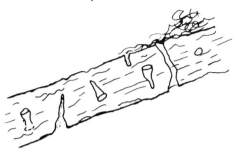

Germ Tube Test for Differentiation of Some Dematiaceous Fungi

Germ tube formation plays an important role in identification of the genera of dematiaceous fungi that form macroconidia with transverse septa, i.e., *Bipolaris*, *Drechslera*, and *Exserohilum* spp.

1. Place a drop of water on a microscope slide.
2. Inoculate the drop of water with a small amount of the actively growing fungus. Examine the slide microscopically to confirm that conidia are present.
3. Place a coverslip over the suspension.
4. Incubate in a moist chamber at room temperature for 8 to 24 h.
5. Examine the slide microscopically to determine the origin and orientation of the germ tubes. See Table 18 (p. 218) for interpretation of results.

Maintenance of Stock Fungal Cultures

OIL OVERLAY TECHNIQUE

Obtain a small but actively growing fungal culture on a short slant of Sabouraud dextrose agar (SDA). Pour over it a good grade of sterile heavy mineral oil (Saybolt viscosity, 330 at 100°F; autoclaved at 15 lb/in² for 45 min in half-filled 250-ml flasks). It is absolutely necessary that the oil cover not only the fungal colony but also the whole agar surface; otherwise, the exposed agar will act as a wick and in time cause the medium to dry out and the colony to die.

The stock cultures are stored upright at room temperature, and most will remain viable for several years. Unfortunately, some fungi must be transferred very often, as they are difficult to keep alive.

To transfer a fungus from an oiled culture, remove a small portion of the colony with a long, disposable inoculating needle or a sterile applicator stick. Drain off the oil along the inside of the tube, and place the inoculum on a fresh agar slant.

WATER CULTURE TECHNIQUE

Rub a sterile moistened swab over the surface of an actively conidiating or sporulating fungus colony; wash the swab off into a screw-cap tube containing approximately 4 ml of sterile distilled water. Tighten the cap, and store at room temperature. Add sterile distilled water periodically if any evaporation occurs.

To prepare a subculture, shake the water culture to resuspend the fungus. Open the tube, flame the mouth, and with a sterile Pasteur pipette transfer 2–3 drops of the suspension to a slant of SDA or other supportive fungal medium. Incubate the agar at 25–30°C.

FREEZING TECHNIQUE

Culture the fungus on a slant of potato dextrose agar in a screw-cap glass test tube. Incubate at 25–30°C until the organism reaches maturity and is actively producing conidia or spores. Close caps tightly, and place tubes in a freezer. Best results are obtained at −70°C, but −20°C has also been used with success. If stored at −20°C, organisms may need to be subcultured annually.

To subculture, remove the tube from the freezer and chip a small portion of the colony from the agar slant. Place the chipped section on a fresh agar slant, and immediately return the frozen slant to the freezer. If the culture is allowed to thaw, it should not be refrozen; the fungus must be transferred to a fresh slant, incubated to maturity, and then frozen.

Controlling Mites

Mites are tiny arachnids that graze on fungi if given the opportunity. Their most common means of entry into the mycology laboratory is on specimens of hair, skin, or nails or in cultures received from other laboratories that have a mite problem. These tiny creatures can cause enormous problems as they walk from one culture to another, contaminating the cultures with the bacteria and fungi they carry on their bodies.

The very best system of mite control is to prevent their initial entry into the laboratory. If there is a risk of mites, culture plates and tubes should be sealed with parafilm or shrink seals. If mites are detected and have spread, it is advisable to autoclave and discard all of the cultures that are not absolutely essential to save and to thoroughly clean the laboratory with a good disinfectant. An attempt to save indispensable cultures can be made by transferring them to slants of media containing 0.1% hexachlorocyclohexane or by exposing the mite-infested fungi to naphthalene (mothball) crystals. Exposure can be attained by placing the cultures in a plastic bag along with naphthalene (or other chemicals poisonous to mites); if the fungi are in tubes, the caps must be loosened. Alternatively, a gauze plug containing the crystals can be put in the neck of each tube. By placing petri plates of naphthalene in incubators and refrigerators for at least a week, those areas can be cleared of mites.

Do not conduct yeast assimilation tests in the vicinity of the chemicals; the vapors may be used as a carbon source by the yeasts, yielding false-positive results.

For further information, see McGinnis, 1980, pp. 454–456, 559

Staining Methods

Positive and negative controls must be run on new lots of stain and periodically thereafter. If the stain is not frequently used, it is advisable to run controls each time the staining procedure is performed on an unknown organism.

Acid-Fast Modified Kinyoun Stain for *Nocardia* spp.

The filaments of *Nocardia* spp. usually appear at least partially acid fast with this staining procedure. Acid-fast organisms stain pink to red.

Procedure

1. Make a smear and fix over flame.
2. Flood slide with Kinyoun carbol-fuchsin for 5 min.
3. Pour off excess stain.
4. Flood slide with 50% alcohol and immediately wash with water.
5. Decolorize with 1% aqueous sulfuric acid (see alternative decolorizer below).
6. Wash with tap water.
7. Counterstain with methylene blue or brilliant green for 1 min.
8. Rinse with water, dry, and examine under oil immersion objective.

Negative and positive controls should be included each time this method is used.

Reagents
Kinyoun carbol-fuchsin (same as for staining mycobacteria)

Basic fuchsin	4 g
Phenol	8 ml
Alcohol, 95%	20 ml
Distilled water	100 ml

Dissolve the dye in the alcohol, and then add the water and phenol.

1% aqueous H_2SO_4 (see alternative decolorizer below)

Concentrated H_2SO_4	1 ml
Distilled water	99 ml

Be sure to add the acid to the water, not vice versa.

Counterstain

Methylene blue	2.5 g
Ethanol, 95%	100.0 ml

or

Brilliant green	0.5 g
Distilled water	100.0 ml

The following decolorizing agent, commonly used in the fluorochrome method for acid-fast bacilli, may be successfully used to substitute for steps 4 and 5 of the above procedure:

Concentrated HCl ....0.5 ml
Ethanol, 70% ....99.5 ml

Acid-Fast Stain for Ascospores

When staining for ascospores, the classic Kinyoun method is used (as for mycobacteria), i.e., decolorize with solution of:

Concentrated HCl ....3 ml
Ethanol, 95% ....97 ml

Add acid to alcohol; mix well.
The ascospores will stain red; other cells will take the counterstain.

Ascospore Stain

1. Culture the fungus on a medium that promotes ascospore formation (see p. 327).
2. Make thin smear and fix in flame.
3. Stain with 5% aqueous malachite green (filter before using) containing Tergitol 7 (Sigma Chemical Co., St. Louis, Mo.) for 3 min.
4. Wash with tap water.
5. Decolorize with 95% ethyl alcohol for 30 s.
6. Wash with tap water.
7. Counterstain with 5% aqueous safranin for 30 s.
8. Wash with water, allow to dry, and examine under oil immersion objective.

Ascospores stain green, and vegetative cells stain red.
The acid-fast stain (above) is also useful for observing ascospores. It should be noted that ascospores may be observed in simple aqueous wet mounts without any stain.

Calcofluor White Stain

Calcofluor White (CFW) has become a valuable and routine reagent in the clinical mycology laboratory. It binds to β-1–3 and 1–4 polysaccharides, such as cellulose and chitin (present in fungal cell walls), and fluoresces when exposed to long-wave UV light. It is exceedingly useful for direct microscopic examination of specimens, as the fungal elements are seen much more easily than with the older traditional potassium hydroxide (KOH) preparations. Additionally, it is exceptional for exhibiting certain morphologic structures of fungi that have been isolated on culture.

Preparation of Stain Solution

CFW M2R (Fluorescent Brightener 28)*.........100 mg
Evans Blue..50 mg
Distilled water ....100 ml

---

    * The powder form is available from Sigma Chemical Co. and Aldrich Chemical Co. Several other companies produce solutions of various formulations. It is imperative to follow manufacturers' instructions for use; excitation wavelengths may vary and require filters other than those described below.

Mix well. Store at room temperature in a dark bottle.

Procedure

1. Smear specimen onto glass slide. The specimen may be stained while wet or allowed to dry on the slide and rehydrated with the CFW solution. If the slide is to be subsequently reprocessed with another stain, it must first be allowed to dry and then heat fixed before applying the CFW.

2. Add 1 drop of CFW solution. One drop of 10% KOH may also be added if clearing is required.

3. Apply coverslip. Allow slide to sit at room temperature at least 5 min (it often takes a few minutes for the CFW to penetrate the organism).

4. Examine slide with a UV microscope equipped with an excitation filter that transmits wavelengths between 300 and 412 nm (the optimum wavelength for excitation of CFW M2R is 365 nm) and a barrier filter (530 nm) that removes UV and blue light while transmitting longer wavelengths.

The required light source is a mercury vapor lamp. Quartz halogen bulbs are usually not suitable, as the energy output is too low.

Fungal elements will stand out as bright apple green on a red background; the barrier filters that allow transmission of shorter wavelengths and yield white elements on a blue background are no longer recommended (for eye safety).

Quality control must be performed on a routine basis to ensure the quality of the reagent, procedure, and microscope.

Positive control is a suspension of a yeast or mould, e.g., *Candida* sp. or *Aspergillus* sp.

Negative control is a solution without fungi.

If the slide is to be saved or restained, remove the coverslip, rinse the slide briefly with distilled water, and air dry. The slide can later be restained with CFW or other stains, such as Gomori methenamine silver, Gram, etc.

Giemsa Stain

The Giemsa stain is used for the detection of intracellular *Histoplasma capsulatum* in bone marrow or blood smears. The blood smears are made from the buffy coat of centrifuged citrated blood or from the bottom of the tube, where heavily infected cells are often found. *H. capsulatum* is seen as small, oval yeast cells that stain light to dark blue with a hyaline halo due to the unstained cell wall (see p. 150). Giemsa stain is commercially available.

Procedure

1. Place slide in 100% methanol for 1 min (to fix smear).
2. Drain off methanol.
3. Flood slide with Giemsa stain (freshly diluted 1:10 with distilled water) for 5 min.
4. Wash with water; air dry.

Gomori Methenamine Silver (GMS) Stain

Of the special stains for fungi, methenamine silver nitrate is considered by many to be the most useful for screening clinical specimens. It provides better contrast and often stains fungal elements that may not be revealed by other procedures. Fungi are sharply delineated in black against a pale green background. The inner parts of hyphae are charcoal gray. Certain bacteria (including *Nocardia* spp.), as well as some tissue elements, also take the stain, so it must be remembered that all that is gray or black is not necessarily a fungus.

Histology laboratories routinely perform some method of Gomori methenamine silver staining. The following are simpler and faster methods that may be used on smeared material or deparaffinized tissue.

METHENAMINE SILVER STAIN (Method of Mahan and Sale (1978))*
Solutions Required (All Are Aqueous Solutions)

> 10% chromic acid (chromium trioxide)
> 5% silver nitrate
> 3% methenamine (hexamethylenetetramine)
> 5% borax (sodium borate)
> 1% gold chloride
> 1% sodium metabisulfite
> 5% sodium thiosulfate

Preparation of Stains
Methenamine silver nitrate solution

> 3% methenamine ....40 ml
> 5% silver nitrate ....2 ml
> 5% borax ....3 ml
> Distilled water ....35 ml

This solution must be freshly prepared before use; it can be used only once. The other solutions may be reused for up to 1 month provided fungal contamination does not occur.

---

* Prepared reagents for an equally rapid method that employs a microwave oven are commercially available from Sigma Diagnostics, St. Louis, Mo.

Light green stock solution

        Light green SF-yellowish ....0.2 g
        Distilled water ....100.0 ml
        Glacial acetic acid ....0.2 ml

Solution is stable for 1 year.

Working solution

        Stock light green solution ....10 ml
        Distilled water ....40 ml

Solution is stable for 1 month.

Procedure

Before starting, heat Coplin jar of methenamine silver nitrate solution in oven or water bath until the solution becomes a deep golden brown (approximately 95°C). Then, proceed as follows.

A. If slide to be stained is paraffin fixed, rehydrate (see procedure, p. 323); other slides must be fixed by heating or submerging in alcohol. Positive-control slides must be included each time the staining procedure is performed.

B. Rinse slides with water.

C. Place slides in reagents in Coplin jars as follows:

   1. Chromic acid (discard after use) ....10 min
   2. Running tap water ....5 s
   3. 1% sodium metabisulfite..1 min
   4. Hot tap water ....1 min
   5. Methenamine silver nitrate solution, approximately 95°C ....5–10 min

   Periodically remove the control slide, wash with water, and observe microscopically to determine when optimal staining has been achieved. The color should never be so intense as to obscure the morphologic detail of a fungus. Prolonged staining time may be required when old and nonviable fungal elements or filaments of actinomycetes are suspected.

   When control shows optimal staining, rinse all slides in hot tap water and then in gradually cooler water.

   6. Distilled water ....Rinse
   7. 1% gold chloride ....10 s
   8. Distilled water ....Rinse
   9. 5% sodium thiosulfate...3 min
   10. Running tap water..30 s
   11. Light green working solution ....30 s

D. Rinse twice with each increasing concentration of ethanol: 70%, 95%, and absolute alcohol.

E. Dip slides twice in xylene.

F. Place drop of mounting medium on slide, and cover with coverslip.

MORE RAPID METHENAMINE SILVER STAIN
(Method of Shimono and Hartman (1986))

The solutions and procedure for the Shimono-Hartman method are identical to those for the method of Mahan and Sale (see above), except that the methenamine solution is not preheated and the slides are stained while on a heating platform.

1. Begin staining procedure as for Mahan and Sale's method above, steps C.1–4.

2. At this point, place slides on a 70°C heating platform or hot plate. The slides can be placed directly on the heated surface or in a large (150-mm-diameter) glass petri plate to handle any spillage.

3. Layer the methenamine silver solution onto the slides.

4. When the control tissue becomes golden brown (approximately 1 min if slide is directly on heating plate, 4–5 min if slide is in a petri plate), remove slides from heat.

5. Continue from step 7 to completion as in Mahan and Sale's method.

   The advantages of this system are that the time required to heat the methenamine solution in volume is eliminated along with the general manipulations and handling of the hot solution. Additionally, a smaller volume of methenamine solution is usually required, resulting in cost saving.

Gram Stain (Hucker Modification)

Fungi are gram positive but often stain poorly.

Procedure

1. Fix the smear by passing it over a flame.
2. Place crystal violet solution on the slide for 20 s.
3. Wash gently with tap water.
4. Apply Gram iodine solution to the slide for 20 s.
5. Wash gently with tap water.
6. Decolorize quickly in solution of equal parts acetone and 95% ethanol.
7. Wash gently with tap water.
8. Counterstain with safranin for 10 s.
9. Wash with tap water; air dry or blot dry.

Reagents
Crystal violet solution

   a. Crystal violet, 85% dye content ....2 g
      Ethyl alcohol, 95% ....10 ml
      Dissolve the dye in alcohol.
      Add distilled water ....100 ml

   b. Ammonium oxalate...................................4 g
      Distilled water..400 ml
      Dissolve the ammonium oxalate in the water.

Mix the crystal violet-alcohol solution (a) with the ammonium oxalate solution (b).

Gram iodine solution

> Iodine ....1 g
> Potassium iodide..............................2 g

Dissolve the iodine and potassium iodide completely in 5 ml of distilled water.

> Add distilled water.......................240 ml
> Sodium bicarbonate,
> 5% aqueous solution ....60 ml
> (i.e., 3 g of $NaHCO_3$ + 57 ml of distilled water)

Mix well; store in amber glass bottle.

Counterstain

> Safranin O ....1 g
> Ethyl alcohol, 95% ....40 ml

Dissolve the dye in the alcohol.

> Add distilled water.......................400 ml

Mix well.

Note: A slide that has been Gram stained can be decolorized by flooding it with acetone for 30–60 s and rinsing it well with water. Special fungus-staining procedures can then be performed on the slide.

Lactophenol Cotton Blue

Lactophenol cotton blue is used as both a mounting fluid and a stain. Lactic acid acts as a clearing agent and aids in preserving the fungal structures, phenol acts as a killing agent, glycerol prevents drying, and cotton blue gives color to the structures.

> Lactic acid.......................................20 ml
> Phenol crystals...............................20 g
> (or phenol, concentrated..........20 ml)
> Glycerol (or glycerine) ....40 ml
> Distilled water...............................20 ml
> Cotton blue ....0.05 g
> (or 1% aqueous solution ....2 ml)

1. Dissolve the phenol in the lactic acid, glycerol, and water by gently heating (if crystals are used).
2. Add cotton blue (Poirrier's blue and aniline blue are analogous to cotton blue).
3. Mix well. For use, see p. 303.

Lactophenol Cotton Blue with Polyvinyl Alcohol (PVA) (Huber's PVA Mounting Medium, Modified*)

This modification of Huber's plastic mount (Huber and Caplin, 1947) is excellent for making permanent mounts of fungal wet preparations or slide cultures. Upon drying for at least 24 h on a flat surface, these mounts are permanent and will not be dissolved in ether, xylene, or alcohols, and the fixed fungal structures remain picture-perfect for years.

Reagents

PVA; molecular weight, 70,000–100,000 (Sigma Chemical Co., catalog no. P-1763)
Phenol, purified grade (Sigma no. P-5566 or Fisher no. A91 1-500)
Lactic acid, ACS reagent (Sigma no. L-1893)
Aniline blue, certified (Aldrich Chemical Co., catalog no. 86,102-2). This is analogous to cotton blue.

Preparation

1. Add 7.5 g of PVA powder to 50 ml of cold deionized water in a beaker.
2. Transfer beaker to a heated stirring plate; add a magnetic rod for mixing.
3. Place a thermometer in the beaker to monitor temperature.
4. Add 22 g of lactic acid (BEFORE adding phenol).
5. Add 22 g of phenol crystals (or 22 ml of melted phenol).
6. Add 0.05 g of aniline blue.
7. Heat and stir the solution until the temperature reaches 90°C. Do not boil or go over 100°C. Remove from hot plate.
8. Dispense into small dropper bottles (washed used ones from blood bank panel cells work well). Tighten dropper bottle caps, and store at room temperature.

Procedure

Place 1 drop of PVA mounting fluid on a slide with a sample of fungal growth. Apply coverslip. Allow to dry on a flat surface.

Huber's modified PVA mounting medium may be used as a replacement for lactophenol cotton blue. Care must be taken to avoid coverslip runover or droppings on the bench top, since they are difficult to remove. While the solution is in liquid form, it can be cleaned from surfaces with water; after it dries, a razor blade is required to remove the hardened material.

Slides can be examined microscopically at low or high dry power as soon as the slides are prepared. After adequate drying time (2–4 days), the slides can be examined under oil immersion, cleansed in xylene, or decontaminated by dipping them in disinfectant.

The solution is available in prepared form from Scientific Device Laboratory Inc., Des Plaines, Ill.

---

* Appreciation is extended to Lawrence M. Bobon of Wilmington, Del., for his invaluable contributions in the updating and reinstatement of Huber's method.

Rehydration of Paraffin-Embedded Tissue

Treat slides as follows.

Xylene (in Coplin jar)....................12 min

Repeat, using two more jars of xylene.

Absolute ethanol.......................Rinse twice
95% ethanol..............................Rinse twice
70% ethanol..............................Rinse twice
Distilled water..........................Rinse twice

Proceed with staining procedure.

Media

Many of the media prepared for mycology are used relatively rarely in the typical clinical microbiology laboratory. Freshness during long storage may be maintained by dispensing agar medium into screw-cap tubes, autoclaving it, allowing it to cool as butts, and storing it in the refrigerator. When needed, the appropriate number of butts are melted in a boiling-water bath and then poured into petri plates or allowed to cool as slants.

Most of the media can be purchased in dehydrated form. Commercially prepared tubes or plates are also available for most, but not all, of the formulations.

Whenever a new batch of medium is placed in use, positive- and negative-control organisms must be tested. If the medium is not often used, it is advisable to run controls each time an unknown organism is tested.

Ascospore Media

ACETATE ASCOSPORE AGAR

Potassium acetate	5.00 g
Yeast extract	1.25 g
Dextrose	0.50 g
Agar	15.00 g
Distilled water	500.00 ml

1. Dissolve by boiling for 1 min; dispense in screw-cap tubes.
2. Autoclave (15 lb/in^2) for 15 min.
3. Allow tubes to cool in slanted position or as butts to be melted and slanted as needed.

GORODKOWA MEDIUM

Dextrose	1.25 g
NaCl	2.60 g
Beef extract	5.00 g
Agar	5.00 g
Distilled water	500.00 ml

1. Dispense into screw-cap tubes.
2. Autoclave (15 lb/in^2) for 15 min.
3. Allow to harden as slants or as butts to be melted and slanted as needed.

V-8 MEDIUM FOR ASCOSPORES

V-8 vegetable juice	500 ml
Dry yeast	10 g
Agar	20 g
Distilled water	500 ml

1. Dissolve agar in water by boiling.
2. Mix vegetable juice and dry yeast, adjust to pH 6.8 with 20% KOH, add to agar-water mixture, and mix well.

3. Dispense into screw-cap tube.

4. Autoclave (15 lb/in^2) for 15 min.

5. Allow to cool as slants or as butts to be melted and slanted as needed.

Assimilation Media (for Yeasts)

Assimilation is the utilization of a carbon (or nitrogen) source by a microorganism in the presence of oxygen. A positive reaction is indicated by the presence of growth or a pH shift in the medium.

WICKERHAM BROTH METHOD
Carbon Assimilation Medium

> Yeast nitrogen base.....................6.70 g
> Appropriate carbohydrate ....5.00 g
> Distilled water ....100.00 ml

1. If necessary, heat to dissolve.

2. Sterilize by Seitz or membrane filter.

3. Add 0.5 ml of the solution to 4.5 ml of sterile distilled water in screw-cap tubes.

These tubes may now be stored in the refrigerator, ready for use, for 1 month.

Note: Care must be taken to ensure that carbon compounds are pure and not mixed with other carbohydrates. It is advisable to check each new lot of a carbon compound with control yeasts that can and cannot assimilate it before using the material in assimilation studies. The sugars most commonly employed are listed in Tables 4, 8, and 9 (pp. 116, 130, and 131, respectively).

Nitrate Assimilation Medium

> Yeast carbon base ....11.70 g
> Potassium nitrate (KNO$_3$) ....0.78 g
> Distilled water ....100.00 ml

1. Warm gently to dissolve.

2. Sterilize by Seitz or membrane filtration.

3. Add 0.5 ml of medium to 4.5 ml of sterile distilled water in screw-cap tubes.

These tubes may be stored in the refrigerator for 1 month.

Tubes of yeast nitrogen base without sugar and yeast carbon base without KNO$_3$ should be prepared and used as controls to check "carryover" of nutrients that may have been stored within the yeast cell when grown on the previous medium.

Test Procedure

1. Make a suspension of the yeast in sterile distilled water. This suspension should not exceed the turbidity of McFarland no. 1 standard (prepared by mixing 0.1 ml of 1% barium chloride with 9.9 ml of 1% sulfuric acid).

2. Add 0.1–0.2 ml of the yeast suspension to each tube of medium. Include a tube of yeast nitrogen base without any carbon source and a tube of yeast carbon base without KNO_3 as controls for carryover.

3. Incubate tubes at the yeast's optimal temperature. If the organism grows at 35–37°C, positive reactions are usually more rapid at this temperature. Shaking the culture tubes will also enhance growth.

4. Examine cultures over a period of 7–14 days for dense turbidity caused by growth.

5. The negative-control tubes without a carbon or nitrogen source should show no growth. If growth is present, the test is invalid because of carryover. In such cases, a small amount of growth from each tube should be transferred to another tube of the same medium and the test should be repeated.

For identification of yeasts, see Tables 4, 8, and 9 (pp. 116, 130, and 131, respectively).

AUXANOGRAPHIC PLATE METHOD (HALEY AND STANDARD MODIFICATION)
For Carbon Assimilation Tests

> Yeast nitrogen base......................0.67 g
> Noble or washed agar ....20.00 g
> Distilled water ....1,000.00 ml

1. Dispense in 20-ml quantities into 18- × 150-mm screw-cap tubes.

2. Autoclave (15 lb/in²) for 15 min.

3. Allow to harden as butts. Store in refrigerator.

Test procedure

1. Melt a tube of nitrogen base medium in a boiling-water bath; allow to cool to 47–48°C.

2. With a sterile cotton-tipped applicator, make a heavy suspension of a 24- to 72-h yeast culture in 4 ml of sterile distilled water. The density should equal that of a McFarland no. 4 or 5 standard.

3. Pour the yeast suspension into the tube of molten yeast nitrogen base agar. Mix very thoroughly by inverting tube several times.

4. Pour the yeast-agar mixture into a sterile 15- × 150-mm petri plate. Allow to solidify at room temperature.

5. Place carbohydrate disks (available from BBL Microbiology Systems, Sparks, Md.), evenly spaced, on the plate.

6. Incubate at 30°C for 18–24 h, and then examine for growth around each disk. Any amount of growth around a disk indicates that the yeast assimilates that sugar. The plates may be reincubated for an additional 24 h, but reincubation is usually not necessary.

For Nitrate Assimilation Tests
Medium

> Yeast carbon base .... 12 g
> Noble or washed agar .... 20 g
> Distilled water .... 1,000 ml

Tube in 20-ml aliquots and autoclave at 15 lb/in² for 15 min. Store in refrigerator.

Peptone solution for positive control

> Peptone .... 10 g
> Distilled water .... 100 ml

Sterilize by filtration; store in refrigerator.

Test procedure

1. Melt a tube of yeast carbon base medium in a boiling-water bath; allow to cool to 47–48°C.
2. Make an aqueous suspension of the yeast to a density equal to a McFarland no. 1 standard.
3. Add 0.1 ml of the yeast suspension to the tube of medium. Mix thoroughly.
4. Pour the yeast-agar mixture into a sterile 15- × 100-mm petri plate. Allow to solidify at room temperature.
5. Place approximately 1 mg of KNO_3 crystals on agar surface away from the center of the plate.
6. Place approximately 0.1 ml of peptone solution (positive control) on agar surface opposite the KNO_3 site.
7. Incubate at 30°C for 48–96 h. Growth must occur in the "peptone area" for test to be valid. If growth is seen in the peptone area, examine for growth in the KNO_3 area (growth indicates assimilation of KNO_3).

AGAR WITH INDICATOR METHOD
For Carbon Assimilation Tests

This modification of the Wickerham medium was devised by Adams and Cooper (1974). It is easier to read than the conventional methods, yet it is equally reliable. The medium is in the form of agar slants with an indicator added. It is less troublesome than other formulations, for it can be sterilized by autoclaving after the carbohydrates have been added. The quality of each batch of medium should be tested with standard reference strains of yeasts.

Basal medium

> Bromcresol purple (1.6%) .... 0.2 ml
> 0.1 N NaOH .... 1.0 ml
> Noble agar .... 2.0 g
> Deionized water .... 90.0 ml

Heat to dissolve.

Stock carbohydrate solution

             Carbohydrate..............................1.00 g
                (if using raffinose...................2.00 g)
             Yeast nitrogen base.....................0.67 g
             Deionized water........................10.00 ml

Mix to dissolve; gently heat if necessary.

Preparation
1. Add the stock carbohydrate solution to the melted agar base.
2. Mix well.
3. Adjust to pH 7.0.
4. Dispense in 5-ml amounts in 16- $\times$ 125-mm screw-cap tubes.
5. Sterilize by autoclaving at exactly 10 lb/in^2 for 10 min.
6. Allow to solidify in a slanted position.
7. Store in refrigerator at 4°C.

Inoculation and incubation
1. Suspend a 2-mm loopful of pure culture in 9 ml of sterile water.
2. Inoculate each assimilation slant with 0.1 ml of the yeast suspension.
3. Incubate at room temperature (25°C), examining at 7 and 14 days for abundant growth and acid production (yellow).

Assimilations are considered negative when there is no significant difference between the growth of the organism on the carbohydrate medium and that on the control medium without carbohydrate.

MODIFIED POTASSIUM NITRATE ASSIMILATION TEST (Pincus et al., 1988)

             Potassium nitrate..........................1.4 g
             Yeast carbon base.......................1.6 g
             Bromthymol blue........................0.12 g
             Noble agar..................................16.0 g
             Distilled water...........................1,000 ml

1. Adjust final pH to 5.9–6.0.
2. Dispense into screw-cap tubes.
3. Autoclave at 15 lb/in^2 for 15 min.
4. Cool tubes in slanted position.

Test Procedure
1. Inoculate the surface of the slant with yeast isolate.
2. Incubate at 25–30°C.
3. Examine daily; most positive results are seen within 24 h.
      Positive: slant becomes blue-green or blue.
      Negative: slant remains greenish yellow.

Birdseed Agar (Niger Seed Agar; Staib Agar)

Guizotia abyssinica seed ....50 g
> (Commonly known as niger seed; it is available at most stores that sell bird feed.)

Distilled water ....100 ml

1. Pulverize in blender.
2. Add 900 ml of distilled water.
3. Boil for 30 min.
4. Cool and filter through four layers of gauze, and then add enough distilled water to make volume 1,000 ml.
5. Add:

KH_2PO_4 ....1 g
Creatinine ....1 g
Agar ....15 g

> (Glucose, 1 g, is added in the formulation for identification of *Candida dubliniensis*, p. 115, but it can inhibit pigment production by *Cryptococcus neoformans*.)

> (Chloramphenicol, 1 g, may be added in the formulation for pigment production by *C. neoformans*, p. 129.)

6. Mix well. Autoclave (15 lb/in^2) for 15 min.
7. Pour into tubes and cool in slanted position or as butts to be melted and slanted or plated as needed.

Test Procedure

A. For pigment production by *C. neoformans*

Inoculate with suspected *Cryptococcus* sp. (fresh isolate) and incubate at 25–30°C for no more than 7 days.

Only *C. neoformans* produces phenoloxidase, which breaks down the substrate, resulting in the production of melanin and the development of dark brown to black colonies. Colonies of other yeasts are cream to beige. (Color Plate 53.)

Chemically defined tests such as the caffeic acid disk test also detect phenoloxidase and have the advantage of rapidity and sensitivity; see p. 308.

B. For differentiation of *C. dubliniensis* versus *C. albicans*

1. Inoculate a plate of the medium with a 48-h-old colony; streak for isolation.
2. Incubate at 30°C for 3–5 days. Examine macroscopic morphology of colonies (see Table 5, p. 118).

Brain Heart Infusion (BHI) Agar

Brain heart infusion agar is classically recommended for the cultivation of fastidious pathogenic fungi, such as *Histoplasma capsulatum* and *Blastomyces dermatitidis*. The ingredients are listed here for ease of comparison with other enriched fungal media that are commonly used.

    Brain heart infusion......................8.0 g
    Peptic digest of animal tissue.......5.0 g
    Pancreatic digest of casein.........16.0 g
    Sodium chloride...........................5.0 g
    Dextrose.......................................2.0 g
    Disodium phosphate....................2.5 g
    Agar...13.5 g
    Distilled water...........................1,000 ml

Antibiotics are often added to inhibit bacteria, and sheep blood is added to further enrich the medium and enhance the growth of fastidious pathogenic fungi.

Candida ID Agar

Candida ID (bioMerieux, Hazelwood, Mo.) is a chromogenic medium for the culture and isolation of yeasts, the identification of *Candida albicans*, and the separation of other yeast species into two groups. Most filamentous fungi will also grow. Bacteria are inhibited. It can be very useful in detecting mixed yeast populations in clinical specimens. The plates are incubated in ambient air for 48 h at 35–37°C; some species of *Geotrichum* and *Candida* require 30°C for optimal growth. (Color Plate 46.)

The colony colors indicate the following:

Blue: *C. albicans* or *C. dubliniensis* (some strains of *Trichosporon* can be blue, but the colony morphology is very different from that of the *Candida* spp.).

Pink: *C. tropicalis*, *C. guilliermondii*, *C. kefyr*, or *C. lusitaniae* (*Cryptococcus* spp. may also be pink).

White or cream: other yeasts and some filamentous moulds.

Notes:
* Plates must always be stored and incubated in the dark.
* Some bacteria (notably *Enterococcus faecalis*) may grow on the medium and have a pink or blue color.

See also CHROMagar Candida Medium (p. 334).

Casein Agar

(For differentiation of aerobic actinomycetes and characterization of some dematiaceous fungi)

Solution A

Skim milk (dehydrated or instant
    nonfat dry milk)........................10 g
Distilled water..............................90 ml

Add milk with constant stirring to avoid lumping.

Solution B

Agar..3 g
Distilled water..............................97 ml

1. Autoclave each solution separately at 15 lb/in^2 for 10 min.
2. Cool both solutions to 45–50°C, and then combine solutions and mix well.
3. Pour into petri plates (or into screw-cap tubes and allow to solidify as butts to be melted and poured as needed).

Inoculate an area about the size of a dime (10 mm) heavily with a pure culture. Include positive- and negative-control cultures. Three or four organisms can be tested on one 100-mm-diameter plate if they are evenly spaced. Incubate at room temperature or 37°C for 2 weeks. Examine every few days for clearing (hydrolysis) of casein around or directly beneath the colony.

For results with aerobic actinomycetes, see Table 2 (p. 103).

For results with dematiaceous fungi, see Table 16 (p. 200).

CHROMagar Candida Medium

CHROMagar Candida medium (Becton Dickinson, Sparks, Md.) is for the isolation of all, and the definitive differentiation of a few, of the most commonly encountered yeasts in the clinical laboratory. It is also extremely effective as a primary medium for detecting mixed yeast populations in clinical specimens. (Color Plate 45.)

Chromogenic substrates produce unique and specific colors for the identification of:

C. albicans (light to medium green; *C. dubliniensis* often forms darker green colonies on primary isolation, but this property is often lost on subcultures)

C. tropicalis (dark blue to metallic blue-purple)

C. krusei (light rose with a whitish border; rough)

Studies have shown that further identification tests for these three species are not necessary.

Other yeasts (cream color or light to dark mauve; *C. glabrata* forms pink colonies but cannot be reliably distinguished on this basis from other yeasts)

Filamentous fungi (colors that may differ from those exhibited on Sabouraud dextrose agar)

Notes:
- Plates produce the best color development in the colonies when incubated at 37°C (they should NOT be incubated below 30°C).
- Incubate in atmospheric air, not in CO_2, for 36–48 h.
- It is advisable to minimize exposure of the plates to light both before and during incubation.
- All yeasts and filamentous fungi will grow, while bacteria are inhibited.

See also Candida ID Agar (p. 333).

Cornmeal Agar

    Cornmeal.......................................40 g
    Agar..20 g
    Tween 80 (polysorbate 80)...........10 ml
    Distilled water..........................1,000 ml

1. Mix cornmeal well with 500 ml of water; heat to 65°C for 1 h.
2. Filter through gauze and then paper until clear; restore to original volume.
3. Adjust to pH 6.6–6.8; add agar dissolved in 500 ml of water.
4. Add Tween 80; autoclave (15 lb/in²) for 15 min.
5. Dispense into petri plates or into screw-cap tubes to form butts to be melted and poured as needed.

Cornmeal with Tween 80 is used in distinguishing the different genera of yeasts and the various species of *Candida* and can also be useful in slide cultures, as it stimulates conidiation in many fungi.

If 10 g of dextrose is added to the medium in place of the Tween 80, the medium can be used to differentiate *Trichophyton mentagrophytes* from *Trichophyton rubrum* on the basis of pigment production (see Table 19, p. 242).

For studying the morphology of yeasts, the **Dalmau method** is recommended. It is performed by using one-fourth or one-third of a cornmeal-Tween 80 agar plate for each organism. (Color Plate 64.)

1. Make one streak of a young, actively growing yeast down the center of the area (do not cut the agar); make three or four streaks across the first to dilute the inoculum.
2. Cover with a 22- × 22-mm coverslip.
3. Incubate at room temperature, in the dark, for 3 days.
4. Examine by placing the plate, without its lid, on the microscope stage and using the low-power (10×) and high-dry (40×) objectives. The most characteristic morphology (especially the terminal chlamydospores of *Candida albicans*) is often found near the edge of the coverslip.

C. albicans should always be included as a control for production of chlamydospores and blastoconidia.

Dermatophyte Test Medium (DTM)

Specimens from hair, skin, or nails may be inoculated directly onto DTM and incubated at room temperature with the cap of the culture tube loose. Dermatophytes change the color of the medium from yellow to red within 14 days. Care must be taken in specimen collection and interpretation of results, as many contaminants and other fungi increase the number of false-positive changes in color. DTM does not interfere with macroscopic morphology and microscopic characteristics of the dermatophytes, but it cannot be used to study pigment production because of the intense red color of the indicator. (Color Plate 125.)

Phytone	10.0 g
Dextrose	10.0 g
Agar	20.0 g
Phenol red solution	40.0 ml
0.8 M HCl	6.0 ml
Cycloheximide	0.5 g
Gentamicin sulfate (Schering)	0.1 g
Chlortetracycline HCl (Lederle)	0.1 g
Distilled water	1,000.0 ml

1. Dissolve the phytone, dextrose, and agar by boiling them in the water.
2. While stirring, add 40 ml of phenol red solution (0.5 g of phenol red dissolved in 15 ml of 0.1 N NaOH made up to 100 ml with distilled water).
3. While stirring, add the 0.8 M HCl.
4. Dissolve cycloheximide in 2 ml of acetone, and add to hot medium while stirring.
5. Dissolve gentamicin sulfate in 2 ml of distilled water, and add to medium while stirring.
6. Autoclave at 12 lb/in^2 for 10 min, and cool to approximately 47°C.
7. Dissolve chlortetracycline in 25 ml of sterile distilled water in sterile container, and add to medium while stirring.
8. Dispense into sterile 1-oz (~30-ml) screw-cap bottles or screw-cap tubes; slant and cool. The final pH of the medium is 5.5 ± 0.1, and the medium should be yellow in color.
9. Store in refrigerator at 4°C.

Fermentation Broth for Yeasts

Broth

Bromthymol blue	0.04 g
Powdered yeast extract	4.50 g
Peptone	7.50 g
Distilled water	1,000 ml

Stock Carbohydrate Solutions

> Carbohydrate.....................................6 g
> Distilled water.............................100 ml

1. Filter sterilize through a 0.22-μm-pore-size filter.
2. Dissolve bromthymol blue in 3 ml of 95% ethanol. Add to other ingredients.
3. Dispense 2-ml aliquots into screw-cap tubes.
4. Place Durham tube (mouth down) into each tube of broth.
5. Autoclave at 15 lb/in² for 15 min. Allow to cool.
6. Add 1 ml of each carbohydrate solution to separate tubes of broth. (After the carbohydrates have been added, the broths may be stored for 1 month in the refrigerator.)

Test Procedure

1. Inoculate each of the carbohydrate broths with a pure culture of the organism grown on a sugar-free medium. Be sure that the Durham tube is completely filled with broth before incubating.
2. Incubate at room temperature for 10–14 days, examining at 48- to 72-h intervals for production of gas (observed in Durham tube).

Gas production is the only reliable evidence of carbohydrate fermentation; acid production may simply indicate that the carbohydrate has been assimilated. All fermented carbohydrates will also be assimilated, but many compounds that are assimilated are not necessarily fermented. For identification of yeasts, see Table 4 (p. 116) and Table 9 (p. 131).

Gelatin Medium

FRAZIER PLATE METHOD

The Frazier plate method is the most rapid and reliable test for the ability of microorganisms to decompose gelatin; it is therefore highly recommended over the old conventional butt method.

Agar

> Standard method agar (Tryptone Glucose
>   Yeast Agar; BBL)
>
>   or
>
> Tryptone glucose extract agar (Standard
>   Plate Count Agar; BBL)....................24 g
> Distilled water.................................1,000 ml

1. Heat to dissolve, mixing well.
2. Remove from heat, cool slightly.
3. Add

> Gelatin...4 g

4. Mix thoroughly until gelatin dissolves.

5. Autoclave at 15 lb/in^2 for 12 min.

6. Dispense into small petri plates or into screw-cap tubes and allow to solidify as butts to be melted and poured as needed.

Developer (Acid Mercuric Chloride)

> Mercuric chloride (HgCl$_2$) ....12 g
> Distilled water...............................80 ml
> Concentrated HCl ....16 ml

Prepare in order listed; HgCl$_2$ will dissolve only after HCl is added. Mix well.
(An aqueous saturated solution of ammonium sulfate may also be used as a developer.)

Test Procedure

1. Inoculate the agar surface in one spot approximately the size of a dime.

2. Incubate at room temperature until growth is mature.

3. Flood surface of plate with developer.

Mercuric chloride (or ammonium sulfate) precipitates gelatin, causing the medium to become cloudy where gelatin is intact.

Gelatin decomposition (a positive test result) is demonstrated by a clear zone around the colony.

See Table 2 (p. 103) and Table 14 (p. 193).

BUTT LIQUEFACTION METHOD

> Brain heart infusion.......................25 g
> Gelatin ....120 g
> Distilled water ....1,000 ml

1. Heat to dissolve ingredients; adjust to pH 7.4–7.6.

2. Dispense 5- to 8-ml aliquots in 16- × 125-mm screw-cap tubes.

3. Autoclave at 15 lb/in^2 for 15 min. Allow to harden as butts.

Test Procedure

1. Inoculate the surface and just below the surface of the medium with the organism to be tested.

2. Incubate tubes at room temperature for 4 weeks.

3. Examine at weekly intervals for proteolytic activity by placing in refrigerator for 1 h and observing for liquefaction. If the medium solidifies in the refrigerator, proteolysis has not occurred and the tube should be returned to room temperature and retested the following week.

See Table 2 (p. 103) and Table 14 (p. 193).

Inhibitory Mold Agar (IMA)

IMA is an enriched medium that contains chloramphenicol (some formulations also contain gentamicin) but no cycloheximide; bacteria are inhibited, while fungi grow well. When specimens are contaminated with bacteria, IMA is especially useful in isolating cycloheximide-sensitive fungi, e.g., *Cryptococcus neoformans*, *Pseudallescheria boydii*, the zygomycetes, many species of *Candida* and *Aspergillus*, and most saprophytic or opportunistic fungi. It is commercially available in dehydrated and prepared form (BBL Microbiology Systems, Sparks, Md.). The ingredients are listed below to allow comparison with other enriched fungal media.

Pancreatic digest of casein	3.0 g
Peptic digest of animal tissue	2.0 g
Yeast extract	5.0 g
Dextrose	5.0 g
Starch	2.0 g
Dextrin	1.0 g
Chloramphenicol	0.125 g
Sodium phosphate	2.0 g
Magnesium sulfate	0.8 g
Ferrous sulfate	0.04 g
Sodium chloride	0.04 g
Manganese sulfate	0.16 g
Agar	15.0 g
Distilled water	1,000.0 ml

Loeffler Medium

(For testing proteolytic activity of *Cladosporium* species and similar organisms) The medium may be obtained in dehydrated form or bought commercially prepared from a number of sources.

Test Procedure

1. Place a fragment of the fungus on the agar slant, taking care not to place the inoculum on the bottom part of the slant that is usually covered with liquid.
2. Incubate all tubes at room temperature for 4 weeks.
3. Examine tubes at weekly intervals for evidence of proteolytic activity, i.e., disintegration of medium.

Usually, saprophytic species of *Cladosporium* are proteolytic, whereas pathogenic species, such as *Cladophialophora carrionii* and *Cladophialophora bantiana*, are not (see Table 14, p. 193).

Lysozyme Medium

Basal Glycerol Broth

```
Peptone ...........................................1.0 g
Beef extract...................................0.6 g
Glycerol .......................................14.0 ml
Distilled water...........................200.0 ml
```

1. Combine ingredients; mix well to dissolve.
2. Pour 95 ml of broth into a separate container.
3. Dispense the remainder into screw-cap tubes in 5-ml quantities. These will be used as control tubes.
4. Autoclave broth at 15 lb/in² for 15 min.

Lysozyme Broth

```
Lysozyme.........................................50 mg
0.01 N HCl......................................50 ml
```

1. Sterilize by filtration.
2. Aseptically add 5 ml of lysozyme solution to the 95 ml of basal glycerol broth.
3. Mix well.
4. Dispense 5-ml aliquots into sterile screw-cap tubes.
5. Store all tubes in the refrigerator.

Test Procedure

1. Inoculate a tube of control broth (glycerol broth without lysozyme) and a tube of lysozyme broth with the organism to be tested.
2. Incubate at room temperature until control tube shows good growth. The organism must grow in the control tube for the test to be valid. Growth in the lysozyme broth indicates resistance to the enzyme.

A known Streptomyces sp. should be used as a susceptible control organism; i.e., growth must occur in the control tube but not in the lysozyme tube to prove the lysozyme is active.

Mycosel Agar

Mycosel agar is a selective medium that is frequently part of the medium battery that is used for primary isolation of fungi. It contains chloramphenicol to inhibit the growth of bacteria and cycloheximide to inhibit fungi that are commonly considered saprobes. However, cycloheximide also inhibits the growth of some known pathogens, e.g., *Cryptococcus neoformans*, *Aspergillus fumigatus*, *Pseudallescheria boydii*, *Penicillium marneffei*, some species of *Candida*, and most zygomycetes, as well as many other opportunistic "saprobes."

The medium is also used to test an organism's ability to grow in the presence of cycloheximide; the interpretive information may state the level of cycloheximide against which the reference organisms were tested. Mycosel agar contains 0.04% cycloheximide.

Mycosel is produced in prepared and dehydrated form by Becton Dickinson (Cockeysville, Md.).

Phytone peptone ....10.0 g
Dextrose ....10.0 g
Agar ....15.5 g
Cycloheximide ....400.0 mg
Chloramphenicol ....50.0 mg
Distilled water ....1,000.0 ml

Potato Dextrose Agar (PDA) and Potato Flake Agar (PFA)

Potato dextrose agar and potato flake agar are available commercially prepared or in dehydrated form and should be prepared according to manufacturers' instructions. They support the growth of most clinically encountered fungi, and some laboratories use one of them as a primary medium. They can sometimes stimulate the production of conidia and pigment when other media fail to do so and are therefore often recommended for slide cultures or for inducing an isolate to exhibit a characteristic pigment.

Rapid Assimilation of Trehalose (RAT) Broth
(Stockman & Roberts, 1985, and personal communication)

The RAT test is used for the rapid identification of *Candida glabrata*. It is ONLY for yeasts that

* form colonies that are relatively slow growing and small
* are microscopically small and oval and have terminal budding
* form neither germ tubes nor pseudohyphae in the germ tube test

The RAT test is based on the utilization of trehalose in the presence of a protein inhibitor, cycloheximide. This broth contains more nitrogen and carbohydrate than the traditional Wickerham broth and incorporates an indicator, bromcresol green, that has a low pH range (3.8–5.4). *C. glabrata* utilizes the trehalose and produces acid more quickly than do other yeast isolates. (Color Plate 51.)

PREPARATION OF REAGENTS
Yeast Nitrogen Base

A. *Stock solution*
1. Add 6.7 g of yeast nitrogen base to 100 ml of distilled water.
2. Dissolve by gently heating.
3. Filter sterilize.

B. *Working solution*

Dilute by combining 20 ml of the stock yeast nitrogen base solution with 80 ml of sterile distilled water.

40% Trehalose

1. Add 4 g of trehalose to 10 ml of distilled water.
2. Dissolve by gently heating at 56°C.
3. Filter sterilize.

Bromcresol Green

1. Add 0.1 g of bromcresol green to 7.1 ml of 0.01 N NaOH. (Prepare 0.01 N NaOH by adding 0.4 g of NaOH to 1,000 ml [1 liter] of distilled water. Mix to dissolve.)
2. Dilute by adding 117.9 ml of distilled water.
3. Filter sterilize.

Cycloheximide

1. Add 0.1 g of cycloheximide to 10 ml of distilled water.
2. Gently heat to dissolve.
3. Filter sterilize.
4. Aliquot in 0.5-ml amounts. Store at −30°C (stable for 6 months).

PREPARATION OF RAT BROTH

Yeast nitrogen base (working solution) ....80 ml
40% trehalose..10 ml
Bromcresol green ....10 ml
Cycloheximide ....0.4 ml

1. Combine ingredients and mix well.
2. Adjust pH to 5.4–5.5.
3. Dispense into sterile screw-cap tubes.

TEST PROCEDURE

1. Dispense 3 drops of RAT broth into as many microtiter wells as are needed for tests and controls.
2. Using a microtiter grid form, label each space as to culture number or control.
3. Emulsify a **<u>HEAVY</u>** inoculum of the yeast into the broth in the appropriate well.
4. Incubate plate for 1 h at 37°C in ambient air; do not cover with tape.

(When the test is finished, the used wells can be covered with tape and held until the remainder of the wells have been used.)

INTERPRETATION

Positive: broth changes from a blue to yellow; *C. glabrata*
Negative: broth remains blue or green; isolate is NOT *C. glabrata* (further testing is required for complete identification)

QUALITY CONTROL

Positive control, *Candida glabrata*
Negative control, *Candida albicans*

Notes:

- Best results are obtained when isolate is taken from Sabouraud dextrose agar (Emmons modification).
- Some reports indicate that incubation at 42°C for 3 h may increase the specificity of the test; this is not necessary if the yeasts to be tested are properly selected as described above. Only those meeting the criteria should be tested by this method.
- Beware: bacteria and *Prototheca* spp. can give positive results.

A RAT slide method that is incubated at 37°C for 1 h is available from Scientific Device Laboratory, Des Plaines, Ill.

Another commercially available RAT test (Remel, Lenexa, Kans.) has a slightly different formulation; it is performed in small tubes and incubated at 42°C for 3 h.

Rapid Sporulation Medium (RSM)

RSM is designed for the isolation and identification of dermatophytes; it contains chloramphenicol and chlortetracycline for the inhibition of bacteria and cycloheximide for the inhibition of saprobic fungi. Bromthymol blue in the formulation changes from yellow to blue-green in the presence of alkaline metabolites that are characteristically produced by dermatophytes; notably, the pH color change does not obscure the natural pigment of the isolate. It is very similar to dermatophyte test medium (DTM; p. 336) but differs in promoting increased production of conidia and enabling better visualization of the isolates' color. RSM is manufactured and distributed by BACTI-LAB, Mountain View, Calif.

SABHI Agar

SABHI agar combines two commonly used media. It has the glucose content of Sabouraud dextrose agar and the calf brain and beef heart infusions (albeit half as much) found in brain heart infusion agar. Antibiotic or sheep blood can be added to the formulation. It is favored as a medium for primary isolation of fungi in a number of clinical mycology laboratories.

Glucose......................................21.00 g
Neopeptone ....5.00 g
Proteose peptone.......................5.00 g
Calf brains, infusion................100.00 g

Beef heart, infusion.................125.00 g
Sodium chloride..........................2.50 g
Disodium phosphate ....1.25 g
Agar ....15.00 g
(Optional: Chloramphenicol ....50 mg
Sheep blood...............100 ml)

1. Mix reagents and bring to boil.
2. Autoclave at 15 lb/in² for 15 min.
3. If antibiotic and/or blood is to be added, cool to 50–52°C.
4. Add chloramphenicol to 10 ml of sterile distilled water.
5. Add the sheep blood.
6. Dispense into tubes; slant and cool.

Sabouraud Dextrose Agar (SDA)

EMMONS MODIFICATION

The Emmons modification differs from the original formula in that it has an approximately neutral pH and contains only 2% dextrose.

Most mycologists no longer consider it necessary or desirable to use 4% sugar, as in the original formula, and a pH near neutrality has been found to be better for some fungi. The very acid original formula once recommended for suppression of bacterial contaminants can now be replaced by media containing antibiotics.

Dextrose.................................20 g
Peptone ....10 g
Agar ....17 g
Distilled water..........................1,000 ml

Final pH, 6.9.

ORIGINAL FORMULA

Some workers still prefer the original formula.

Dextrose.................................40 g
Peptone ....10 g
Agar ....15 g
Distilled water..........................1,000 ml

Final pH, 5.6.

1. To prepare either of the formulas, dissolve the ingredients by boiling, dispense in tubes, and autoclave at 15 lb/in² for 10 min.
2. Allow tubes to cool in slanted position.
3. Store in refrigerator.

Both formulations of SDA are commercially available in prepared or dehydrated form.

Sabouraud Dextrose Agar with 15% NaCl

Testing for tolerance to 15% sodium chloride (NaCl) can be valuable for identifying some dematiaceous (black) fungi.

SDA .... 500 ml
NaCl .... 75 g

1. Heat to dissolve.
2. Dispense in tubes; autoclave at 15 lb/in^2 for 10 min.
3. Allow to solidify as butts to be melted and slanted as needed.

Test Procedure

1. Place a pinpoint inoculum of the organism to be tested on a slant of the agar.
2. Incubate at room temperature.

The organism is considered to be strongly inhibited if its colony diameter is less than 2 mm at 21 days. If the colony surpasses 2 mm, the organism is considered tolerant of 15% NaCl.

Sabouraud Dextrose Broth

Dextrose .... 20 mg
Peptone .... 10 mg
Distilled water .... 1,000 ml

Final pH, 5.7.

1. Dissolve ingredients; dispense into tubes.
2. Autoclave (15 lb/in^2) for 10 min.

Noting the manner in which yeasts grow in this broth can assist in their identification (see Table 3, p. 114, and Table 4, p. 116). Sabouraud dextrose broth is also used for the detection of fungal contaminants in pharmaceutical products.

Starch Hydrolysis Agar

(For aerobic actinomycetes)

Nutrient agar .... 23 g
Potato starch................................. 10 g
Demineralized water................ 1,000 ml

1. Dissolve agar in 500 ml of water by boiling.
2. Dissolve starch in 250 ml of water by boiling.
3. Combine and add 250 ml of water.
4. Dispense into screw-cap tubes.
5. Autoclave (15 lb/in^2) for 30 min.
6. Allow to cool as butts; melt down and pour into petri plates as needed.

Test Procedure

1. Inoculate a 10-mm-diameter round area of agar heavily with a pure culture of the organism to be tested.
2. Incubate at optimal growth temperature until good growth occurs.
3. Flood the area around the growth with Gram iodine.

Starch hydrolysis is demonstrated by a colorless (complete hydrolysis) or red (partial hydrolysis) area around the growth.

Unhydrolyzed starch in the medium will produce a deep blue to purple color in the presence of iodine (see Table 2, p. 103).

Trichophyton Agars

(Nutritional requirement tests for the differentiation of *Trichophyton* spp.)

Trichophyton agars are available commercially, either prepared or in dehydrated form. Rehydration is performed according to manufacturers' instructions.

The set of seven media tests the growth factor requirements of the species of *Trichophyton*. They are often helpful in differentiating the species. Their compositions are as follows:

    No. 1, casein agar base (vitamin free)
    No. 2, casein agar base plus inositol
    No. 3, casein agar base plus inositol and thiamine
    No. 4, casein agar base plus thiamine
    No. 5, casein agar base plus nicotinic acid
    No. 6, ammonium nitrate agar base
    No. 7, ammonium nitrate agar base plus histidine

Inoculation of Media

The center of a slant of each medium must be inoculated with a small and equal-size amount of pure culture grown on SDA (or other primary medium) with or without antibiotics. It is important that the culture be free of bacteria, for many bacteria synthesize vitamins which may invalidate the test. Care must also be taken not to transfer any of the primary medium with the organism, as this may supply carryover nutrients and cause false reactions.

The following method of inoculation dilutes possible carryover nutrients and ensures that each slant receives an equal inoculum:

1. Make a homogeneous suspension of fuzzy or granular colonies in sterile saline or water.
2. Place 2 drops of the suspension on each slant of medium.

Test Procedure

1. Incubate tubes at 25–30°C for 2 weeks, preferably in a reclining position for the first few days so that the inoculum remains evenly dispensed over the surface of the agar.
2. Examine periodically for growth.
3. The tube that shows maximum growth is recorded as 4+. Other tubes are graded by comparison.

   For interpretation of results, see Table 19 (p. 242) and Table 20 (p. 248).

Tyrosine or Xanthine Agar

(For differentiation of aerobic actinomycetes and characterization of *Exophiala*, *Wangiella*, and *Phaeoannellomyces* spp.)

> Nutrient agar .... 23 g
> Tyrosine .... 5 g
>   (or xanthine .... 4 g)
> Distilled water .... 1,000 ml

1. Dissolve the agar in the distilled water by boiling (swirl frequently).
2. Add tyrosine or xanthine, taking care to distribute the crystals evenly throughout the agar.
3. Adjust to pH 7.0; autoclave at 15 lb/in² for 15 min.

If the agar is too hot when poured, the time required for solidification will be long enough to permit settling out of the tyrosine or xanthine granules. To avoid this, the medium should be allowed to cool to 45–48°C before being poured, and the flask should be mixed well while the plates are poured to ensure an even distribution of the crystals. If the medium is to be stored for a long period, pour well-mixed medium, with evenly distributed crystals, into tubes. Allow to solidify as butts and refrigerate.

Test Procedure

1. When needed, place tubes of agar in boiling-water bath to melt, cool to 45–48°C, mix well to resuspend crystals, pour into petri plates, and allow to solidify.
2. Heavily inoculate an area of agar 10 mm in diameter with a pure culture.
3. Incubate at room temperature or at 35–37°C for 2–3 weeks.
4. Examine every 3 or 4 days for clearing of the medium around or directly beneath the colony, which indicates hydrolysis. (Color Plate 161.)

   For interpretation of results, see Table 2 (p. 103) and Table 16 (p. 200).

Urea Agar

A.   Urea agar base (Christensen) ...29 g
Distilled water ....100 ml

Dissolve the powder in the water and sterilize by filtration.

B.   Agar ....15 g
Distilled water ....900 ml

1. Dissolve the agar in the water, and sterilize by autoclaving it at 15 lb/in² for 15 min.
2. Cool the agar to approximately 50°C.
3. Add the 100 ml of sterile urea agar base.
4. Mix well; dispense aseptically into sterile tubes.
5. Allow to cool in slanted position to form butt about 1 in. (2.5 cm) deep and slant approximately 1.5 in. (3.8 cm) long.

Urease-positive organisms produce an alkaline reaction indicated by a pink-red color.

This medium is used for the differentiation of the yeastlike fungi and also in the identification of aerobic actinomycetes and *Trichophyton* species. It is commercially available in prepared or dehydrated form.

Water Agar

Nutritionally deficient media are known to enhance production of spores and conidia. Water agar is used for that purpose.

Agar ....20 g
Distilled water ....1 liter

1. Mix reagents; bring to boil.
2. Dispense into tubes.
3. Autoclave at 15 lb/in² for 15 min.
4. Cool in slanted position or store as butts to be melted down and used as slants or plates when needed.

Yeast Extract-Phosphate Agar with Ammonia

(For isolation of *Histoplasma capsulatum* and *Blastomyces dermatitidis* from contaminated specimens)

Phosphate Buffer

Na_2HPO_4 ....4 g
KH_2PO_4 ....6 g
Distilled water ....30 ml

Mix well to dissolve; adjust pH to 6.0 with 1 N HCl or 1 N NaOH.

Yeast Extract Solution

Yeast extract.......................................1 g
Agar ....20 g
Chloramphenicol (optional)..........50 mg
Distilled water ....1,000 ml

1. Mix; bring to boil while stirring frequently.
2. Add 2 ml of phosphate buffer to the liter of yeast extract solution. Mix well.
3. Dispense 17–18 ml into screw-cap tubes.
4. Autoclave at 15 lb/in² for 15 min.

Test Procedure

1. As needed, melt and pour two tubes of medium (total, ca. 35 ml) into a sterile petri plate.
2. Spread approximately 0.5 ml of specimen over surface of solidified agar.
3. Place 1 drop (0.05 ml) of concentrated NH_4OH off center on the agar surface. Allow it to diffuse.
4. Incubate at 25–30°C.

The diffusing NH_4OH inhibits bacteria, yeasts, and many moulds while allowing slow-growing dimorphic fungi to grow.

Color Plates

The photographs on the following pages are presented to exhibit color where it will help in gaining a better visual image and understanding of descriptions that appear in the text of this book. The first 37 images pertain to direct microscopic examination of specimens. The remaining 124 pertain to fungal cultures and tests that contribute to identification.

Many of the photographs of fungal colonies are from stock cultures. It is imperative that the reader be cognizant of the fact that many fungi may vary somewhat in their colony pigment and texture, depending mainly on the strain of the organizm and sometimes on the medium on which it is cultured. Initial isolates from patient specimens usually produce the most classic colony morphology. Stock cultures may lose some of the typifying characteristics, especially outstanding pigment production; proficiency test samples, unfortunately, often demonstrate this loss.

The colonies represented are either on Sabouraud dextrose agar (SDA) or potato dextrose agar (PDA); the medium is indicated in each instance.

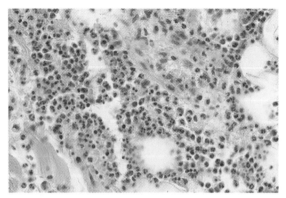

1. Suppurative inflammation/microabscess. Low magnification. H&E.

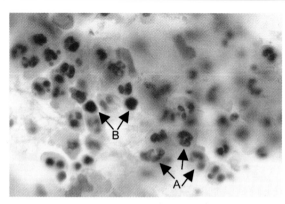

2. Suppurative inflammation: (A) polymorphonuclear leukocytes (neutrophils); (B) few lymphocytes. High magnification. H&E.

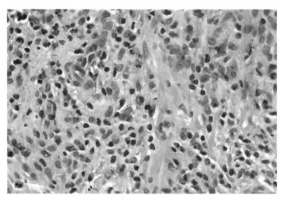

3. Chronic inflammation. Low magnification. H&E.

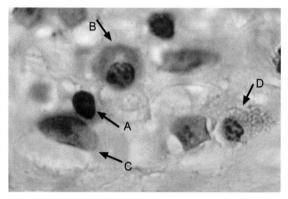

4. Chronic inflammation showing (A) lymphocyte, (B) plasma cell, (C) histiocyte, (D) eosinophil. High magnification. H&E.

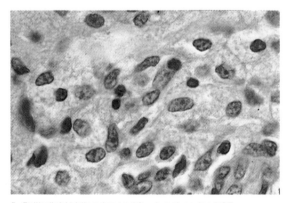

5. Epithelioid histiocytes and few lymphocytes. H&E.

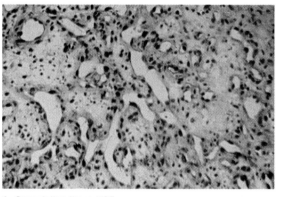

6. Granulation tissue. H&E.

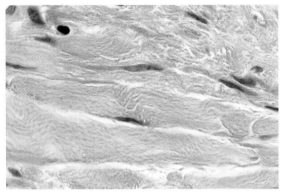

7. Collagen and fibroblasts. High magnification. H&E.

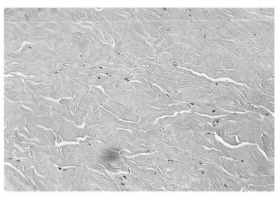

8. Fibrosis. Low magnification. H&E.

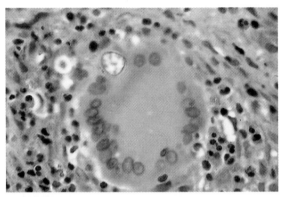

9. Langhans giant cell with engulfed spherule of *Coccidioides*. H&E. (Courtesy of Joan Barenfanger.)

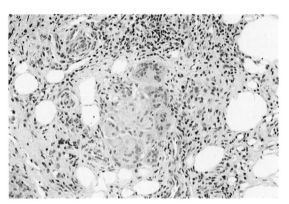

10. Granuloma composed of giant cells. H&E.

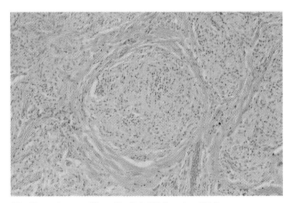

11. Granuloma with epithelioid histiocytes. H&E.

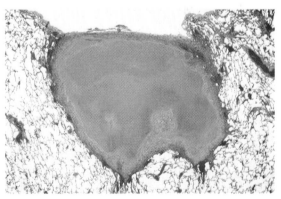

12. Granuloma with caseous necrosis in center. H&E. Low magnification. (Courtesy of Douglas Flieder.)

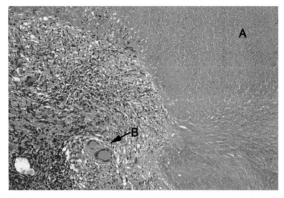

13. Granuloma with caseous necrosis (A); higher magnification of Color Plate 12. Giant cell (B, at arrow) in rim. H&E. (Courtesy of Douglas Flieder.)

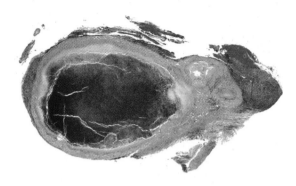

14. Calcified granuloma in a case of histoplasmosis. Low magnification. H&E. (Courtesy of Douglas Flieder.)

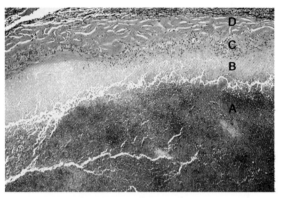

15. Calcified granuloma; higher magnification of Color Plate 14. (A) Calcification; (B) necrosis; (C) histiocytes; (D) fibrosis. H&E. (Courtesy of Douglas Flieder.)

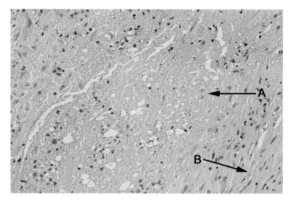

16. (A) Necrotic tissue. (B) Nonnecrotic tissue. H&E.

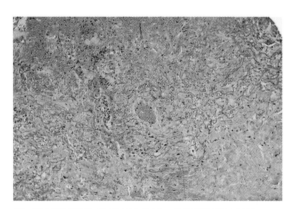

17. Angioinvasion and necrosis. Low magnification. H&E.

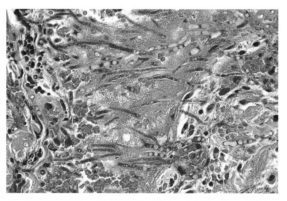

18. Angioinvasion and infarction. High magnification of Color Plate 17. H&E.

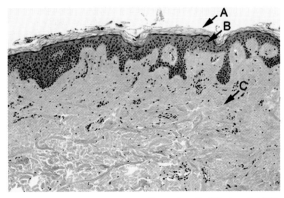

19. Skin: (A) stratum corneum; (B) epidermis; (C) dermis. H&E.

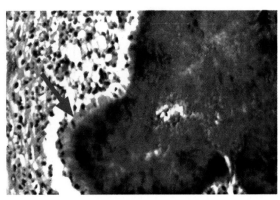

20. Splendore-Hoeppli phenomenon (at arrow) surrounding an actinomycotic granule. (Courtesy of Joan Barenfanger.)

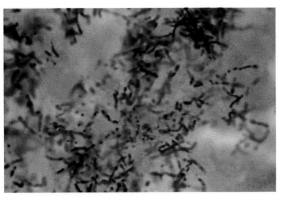

21. *Actinomyces* in liver aspirate. Gram stain. (Courtesy of Joan Barenfanger.)

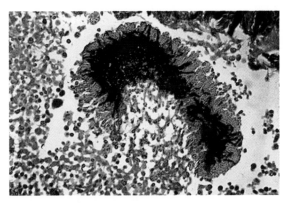

22. Eumycotic mycetoma granule. GMS. (Courtesy of Evelyn Koestenblatt.)

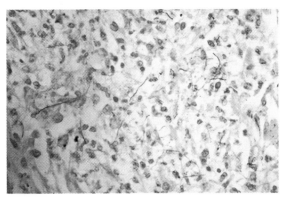

23. *Nocardia* in lung. Coates-Fite acid-fast stain. (Courtesy of Ron C. Neafie.)

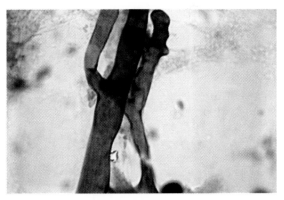

24. Zygomycete in tissue. GMS. (Courtesy of Joan Barenfanger.)

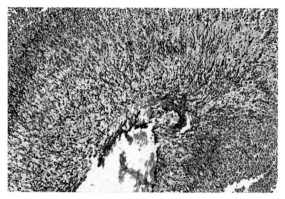

25. *Aspergillus* in lung. Low magnification. GMS.

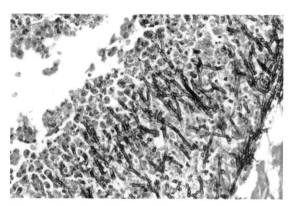

26. *Aspergillus* in lung. High magnification. GMS.

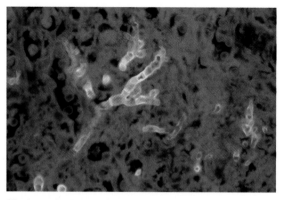

27. *Aspergillus* in lung. Oil immersion magnification. Calcofluor White stain.

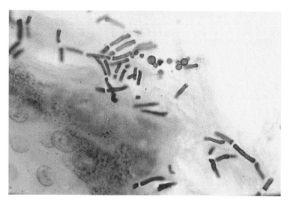

28. Tinea versicolor. PAS.

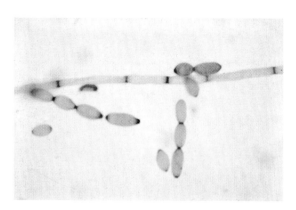

29. Fontana-Masson stain. *Cladosporium* in sputum smear.

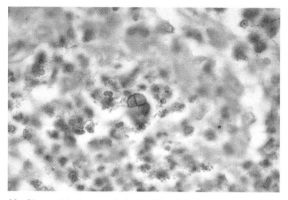

30. Chromoblastomycosis; brownish sclerotic body in center. H&E. (Courtesy of Ron C. Neafie.)

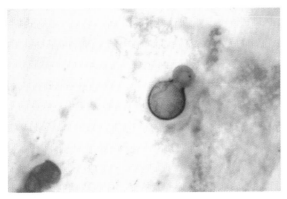

31. *Blastomyces dermatitidis.* GMS. (Courtesy of Joan Barenfanger.)

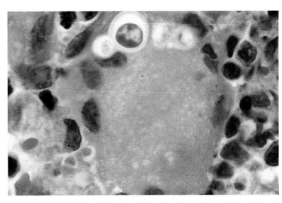

32. *Blastomyces dermatitidis* in giant cell. H&E. (Courtesy of Joan Barenfanger.)

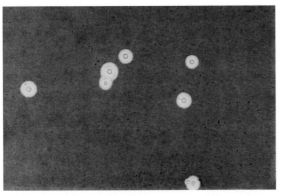

33. *Cryptococcus neoformans* in cerebrospinal fluid. India ink preparation.

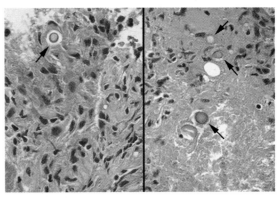

34. *Cryptococcus neoformans* (at arrows) in tissue. H&E (left). Mucicarmine (right). (Courtesy of Douglas Flieder.)

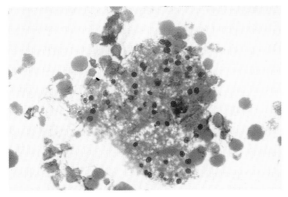

35. *Pneumocystis carinii* in lung. GMS.

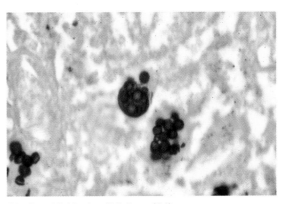

36. *Coccidioides immitis* in lung. GMS.

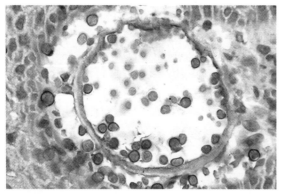

37. *Rhinosporidium seeberi* in nasal tissue. Mucicarmine. (Courtesy of Douglas Flieder.)

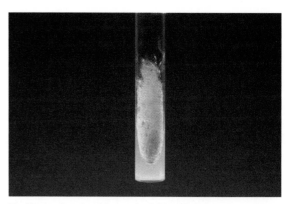

38. *Nocardia asteroides* on slant. SDA, 30°C, 9 days.

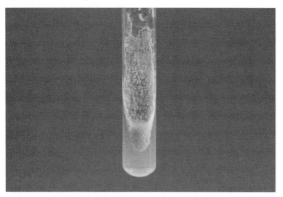

39. *Nocardia brasiliensis* on slant. SDA, 30°C, 9 days.

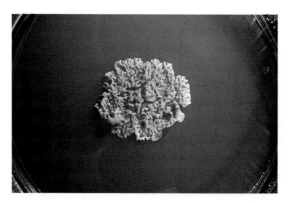

40. *Nocardia brasiliensis.* SDA, 30°C, 9 days.

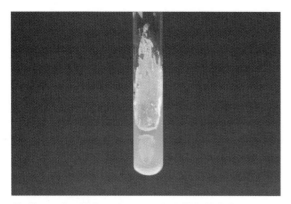

41. *Nocardia otitidiscaviarum* on slant. SDA, 30°C, 9 days.

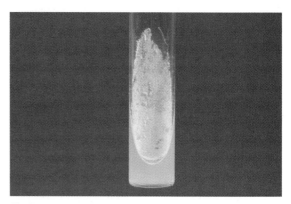

42. *Streptomyces* sp. on slant. SDA, 30°C, 9 days.

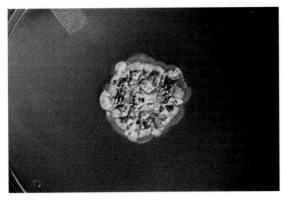

43. *Streptomyces* sp. SDA, 30°C, 9 days.

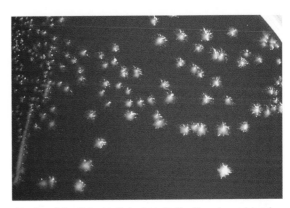

44. *Candida albicans.* Colonies with "feet" on sheep blood agar, 35°C, 2 days.

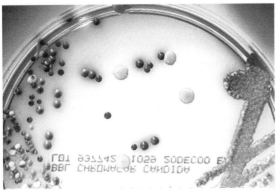

45. CHROMagar: green colonies, *C. albicans;* blue colonies, *C. tropicalis;* pink, dry colonies, *C. krusei.*

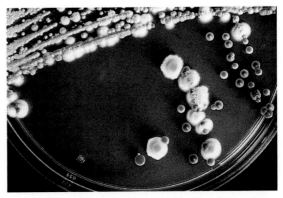

46. Candida ID agar: blue colonies, *C. albicans;* large, pink, dry colonies, *C. krusei;* pink, smooth colonies may be any of a variety of other yeasts.

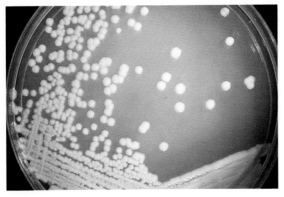

47. *Candida tropicalis.* SDA, 30°C, 2 days.

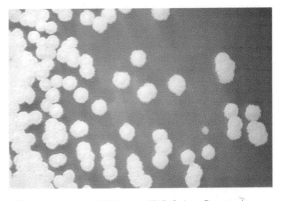

48. *Candida krusei.* SDA plate, 30°C, 2 days. Dry, rough colonies.

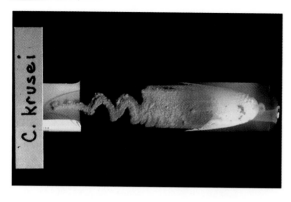

49. *Candida krusei.* SDA slant, 30°C, 3 days. Note film of growth on side of tube.

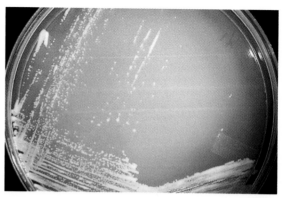

50. *Candida glabrata.* SDA, 30°C, 3 days. Note tiny colonies as compared to *C. tropicalis.*

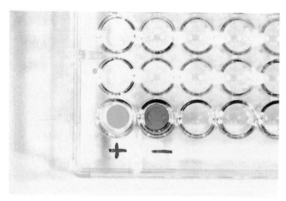

51. Rapid assimilation of trehalose (RAT) test, Mayo Clinic method: *C. glabrata* (positive) and *C. tropicalis* (negative); 37°C, 1 h (see p. 341).

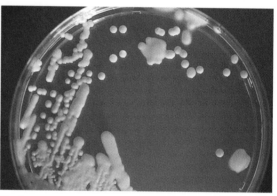

52. *Cryptococcus neoformans.* SDA plate, 30°C, 3 days. Note mucoid nature of colonies.

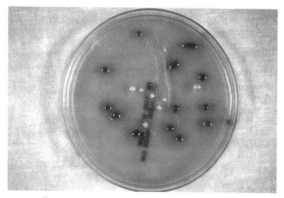

53. Birdseed agar. Room temperature, 3 days. The brown colonies are *C. neoformans* (see p. 332).

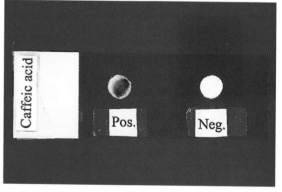

54. Caffeic acid test, 30°C, 4 h. *C. neoformans* (positive) and other *Cryptococcus* sp. (negative); see p. 309.

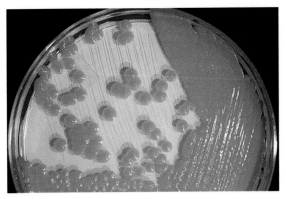

55. *Rhodotorula* sp. SDA, 30°C, 3 days.

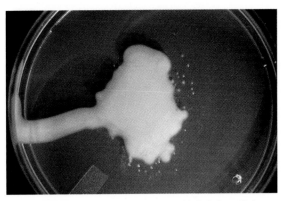

56. *Sporobolomyces salmonicolor.* SDA, 30°C, 5 days. Note small satelliting colonies (due to ballistoconidia).

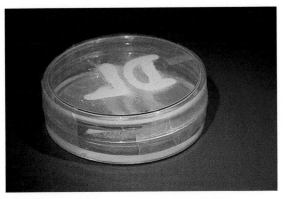

57. SDA plates taped together to best demonstrate ballistoconidia formation (see p. 133).

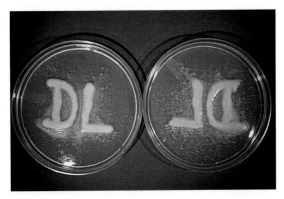

58. SDA plates separated after being taped together for 5 days at room temperature. Note mirror-image colonies of *S. salmonicolor* formed by ballistoconidia.

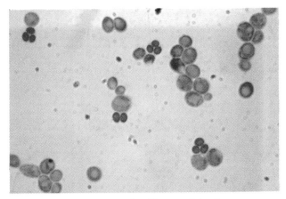

59. *Saccharomyces cerevisiae.* Kinyoun stain of ascospores (red) after growth on ascospore agar.

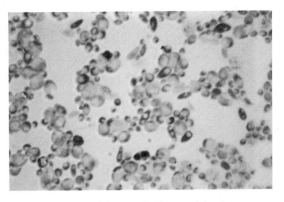

60. *Pichia (Hansenula) anomala.* Kinyoun stain of ascospores (red) after growth on ascospore agar. Note brimmed-hat shape of ascospores.

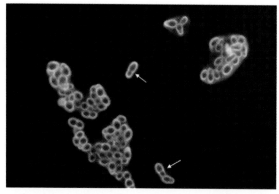

61. *Malassezia furfur.* Calcofluor White stain of organism from culture. Arrows indicate bluntly cut-off neck at point of conidiation.

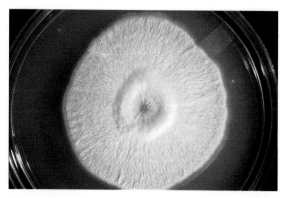

62. *Geotrichum candidum.* SDA plate, 30°C, 3 days. Powdery to cottony strain.

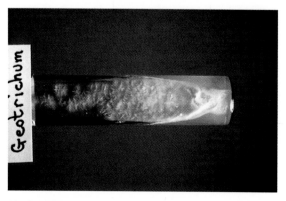

63. *Geotrichum candidum.* SDA slant, 30°C, 3 days. Rough, yeastlike strain.

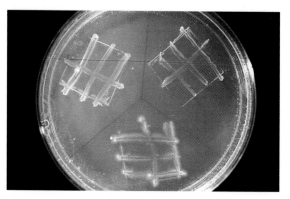

64. Dalmau plate. Three yeastlike fungi inoculated onto cornmeal-Tween 80 agar (see p. 335).

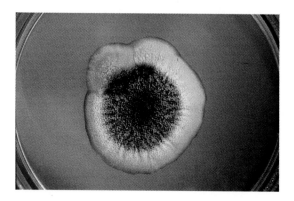

65. *Sporothrix schenckii.* Mould phase, SDA, 30°C, 6 days. Surface of colony.

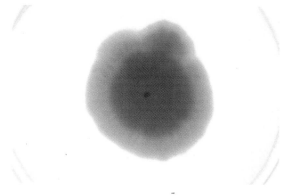

66. *Sporothrix schenckii.* Mould phase, SDA, 30°C, 6 days. Reverse of colony.

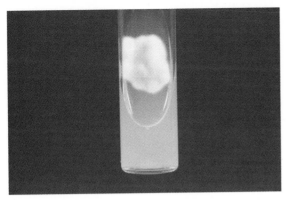

67. *Histoplasma capsulatum* slant. SDA, 30°C, 18 days.

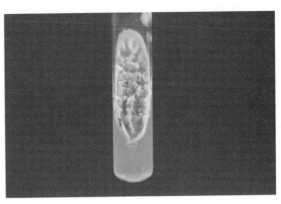

68. *Blastomyces dermatitidis* slant. SDA, 30°C, 18 days.

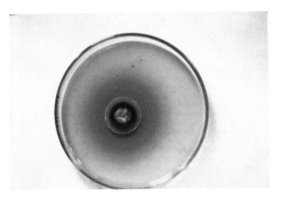

69. *Penicillium marneffei.* SDA, 30°C, 4 days. Surface of colony. Note strong red diffusing pigment of primary isolate. (Courtesy of William Merz.)

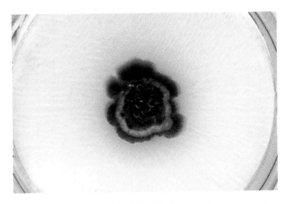

70. *Penicillium marneffei.* PDA, 30°C, 3 days. Surface of colony. Note pale red diffusing pigment of stock culture.

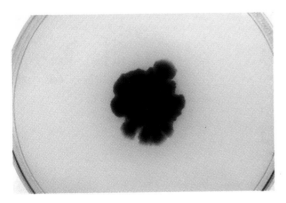

71. *Penicillium marneffei.* PDA, 30°C, 3 days. Reverse of colony. Note pale red diffusing pigment of stock culture.

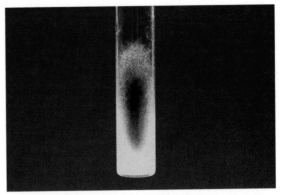

72. *Rhizopus* sp. slant. SDA, 30°C, 4 days. Note robust cotton candy-like growth, typical of many zygomycetes, order Mucorales.

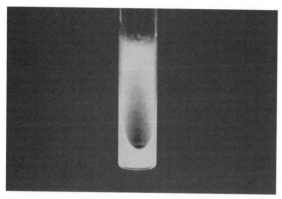

73. *Absidia corymbifera.* SDA, 30°C, 4 days. Cotton candy-like growth.

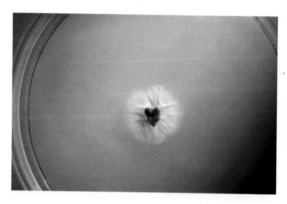

74. *Cokeromyces recurvatus.* PDA, 30°C, 5 days. Note lack of woolly growth.

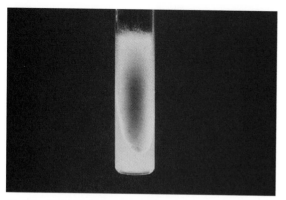

75. *Cunninghamella bertholletiae* slant. SDA, 30°C, 4 days. Cotton candy-like growth.

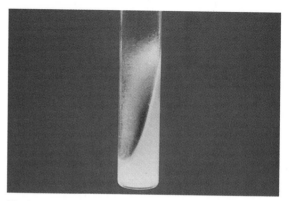

76. *Syncephalastrum racemosum* slant. SDA, 30°C, 3 days. Cotton candy-like growth.

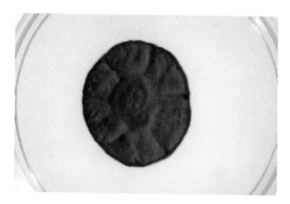

77. *Fonsecaea pedrosoi.* SDA, 30°C, 14 days. Surface of colony.

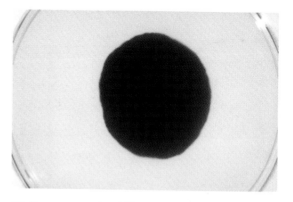

78. *Fonsecaea pedrosoi.* SDA, 30°C, 14 days. Reverse of colony, typical of completely dark, dematiaceous fungi.

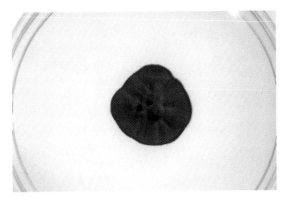

79. *Phialophora verrucosa.* SDA, 30°C, 12 days.

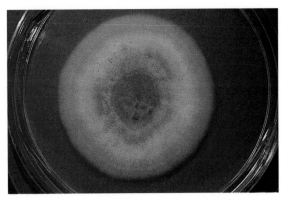

80. *Phaeoacremonium parasiticum.* PDA, 30°C, 7 days.

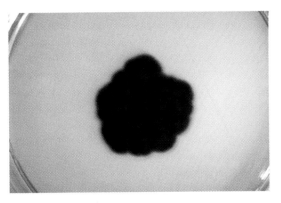

81. *Cladosporium* sp. SDA, 30°C, 7 days.

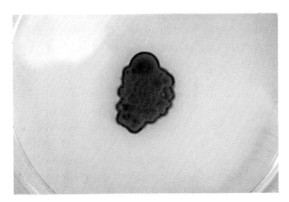

82. *Cladophialophora carrionii.* SDA, 30°C, 14 days. Surface of colony.

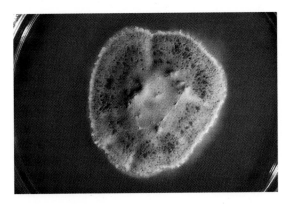

83. *Pseudallescheria boydii/Scedosporium apiospermum.* SDA, 30°C, 7 days. Surface of colony.

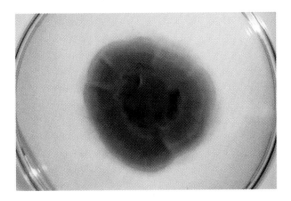

84. *Pseudallescheria boydii/Scedosporium apiospermum.* SDA, 30°C, 7 days. Reverse of colony.

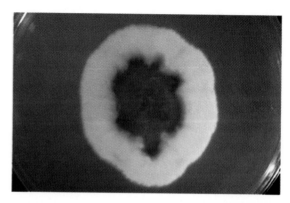

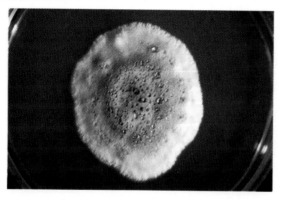

85. *Scedosporium prolificans.* SDA, 30°C, 7 days. Surface of colony.

86. *Scedosporium prolificans.* SDA, 30°C, 7 days. Reverse of colony.

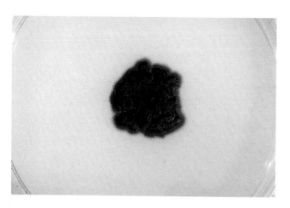

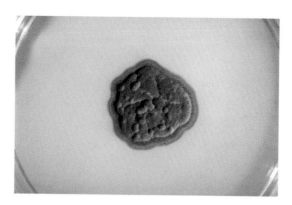

87. *Dactylaria constricta.* SDA, 30°C, 7 days.

88. *Exophiala jeanselmei.* SDA, 30°C, 14 days. Surface of colony.

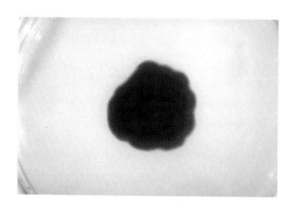

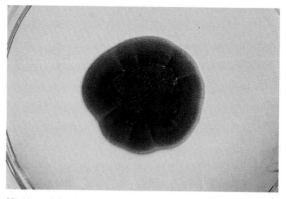

89. *Exophiala jeanselmei.* SDA, 30°C, 14 days. Reverse of colony.

90. *Wangiella dermatitidis.* SDA, 30°C, 21 days. Surface of colony.

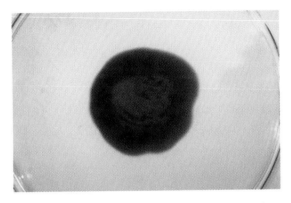

91. *Wangiella dermatitidis.* SDA, 30°C, 21 days. Reverse of colony.

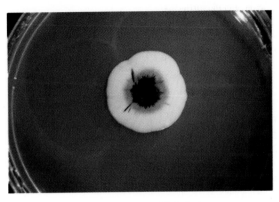

92. *Aureobasidium pullulans.* SDA, 30°C, 7 days.

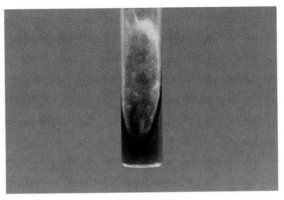

93. *Scytalidium* sp. slant. SDA, 30°C, 3 days.

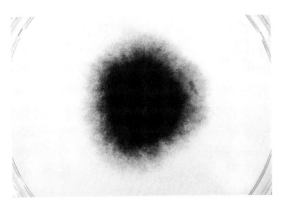

94. *Curvularia* sp. SDA, 30°C, 5 days.

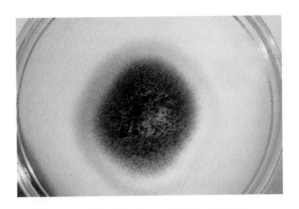

95. *Bipolaris* sp. SDA, 30°C, 5 days. Surface of colony.

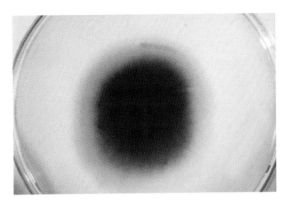

96. *Bipolaris* sp. SDA, 30°C, 5 days. Reverse of colony.

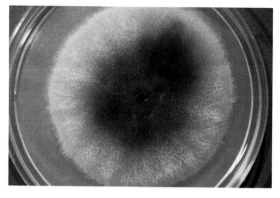

97. *Exserohilum* sp. SDA, 30°C, 7 days.

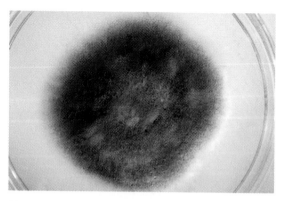

98. *Alternaria* sp. SDA, 30°C, 5 days. Surface of colony.

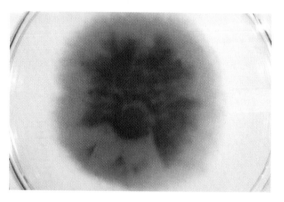

99. *Alternaria* sp. SDA, 30°C, 5 days. Reverse of colony.

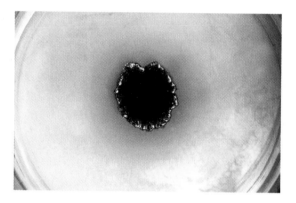

100. *Epicoccum* sp. PDA, 30°C, 7 days. Surface of colony. Note yellow-orange diffusing pigment.

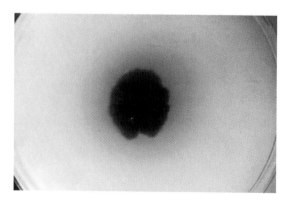

101. *Epicoccum* sp. PDA, 30°C, 7 days. Reverse of colony. Note yellow-orange diffusing pigment.

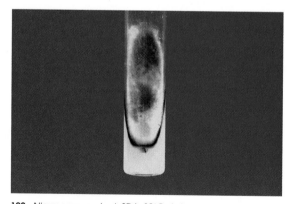

102. *Nigrospora* sp. slant. SDA, 30°C, 4 days.

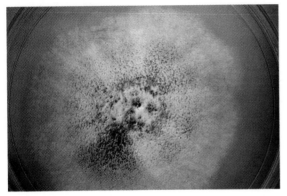

103. *Chaetomium* sp. PDA, 30°C, 5 days. Surface of colony.

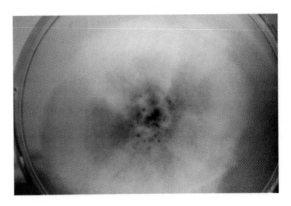

104. *Chaetomium* sp. PDA, 30°C, 5 days. Reverse of colony.

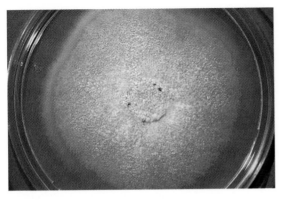

105. *Phoma* sp. SDA, 30°C, 5 days.

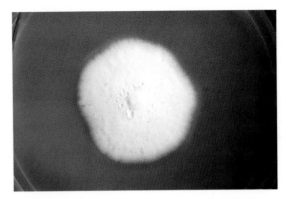

106. *Microsporum audouinii.* PDA, 30°C, 7 days. Surface of colony.

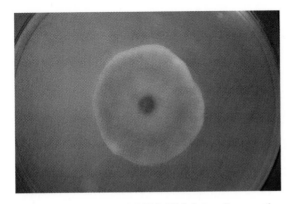

107. *Microsporum audouinii.* PDA, 30°C, 7 days. Reverse of colony.

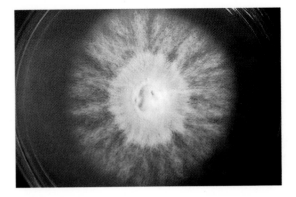

108. *Microsporum canis* var. *canis.* PDA, 30°C, 7 days. Surface of colony.

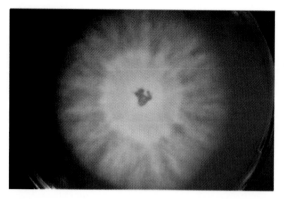

109. *Microsporum canis* var. *canis*. PDA, 30°C, 7 days. Reverse of colony.

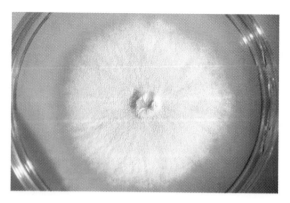

110. *Microsporum gypseum* complex. PDA, 30°C, 6 days. Surface of colony.

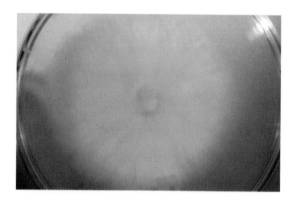

111. *Microsporum gypseum* complex. SDA, 30°C, 6 days. Reverse of colony.

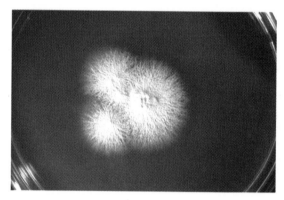

112. *Microsporum nanum*. SDA, 30°C, 7 days. Surface of colony.

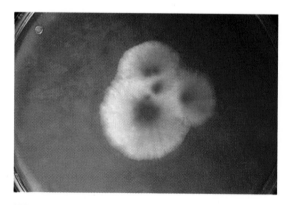

113. *Microsporum nanum*. SDA, 30°C, 7 days. Reverse of colony.

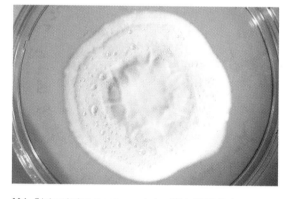

114. *Trichophyton mentagrophytes*. PDA, 30°C, 7 days. Surface of colony.

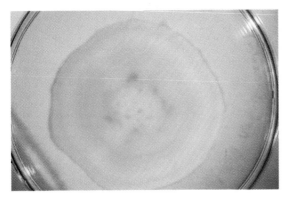

115. *Trichophyton mentagrophytes.* PDA, 30°C, 7 days. Reverse of colony.

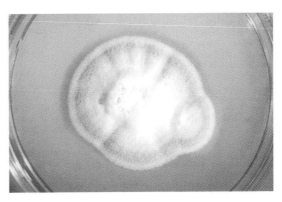

116. *Trichophyton rubrum.* PDA, 30°C, 7 days. Surface of colony.

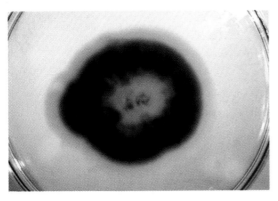

117. *Trichophyton rubrum.* PDA, 30°C, 7 days. Reverse of colony.

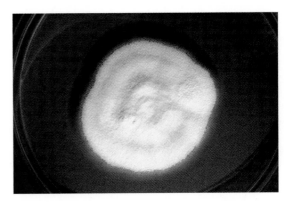

118. *Trichophyton tonsurans.* SDA, 30°C, 7 days. Surface of colony, yellowish rose strain.

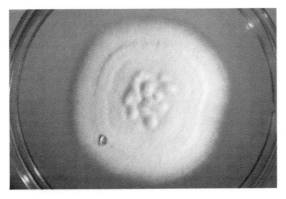

119. *Trichophyton tonsurans.* SDA, 30°C, 7 days. Surface of colony, white and yellow strain.

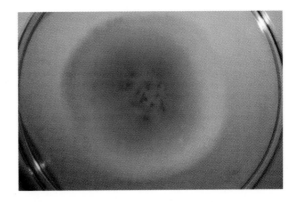

120. *Trichophyton tonsurans.* SDA, 30°C, 7 days. Reverse of colony.

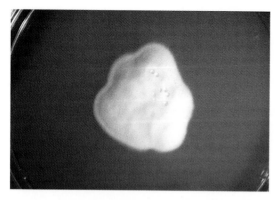

121. *Trichophyton terrestre.* SDA, 30°C, 7 days. Surface of colony.

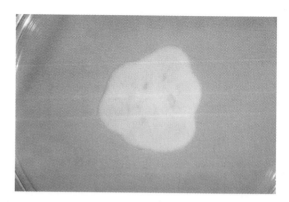

122. *Trichophyton terrestre.* SDA, 30°C, 7 days. Reverse of colony.

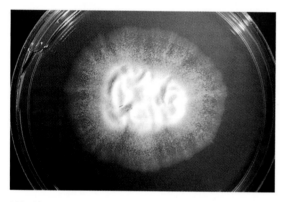

123. *Epidermophyton floccosum.* PDA, 30°C, 12 days. Surface of colony.

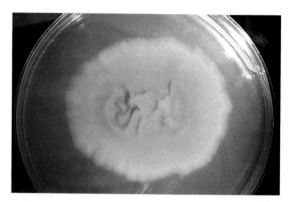

124. *Epidermophyton floccosum.* PDA, 30°C, 12 days. Reverse of colony.

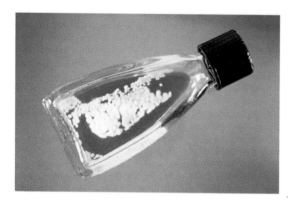

125. Dermatophyte test medium. Dermatophytes turn medium red (see p. 336).

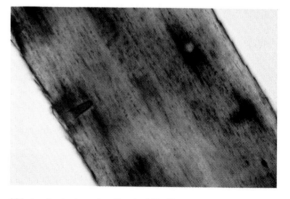

126. In vitro hair perforation test. Positive result. Note wedge-shaped perforations (see p. 310).

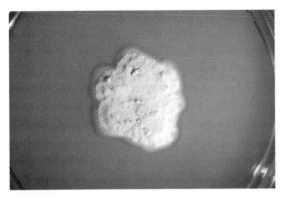

127. *Malbranchea* sp. PDA, 30°C, 7 days. Surface of colony.

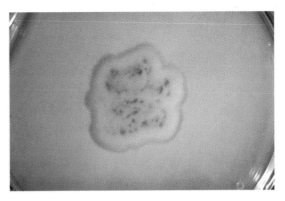

128. *Malbranchea* sp. PDA, 30°C, 7 days. Reverse of colony.

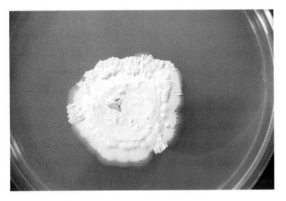

129. *Arthrographis kalrae*. PDA, 30°C, 8 days.

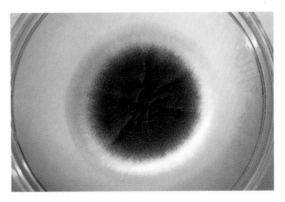

130. *Aspergillus fumigatus*. SDA, 30°C, 4 days. Surface of colony.

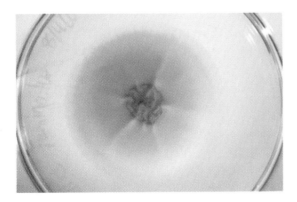

131. *Aspergillus fumigatus*. SDA, 30°C, 4 days. Reverse of colony.

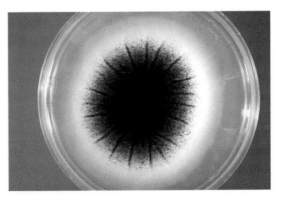

132. *Aspergillus niger*. SDA, 30°C, 4 days. Surface of colony.

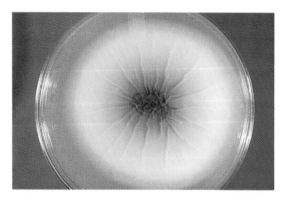

133. *Aspergillus niger.* SDA, 30°C, 4 days. Reverse of colony.

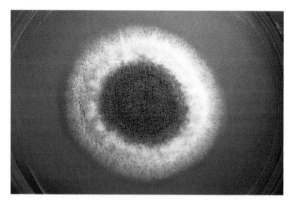

134. *Aspergillus flavus.* PDA, 30°C, 4 days. Surface of colony.

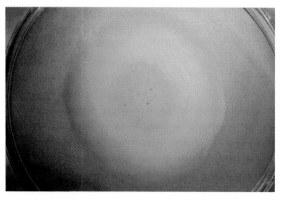

135. *Aspergillus flavus.* PDA, 30°C, 4 days. Reverse of colony.

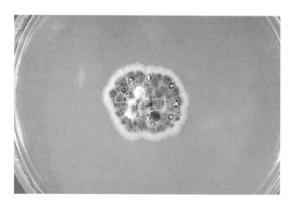

136. *Aspergillus versicolor.* SDA, 30°C, 4 days. Surface of colony.

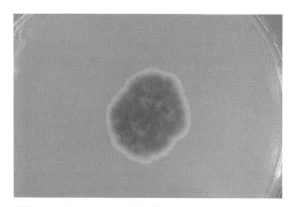

137. *Aspergillus versicolor.* SDA, 30°C, 4 days. Reverse of colony.

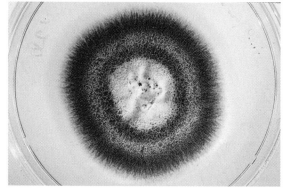

138. *Aspergillus nidulans.* SDA, 30°C, 4 days. Surface of colony.

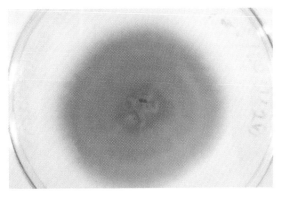

139. *Aspergillus nidulans.* SDA, 30°C, 4 days. Reverse of colony.

140. *Aspergillus nidulans.* Red ascospores and hyaline Hülle cells.

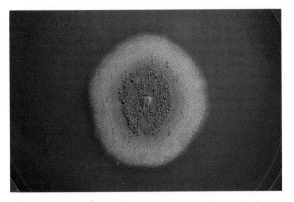

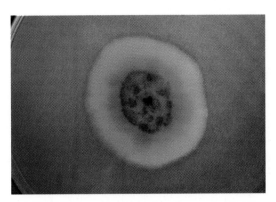

141. *Aspergillus terreus.* PDA, 30°C, 4 days. Surface of colony.

142. *Aspergillus terreus.* PDA, 30°C, 4 days. Reverse of colony.

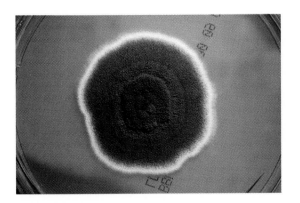

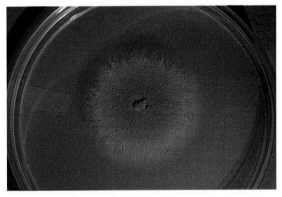

143. *Penicillium* sp. SDA, 30°C, 4 days.

144. *Paecilomyces* sp. SDA, 30°C, 4 days.

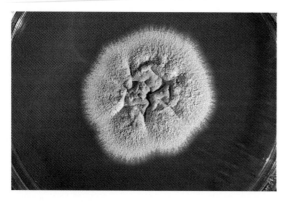

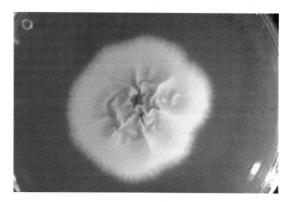

145. *Scopulariopsis brevicaulis* sp. SDA, 30°C, 5 days. Surface of colony.

146. *Scopulariopsis brevicaulis* sp. SDA, 30°C, 5 days. Reverse of colony.

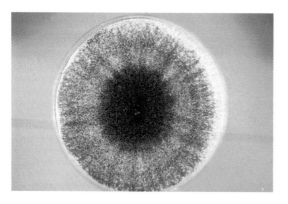

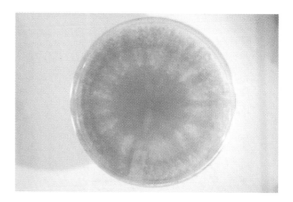

147. *Gliocladium* sp. SDA, 30°C, 5 days. Surface of colony.

148. *Gliocladium* sp. SDA, 30°C, 5 days. Reverse of colony.

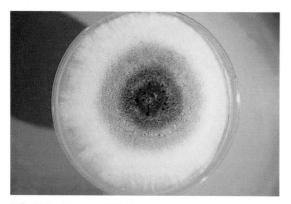

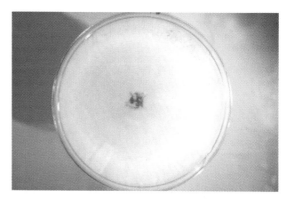

149. *Trichoderma* sp. SDA, 30°C, 5 days. Surface of colony.

150. *Trichoderma* sp. SDA, 30°C, 5 days. Reverse of colony.

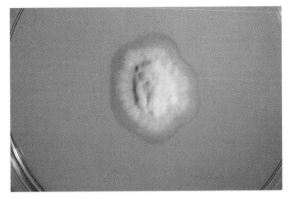

151. *Beauveria* sp. SDA, 30°C, 4 days.

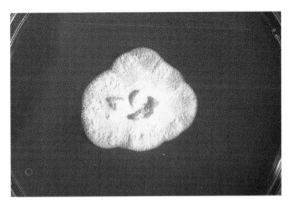

152. *Verticillium* sp. SDA, 30°C, 4 days.

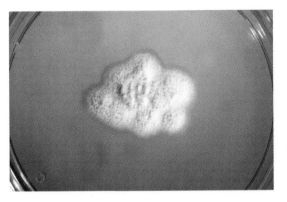

153. *Acremonium* sp. SDA, 30°C, 5 days. Surface of colony.

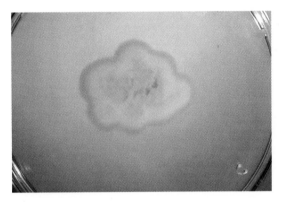

154. *Acremonium* sp. SDA, 30°C, 5 days. Reverse of colony.

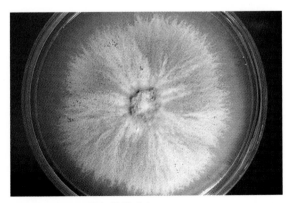

155. *Fusarium* sp. SDA, 30°C, 4 days.

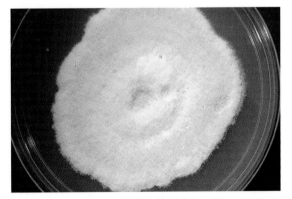

156. *Trichothecium roseum.* PDA, 30°C, 8 days. The extended incubation was required for pigment production.

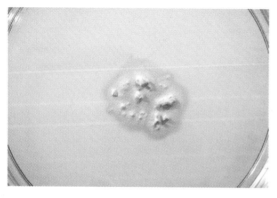

157. *Chrysosporium* sp. PDA, 30°C, 6 days. Surface of colony.

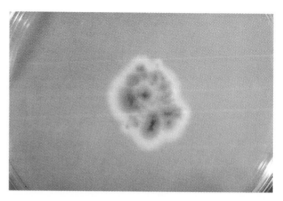

158. *Chrysosporium* sp. PDA, 30°C, 6 days. Reverse of colony.

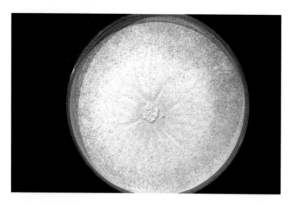

159. *Sporotrichum pruinosum.* SDA, 30°C, 6 days. Colony spreads to cover entire agar surface.

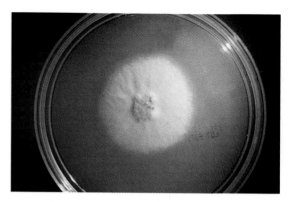

160. *Sepedonium* sp. SDA, 30°C, 6 days.

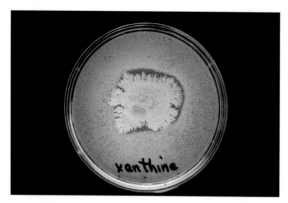

161. Xanthine hydrolysis test. Positive result (see p. 347).

Glossary

Abscess   Localized collection of pus in cavity formed by dissolution of tissue.

Aerial hyphae   Hyphae above the agar surface.

Aerobic   Able to grow in the presence of atmospheric oxygen.

Annellide   A cell that produces and extrudes conidia; the tip tapers, lengthens, and acquires a ring of cell wall material as each conidium is released; oil immersion magnification may be required to see the rings.

Apex (pl. *apices*)   The tip.

Apophysis   The swelling of a sporangiophore immediately below the columella.

Arthroconidium   An asexual propagule formed by the breaking up of a hypha at the point of septation. The resulting cell may be rectangular or barrel shaped and thick or thin walled, depending on the genus.

Ascospore   A sexual spore produced in a sac-like structure known as an *ascus*.

Anomorph.

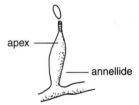

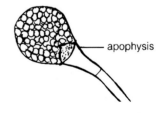

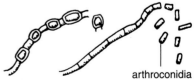

Ascus (pl. *asci*) A round or elongate sac-like structure usually containing 2 to 8 ascospores. The asci are often formed within a fruiting body, such as a cleistothecium or perithecium.

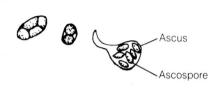

Ascus
Ascospore

Asexual Reproduction of an organism by division or redistribution of nuclei, but without nuclear fusion, i.e., not by the union of two nuclei. Also known as the *imperfect state*.

Assimilation The ability to use a carbon or nitrogen source for growth.

Basidiospore A sexual spore formed on a structure known as a *basidium*. Characteristic of the class Basidiomycetes.

Biseriate With reference to the genus *Aspergillus*, the phialide is supported by a metula as opposed to a uniseriate phialide, which forms directly on the vesicle. (*See* Uniseriate.)

Blastoconidium A conidium formed by budding along a hypha, pseudohypha, or single cell, as in the yeasts.

blastoconidia

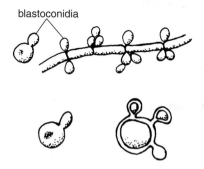

Budding A process of asexual reproduction in which the new cell develops as a smaller outgrowth from the older parent cell. Characteristic of yeasts or yeastlike fungi.

Capsule A colorless, transparent mucopolysaccharide sheath on the wall of a cell.

Chlamydoconidium An enlarged, rounded conidium that is thick walled and contains stored food, enabling it to assist in survival. It may be located at the end of the hypha (terminal) or inserted along the hypha (intercalary), singly or in chains. Characteristically, it is greater in diameter than the hypha on which it is borne. Unlike other conidia, it does not readily separate from the hypha.

Survival type of structure

Terminal
chlamydoconidium

Intercalary
chlamydoconidium

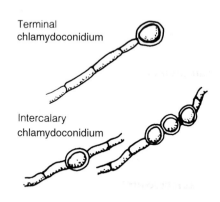

Chlamydospore The misnomer applied to the thick-walled vesicle formed by *Candida albicans*. It neither germinates nor produces conidia when mature.

Chloramphenicol An antibiotic produced by *Streptomyces venezuelae* but usually prepared synthetically. It is a useful additive to mycology media, as it inhibits the growth of many bacteria that might contaminate the cultures.

Clamp connection   A specialized bridge over a hyphal septum in the Basidiomycetes. During the formation of a new cell, it allows postmitosis nuclear migration.

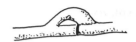

Cleistothecium   A large, fairly round, closed, many-celled structure in which asci and ascospores are formed and held until the structure bursts.

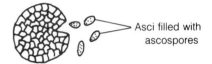

Asci filled with ascospores

Columella   The enlarged, dome-shaped tip of a sporangiophore that extends into the sporangium. Often the sporangium bursts, leaving the columella bare and readily visible upon microscopic examination.

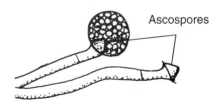

Ascospores

Conidiogenous cell   The cell that produces the conidia.

Conidiophore   A specialized hyphal structure that serves as a stalk on which conidia are formed. The shape and arrangement of the conidiophores and the conidia are generally characteristic of a genus. The suffix -*phore* means "bearer" or "producer" and is added to the word that denotes what it is bearing, e.g., conidiophores bear conidia and sporangiophores bear sporangia.

Conidium (pl. *conidia*)   An asexual propagule that forms on the side or the end of the hypha or conidiophore. It may consist of one or more cells, and the size, shape, and arrangement in groups are generally characteristic of the organism. It is always borne externally, i.e., not enclosed within a sac-like structure such as a sporangium. If a fungus produces two types of conidia, those that are small and usually single celled are referred to as *microconidia*, whereas the larger *macroconidia* are usually segmented into two or more cells.

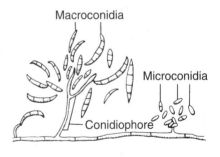

Macroconidia

Microconidia

Conidiophore

Cutaneous   Pertaining to the skin.

Cycloheximide   An antibiotic (proprietary name, Actidione) used in selective mycology media to inhibit the growth of saprophytic fungi. Because it is also known to inhibit some pathogenic fungi, it must be used in conjunction with a medium without antibiotics.

Dematiaceous   Having structures that are brown to black; this is due to a melanotic pigment in the cell walls.

Denticle   Short, narrow projection bearing a conidium.

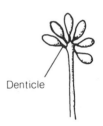

Denticle

Dermatophyte A fungus belonging to the genus *Trichophyton*, *Microsporum*, or *Epidermophyton* with the ability to obtain nutrients from keratin and infect skin, hair, or nails of humans or animals.

Dichotomous Branching (of hyphae) into two equal branches that are each equal in diameter to the hypha from which they originated.

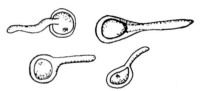

Dimorphic Having two distinct morphological forms. In this guide, it refers to temperature-dependent changes in the organism on artificial culture media, i.e., fungi having a mould phase when cultured at 25–30°C and a yeast phase when cultured at 35–37°C.

Favic chandeliers Terminal hyphal branches that are irregular, broad, and antler-like in appearance. Especially characteristic of *Trichophyton schoenleinii*.

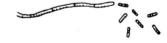

Filamentous Long, cylindrical, and threadlike; hyphae forming.

Floccose Cottony; like raw, fuzzy cotton.

Foot cell The base of the conidiophore, where it merges with the hyphae, giving the impression of a foot; typically seen in *Aspergillus* spp.

Fragmentation Breaking of the hyphae into pieces, each of which is capable of forming a new organism. Arthroconidia are formed in this manner.

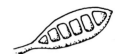

Fungus (pl. *fungi*) An organism that is either filamentous or unicellular and lacks chlorophyll. It has a true nucleus enclosed in a membrane and chitin in the cell wall.

Fusiform Spindle shaped, i.e., being wider in the middle and narrowing toward the ends.

Geniculate Bent like a knee. (*See* Sympodial growth.)

Germ tube A tubelike outgrowth from a conidium or spore; the beginning of a hypha.

Glabrous Smooth; without or almost without aerial hyphae.

Hilum (pl. *hila*)   Scar of attachment; it appears at the point(s) where the conidium was formerly attached to the conidiophore and/or another conidium.

Host   The animal or plant that supports a parasite.

Hülle cells   Thickened large sterile cells with a small lumen; they are associated with cleistothecia produced by the sexual stage of some *Aspergillus* spp.

Hyaline   Clear, transparent, colorless.

Hypha (pl. *hyphae*)   A filamentous structure of a fungus. Many together compose the mycelium.

Hyphomycete   An asexual fungus that produces septate mycelium that may be colorless (hyaline) or darkly pigmented (dematiaceous).

Inflammation   A local protective response of the body; characterized by redness, pain, heat, and swelling.

Intercalary   Situated along the hypha, not at its end.

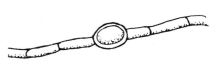

Intracellular   Within cells.

Keratin   A scleroprotein containing large amounts of sulfur, such as cystine; the primary component of skin, hair, and nails.

Keratitis   Inflammation of the cornea of the eye.

Macroconidium (pl. *macroconidia*)   The larger of two types of conidia in a fungus that produces both large and small conidia; may be single celled but usually is multicelled. (See *Conidium*.)

Metula (pl. *metulae*)   The separate structural portion of the conidiophore that supports (much like a pedestal) the phialide in genera such as *Aspergillus*, *Penicillium*, and *Paecilomyces*.

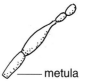
metula

Microconidium (pl. *microconidia*)   The smaller of two types of conidia in a fungus that produces both large and small conidia; usually single celled and round, ovoid, pear shaped, or club shaped. (See *Conidium*.)

Monomorphic   In this guide, refers to fungi having the same type of morphology in culture at both 25–30°C and 35–37°C (i.e., if growth occurs at both temperature ranges; some saprophytes are inhibited at 35–37°C).

Mould   A filamentous fungus composed of filaments that generally form a colony that may be either fuzzy, powdery, woolly, velvety, or relatively smooth.

Muriform   Having transverse and longitudinal septations.

Mycelium (pl. *mycelia*)   A mat of intertwined hyphae that constitutes the colony surface of a mould.

Mycetoma   A localized, chronic cutaneous or subcutaneous infection classically characterized by draining sinuses, granules, and swelling.

Mycology   The study of fungi and their biology.   *oncomycosis*

Mycosis (pl. *mycoses*)   A disease caused by a fungus.

Nodular body   A round knot-like structure formed by intertwined hyphae; seen especially in some dermatophytes.

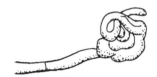

Ostiole   A mouth or opening.

Pathogen   Any disease-producing microorganism.

Pectinate   Resembling a comb.

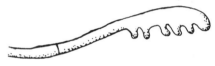

Pellicle   A firm or button-like mass formed on liquid medium by some fungi.

Perithecium (pl. *perithecia*)   A large round or pear-shaped structure usually having a small rounded opening (which differentiates it from a cleistothecium; the opening is called an *ostiole*) and containing asci and ascospores.

ascospores

ostiole

perithecium

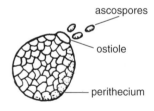

Phaeo-   A prefix meaning dark (brownish or blackish).

Phaeohyphomycosis   A subcutaneous or systemic disease caused by a variety of black fungi that develop in tissue as dark hyphae and/or yeastlike cells.   *dematis fungia*

Phialide   A cell that produces and extrudes conidia without tapering or increasing in length with each new conidium produced. It is usually shaped like a flask, vase, or tenpin.

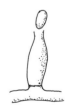

Pleomorphism   The occurrence of two or more forms in the life cycle of an organism. Also refers to the occurrence of a form of dermatophyte that ceases to produce conidia (becomes sterile).

Propagule   A unit that can give rise to another organism.

Pseudohypha   Chain of cells formed by budding which, when elongated, resembles a true hypha; differs from true hyphae by being constricted at the septa, forming branches that begin with a septation, and having terminal cells smaller than the other cells.

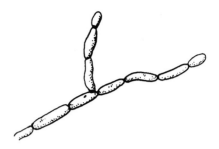

Pycnidium (pl. *pycnidia*)   A large round or flask-shaped fruiting body containing conidia. Pycnidia usually have an opening (an ostiole).

Pyriform   Pear shaped.

Racquet hypha   A hypha with club-shaped cells, the larger end of one cell being attached to the smaller end of an adjacent cell.

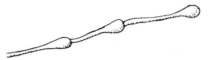

Rhizoid   Rootlike, branched hypha extending into the medium.

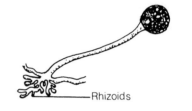

Rhizoids

Ringworm   Superficial skin disease caused by dermatophytes. Term derived from the ringlike, circular form of the lesions and from the belief that these infections were caused by wormlike organisms. The current accepted term is *tinea*.

Saprobe/Saprophyte   An organism that uses dead organic matter as a source of nutrients.

Septate   Having cross walls.

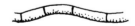

Sexual state   The portion of the life cycle in which the organism reproduces by the union of two nuclei. Also known as the *perfect state*.

Spherule   Large, round, thick-walled structure containing spores; characteristic of *Coccidioides immitis* in infected host material under direct microscopic examination. Spherules do not grow on routine artificial mycology media.

Spiral hypha   Hypha forming coiled or corkscrew-like turns.

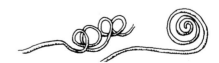

Sporangiophore A specialized hyphal branch or stalk bearing a sporangium.

Sporangiospore An asexual spore produced in a sporangium.

Sporangium (pl. *sporangia*) A closed sac-like structure in which asexual spores (sporangiospores) are formed by cleavage.

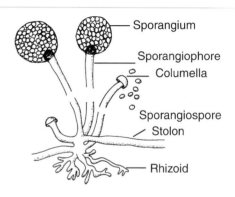

Spore Propagule that develops by sexual reproduction (ascospore, basidiospore, or zygospore) or by asexual means within a sporangium (sporangiospore). Those most commonly seen in the clinical laboratory are usually enclosed in a sac-like structure (as opposed to conidia, which are free, not enclosed).

Sterigmata Term formerly used to denote phialides of *Aspergillus* and other genera. More accurately refers to denticles produced by Basidiomycetes.

Stolon A horizontal hypha, or runner, that grows along the surface of the medium, often bearing rhizoids that penetrate the medium and sporangiophores that ascend into the air.

Subcutaneous Situated or occurring directly under the skin.

Suppurative Producing pus.

Sympodial growth Conidiogenous structure that continues to increase in length by forming a new growing point just below each new terminal conidium, often resulting in a geniculate (bent) appearance.

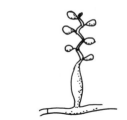

Terminal At the end.

Taliomarph

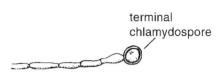

Thallus The vegetative body of a fungus.

Truncate Cut off sharply; ending abruptly with a flattened edge.

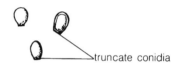

Tuberculate Having knob-like projections.

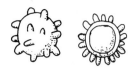

Uniseriate With reference to the genus *Aspergillus*, the phialide forms directly on the vesicle; a biseriate phialide is supported by a metula. (*See* Biseriate.)

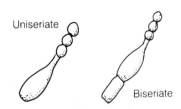

Vesicle Enlarged structure at the end of a conidiophore or sporangiophore. In *Aspergillus* spp. it bears the phialides, which in turn bear the conidia.

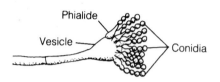

Whorl A group of cells radiating from a common point.

Yeastlike colony A soft, pasty, smooth colony; usually no filamentous (fuzzy) growth can be observed macroscopically.

Anamorph: A asexual form of a fungus

Teleomorph: the sexual form of a fungus
demonstrate sexual structure. such as
ascospore or large fruiting bodies
eg cleistothecia.

Bibliography

Suggested for Further Information

Adams, E. D., and B. H. Cooper. 1974. Evaluation of a modified Wickerham medium for identifying medically important yeasts. *Am. J. Med. Technol.* **40:**377–388.

Barron, G. L. 1977. *The Genera of Hyphomycetes from Soil.* Robert E. Krieger Publishing Co., Huntington, N.Y.

Blinkhorn, R. J., D. Adelstein, and P. J. Spagnuolo. 1989. Emergence of a new opportunistic pathogen, *Candida lusitaniae. J. Clin. Microbiol.* **27:**236–240.

Chandler, F. W., and J. C. Watts. 1987. *Pathologic Diagnosis of Fungal Infections.* American Society of Clinical Pathology Press, Chicago, Ill.

Connor, D. H., F. W. Chandler, D. Schwartz, H. Manz, and E. Lack. 1997. *Pathology of Infectious Diseases.* Appleton & Lange, Stamford, Conn.

Cooper, C. R., and N. G. Haycocks. 2000. *Penicillium marneffei:* an insurgent species among the penicillia. *J. Eukaryot. Microbiol.* **47:**24–28.

Crous, P. W., W. Gams, M. J. Wingfield, and P. S. van Wyk. 1996. *Phaeoacremonium* gen. nov. associated with wilt and decline diseases of woody hosts and human infections. *Mycologia* **88:**786–796.

de Hoog, G. S., J. Guarro, J. Gené, and M. J. Figueras. 2000. *Atlas of Clinical Fungi,* 2nd ed. Centraalbureau voor Schimmelcultures, Utrecht, The Netherlands.

Dixon, D. M., and I. F. Salkin. 1986. Morphologic and physiologic studies of three dematiaceous pathogens. *J. Clin. Microbiol.* **24:**12–15.

Etzel, R. A., E. Montana, W. G. Sorenson, G. J. Kullman, T. M. Allan, and D. G. Dearborn. 1998. Acute pulmonary hemorrhage in infants associated with exposure to *Stachybotrys atra* and other fungi. *Arch. Pediatr. Adolesc. Med.* **152:**757–762.

Evans, E. G. V., and M. D. Richardson (ed.). 1989. *Medical Mycology; a Practical Approach.* IRL Press, Oxford, United Kingdom.

Fung, F., R. Clark, and S. Williams. 1998. *Stachybotrys,* a mycotoxin-producing fungus of increasing toxicologic importance. *Clin. Toxicol.* **36:**79–86.

Gams, W., and M. R. McGinnis. 1983. *Phialemonium,* a new anamorph genus intermediate between *Phialophora* and *Acremonium. Mycologia* **75:**977–987.

Gromadzki, S. G., and V. Chaturvedi. 2000. Limitation of the AccuProbe *Coccidioides immitis* culture identification test: false-negative results with formaldehyde-killed cultures. *J. Clin. Microbiol.* **38:**2427–2428.

Guarro, J., W. Gams, I. Pujol, and J. Gené. 1997. *Acremonium* species: new emerging fungal opportunists—in vitro antifungal susceptibilities and review. *Clin. Infect. Dis.* **25:**1222–1229.

Guarro, J., M. Nucci, T. Akiti, J. Gené, J. Cano, M. Da Gloria, C. Barreiro, and C. Aguilar. 1999. *Phialemonium* fungemia; two documented nosocomial cases. *J. Clin. Microbiol.* **37:**2493–2497.

Guého, E., M. T. Smith, G. S. de Hoog, G. Billon-Grand, R. Christen, and W. H. Batenburg-van der Vegte. 1992. Contributions to a revision of the genus *Trichosporon. Antonie Leeuwenhoek* **61:**289–316.

Harris, J. L. 2000. A safe, low-distortion tape touch method for fungal slide mounts. *J. Clin. Microbiol.* **38:**4683–4684.

Huber, W. M., and S. M. Caplin. 1947. Simple and plastic mount for permanent preservation of fungi and small arthropods. *Arch. Dermatol. Syphilol.* **56:**763–765.

Ibrahim-Granet, O., and C. de Bievere. 1984. Study of the conidial development and cleistothecium-like structure of some strains of *Fonsecaea pedrosoi. Mycopathologia* **84:**181–186.

Isenberg, H. D. (ed.). 1992. *Clinical Microbiology Procedures Handbook.* American Society for Microbiology, Washington, D.C.

Kane, J., R. Summerbell, L. Sigler, S. Krajden, and G. Land. 1997. *Laboratory Handbook of Dermatophytes.* Star Publishing Co., Belmont, Calif.

Kemna, M. E., R. C. Neri, R. Ali, and I. F. Salkin. 1994. *Cokeromyces recurvatus,* a mucoraceous zygomycete rarely isolated in clinical laboratories. *J. Clin. Microbiol.* **32:**843–845.

Kimura, M., and M. R. McGinnis. 1998. Fontana-Masson-stained tissue from culture-proven mycoses. *Arch. Pathol. Lab. Med.* **122:**1107–1111.

Kimura, M., M. B. Smith, and M. R. McGinnis. 1999. Zygomycosis due to *Apophysomyces elegans. Arch. Pathol. Lab. Med.* **123:**386–390.

Koneman, E. W., and G. D. Roberts. 1991. Mycotic disease, p. 1099–1130. *In* J. B. Henry (ed.), *Clinical Diagnosis and Management by Laboratory Methods,* 18th ed. W. B. Saunders Co., Philadelphia, Pa.

Kwon-Chung, K. J., and J. E. Bennett. 1992. *Medical Mycology.* Lea and Febiger, Philadelphia, Pa.

Kurtzman, C. P., and J. W. Fell (ed.). 2000. *The Yeasts, a Taxonomic Study,* 4th ed. Elsevier, Amsterdam, The Netherlands.

Levenson, D., M. A. Pfaller, M. A. Smith, R. Hollis, T. Gerarden, C. B. Tucci, and H. D. Isenberg. 1991. *Candida zeylanoides:* an opportunistic yeast. *J. Clin. Microbiol.* **29:**1689–1692.

Liu, K., D. N. Howell, J. R. Perfect, and W. A. Schell. 1998. Morphologic criteria for the preliminary identification of *Fusarium, Paecilomyces,* and *Acremonium* species by histopathology. *Am. J. Clin. Pathol.* **109:**45–54.

Mahan, C. T., and G. E. Sale. 1978. Rapid methenamine silver stain for *Pneumocystis* and fungi. *Arch. Pathol. Lab. Med.* **102:**351–352.

Marcon, M. J., and D. A. Powell. 1992. Human infections due to *Malassezia* spp. *Clin. Microbiol. Rev.* **5:**101–119.

McGinnis, M. R. 1980. *Laboratory Handbook of Medical Mycology.* Academic Press, New York, N.Y.

McGinnis, M. R., M. G. Rinaldi, and R. E. Winn. 1986. Emerging agents of phaeohyphomycosis: pathogenic species of *Bipolaris* and *Exserohilum. J. Clin. Microbiol.* **24:**250–259.

McGough, D. A., A. W. Fothergill, and M. G. Rinaldi. 1990. *Cokeromyces recurvatus* Poitras, a distinctive zygomycete and potential pathogen: criteria for identification. *Clin. Microbiol. Newsl.* **12:**113–117.

McNeil, M. M., and J. M. Brown. 1994. The medically important aerobic actinomycetes: epidemiology and microbiology. *Clin. Microbiol. Rev.* **7:**357–417.

Miller, J. M. 1999. *Specimen Management in Clinical Microbiology,* 2nd ed. ASM Press, Washington, D.C.

Misra, P. C., K. J. Srivastava, and K. Lata. 1979. *Apophysomyces,* a new genus of the Mucorales. *Mycotaxon* **8:**377–382.

Murray, P. R., E. J. Baron, M. A. Pfaller, F. C. Tenover, and R. H. Yolken (ed.). 1999. *Manual of Clinical Microbiology,* 7th ed. ASM Press, Washington, D.C.

Padhye, A. A., and L. Ajello. 1988. Simple method of inducing sporulation by *Apophysomyces elegans* and *Saksenaea vasiformis. J. Clin. Microbiol.* **26:**1861–1863.

Pincus, D. H., D. C. Coleman, W. R. Pruitt, A. A. Padhye, I. F. Salkin, M. Geimer, A. Bassel, D. J. Sullivan, M. Clarke, and V. Hearn. 1999. Rapid identification of *Candida dubliniensis* with commercial yeast identification systems. *J. Clin. Microbiol.* **37:**3533–3539.

Pincus, D. H., I. F. Salkin, N. J. Hurd, I. J. Levy, and M. A. Kemna. 1988. Modification of potassium nitrate assimilation test for identification of clinically important yeasts. *J. Clin Microbiol.* **26:**366–368.

Polacheck, I., I. F. Salkin, R. Kitzes-Cohen, and R. Raz. 1992. Endocarditis caused by *Blastoschizomyces capitatus* and taxonomic review of the genus. *J. Clin. Micro-biol.* **30:**2318–2322.

Raper, K. B., and D. L. Fennell. 1973. *The Genus Aspergillus.* Robert E. Krieger Publishing Co., Huntington, N.Y.

Rebell, G., and D. Taplin. 1970. *Dermatophytes, Their Recognition and Identification,* 2nd ed. University of Miami Press, Coral Gables, Fla.

Ribes, J. A., C. L. Vanover-Sams, and D. J. Baker. 2000. Zygomycetes in human disease. *Clin. Microbiol. Rev.* **13:**236–301.

Rippon, J. W. 1988. *Medical Mycology: the Pathogenic Fungi and the Pathogenic Actinomycetes,* 3rd ed. W. B. Saunders Co., Philadelphia, Pa.

Roilides, E., L. Sigler, E. Bibashi, H. Katsifa, N. Flaris, and C. Panteliadis. 1999. Disseminated infection due to *Chrysosporium zonatum* in a patient with chronic granulomatous disease and review of non-*Aspergillus* fungal infections with this disease. *J. Clin. Microbiol.* **37:**18–25.

Salkin, I. F., M. A. Gordon, W. A. Samsonoff, and C. L. Reider. 1985a. *Blastoschizomyces capitatus,* a new combination. *Mycotaxon* **22:**373–380.

Salkin, I. F., G. E. Hollick, N. J. Hurd, and M. E. Kemna. 1985b. Evaluation of human hair sources for the in vitro hair perforation test. *J. Clin. Microbiol.* **22:**1048–1049.

Saubolle, M. A., and J. Sutton. 1994. Coccidioidomycosis: centennial year on the North American continent. *Clin. Microbiol. Newsl.* **16:**137–144.

Shimono, L. H., and B. Hartman. 1986. A simple and reliable rapid methenamine silver stain for *Pneumocystis carinii* and fungi. *Arch. Pathol. Lab. Med.* **110:**855–856.

Shin, J. H., S. K. Lee, S. P. Suh, D. W. Ryang, N. H. Kim, M. G. Rinaldi, and D. A. Sutton. 1998. Fatal *Hormonema dematioides* peritonitis in a patient on continuous ambulatory peritoneal dialysis: criteria for organism identification and review of other known fungal etiologic agents. *J. Clin. Microbiol.* **36:**2157–2163.

Sigler, L., and J. W. Carmichael. 1976. Taxonomy of *Malbranchea* and some other hyphomycetes with arthroconidia. *Mycotaxon* **4:**349–488.

Sigler, L., and J. W. Carmichael. 1983. Redisposition of some fungi referred to *Oidium microspermum* and a review of *Arthrographis. Mycotaxon* **18:**495–507.

Sigler, L., R. C. Summerbell, L. Poole, M. Wieden, D. A. Sutton, M. G. Rinaldi, M. Aguirre, G. W. Estes, and J. N. Galgiani. 1997. Invasive *Nattrassia mangiferae* infections: case report, literature review, and therapeutic and taxonomic appraisal. *J. Clin. Microbiol.* **35:**433–440.

Stockman, L., and G. Roberts. 1985. Rapid screening method for the identification of *C. glabrata,* abstr. F-80, p. 377. *Abstr. 85th Annu. Meet. Am. Soc. Microbiol. 1985.* American Society for Microbiology, Washington, D.C.

Sullivan, D., and D. Coleman. 1998. *Candida dubliniensis:* characteristics and identification. *J. Clin. Microbiol.* **36:**329–334.

Sullivan, D. J., G. Moran, S. Donnelly, S. Gee, E. Pinjon, B. McCartan, D. B. Shanley, and D. C. Coleman. 1999. *Candida dubliniensis:* an update. *Rev. Iberoam. Micol.* **16:**72–76.

Supparatpinyo, K., C. Khamwan, V. Baosoung, K. E. Nelson, and T. Sirisanthana. 1994. Disseminated *Penicillium marneffei* infection in southeast Asia. *Lancet* **344:**110–113.

Vossler, J. L. 2001. *Penicillium marneffei:* an emerging fungal pathogen. *Clin. Microbiol. Newsl.* **23:**25–29.

Walsh, T. J., G. Renshaw, J. Andrews, J. Kwon-Chung, R. C. Cunnion, H. I. Pass, J. Taubenberger, W. Wilson, and P. A. Pizzo. 1994. Invasive zygomycosis due to *Conidiobolus incongruus. Clin. Infect. Dis.* **19:**423–430.

Wentworth, B. B. (ed.). 1988. *Diagnostic Procedures for Mycotic and Parasitic Infections,* 7th ed. American Public Health Association, Washington, D.C.

Wilson, J. W., and O. A. Plunkett. 1970. *The Fungous Diseases of Man.* University of California Press, Berkeley.

Additional References

Aly, R. 1994. Culture media for growing dermatophytes. *J. Am. Acad. Dermatol.* **31:**S107–S108.

Baker, J. G., H. L. Nadler, P. Forgacs, and S. R. Kurtz. 1984. *Candida lusitaniae:* a new opportunistic pathogen of the urinary tract. *Diagn. Microbiol. Infect. Dis.* **2:**145–149.

Barnett, J. A., R. W. Payne, and D. Yarrow. 1991. *Yeasts: Characteristics and Identification,* 2nd ed. Cambridge University Press, New York, N.Y.

Bottone, E. J., I. Weitzman, and B. A. Hanna. 1979. *Rhizopus rhizopodiformis:* emerging etiological agent of mucormycosis. *J. Clin. Microbiol.* **9:**530–537.

Bottone, E. J., and G. P. Wormser. 1985. Capsule-deficient cryptococci in AIDS. *Lancet* **ii:**553.

Carmichael, J. W. 1962. *Chrysosporium* and some other alleuriosporic hyphomycetes. *Can. J. Bot.* **40:**1137–1173.

Carmichael, J. W., W. B. Kendrick, I. L. Conners, and L. Sigler. 1980. *Genera of Hyphomycetes.* University of Alberta Press, Alberta, Canada.

Crozier, W. J. 1993. Two cases of onychomycosis due to *Candida zeylanoides. Aust. J. Dermatol.* **34:**23–25.

de Hoog, G. S. 1983. On the potentially pathogenic dematiaceous hyphomycetes, p. 149–217. *In* D. H. Howard (ed.), *Fungi Pathogenic for Humans and Animals,* part A. Marcel Dekker, New York, N.Y.

Dixon, D. M., and A. Polak-Wyss. 1991. The medically important dematiaceous fungi and their identification. *Mycoses* **34:**1–18.

Fincher, R.-M. E., J. F. Fisher, R. D. Lovell, C. L. Newman, A. Espinel-Ingroff, and H. J. Shadomy. 1991. Infection due to the fungus *Acremonium (Cephalosporium). Medicine* **70:**398–409.

Fricker-Hidalgo, H., S. Orenga, G. Lebeau, H. Pelloux, M. P. Brenier-Pinchart, P. Ambroise-Thomas, and R. Grillot. 2001. Evaluation of Candida ID, a new chromogenic medium for fungal isolation and preliminary identification of some yeast species. *J. Clin. Microbiol.* **39:**1647–1649.

Halaby, T., H. Boots, A. Vermuelen, A. Van Der Ven, H. Beguin, H. Van Hooff, and J. Jacobs. 2001. Phaeohyphomycosis caused by *Alternaria infectoria* in a renal transplant recipient. *J. Clin Microbiol.* **39:**1952–1955.

Jabra-Rizk, M. A., W. A. Falkler, Jr., W. G. Merz, A. A. M. A. Baqui, J. I. Kelley, and T. F. Meiller. 2000. Retrospective identification and characterization of *Candida dubliniensis* isolates among *Candida albicans* clinical laboratory isolates from human immunodeficiency virus (HIV)-infected and non-HIV-infected individuals. *J. Clin. Microbiol.* **38:**2423–2426.

Jones, J. M. 1990. Laboratory diagnosis of invasive candidiasis. *Clin. Microbiol. Rev.* **3:**32–45.

Kemna, M. E., M. Weinberger, L. Sigler, R. Zeltser, I. Polacheck, and I. F. Salkin. 1994. A primary oral blastomycosis-like infection in Israel, abstr. F-75, p. 601. *Abstr. 94th Gen. Meet. Am. Soc. Microbiol. 1994.* American Society for Microbiology, Washington, D.C.

King, D., L. Pasarell, D. M. Dixon, M. R. McGinnis, and W. G. Merz. 1993. A phaeohyphomycotic cyst and peritonitis caused by *Phialemonium* species and a reevaluation of its taxonomy. *J. Clin. Microbiol.* **31:**1804–1810.

Koehler, A. P., K.-C. Chu, E. T. S. Houang, and A. F. B. Cheng. 1999. Simple, reliable, and cost-effective yeast identification scheme for the clinical laboratory. *J. Clin. Microbiol.* **37:**422–426.

Larone, D. H. 1989. The identification of dematiaceous fungi. *Clin. Microbiol. Newsl.* **11:**145–150.

Larone, D., and I. Beaty. 1988. Evaluation and modification of tests for phenoloxidase activity in *Cryptococcus neoformans,* abstr. F-111, p. 410. *Abstr. 88th Annu. Meet. Am. Soc. Microbiol. 1988.* American Society for Microbiology, Washington, D.C.

Liao, W. Q., Z. G. Li, M. Guo, and J. Z. Zhang. 1993. *Candida zeylanoides* causing candidiasis as tinea cruris. *Chin. Med. J.* **106:**542–545.

Libertin, C. R., W. R. Wilson, and G. D. Roberts. 1985. *Candida lusitaniae:* an opportunistic pathogen. *Diagn. Microbiol. Infect. Dis.* **3:**69–71.

Marriott, D. J. E., K. H. Wong, E. Aznar, J. L. Harkness, D. A. Cooper, and D. Muir. 1997. *Scytalidium dimidiatum* and *Lecythophora hoffmannii:* unusual causes of fungal infections in a patient with AIDS. *J. Clin. Microbiol.* **35:**2949–2952.

Martino, P., M. Venditti, A. Micozzi, G. Morace, L. Polonelli, M. P. Mantovani, M. C. Petti, V. L. Burgio, C. Santini, P. Serra, and F. Mandelli. 1990. *Blastoschizomyces capitis:* an emerging cause of invasive fungal disease in leukemia patients. *Rev. Infect. Dis.* **12:**570–582.

McGinnis, M. R. 1983. Chromoblastomycosis and phaeohyphomycosis: new concepts, diagnosis, and mycology. *J. Am. Acad. Dermatol.* **8:**1–16.

McGinnis, M. R., L. Ajello, and W. A. Schell. 1985. Mycotic diseases: a proposed nomenclature. *Int. J. Dermatol.* **24:**9–15.

Mok, W. Y. 1982. Nature and identification of *Exophiala werneckii. J. Clin. Microbiol.* **16:**976–978.

Morris, J. T., M. Beckius, and C. K. McAllister. 1991. *Sporobolomyces* infection in an AIDS patient. *J. Infect. Dis.* **164:**623–624.

Mosaid, A. A., D. Sullivan, I. F. Salkin, D. Shanley, and D. C. Coleman. 2001. Differentiation of *Candida dubliniensis* from *Candida albicans* on Staib agar and caffeic acid-ferric citrate agar. *J. Clin. Microbiol.* **39:**323–327.

Nahass, G. T., S. P. Rosenberg, C. L. Leonardi, and N. S. Penneys. 1993. Disseminated infection with *Trichosporon beigelii.* Report of a case and review of the cutaneous and histologic manifestations. *Arch. Dermatol.* **129:**1020–1023.

Padhye, A. A., J. G. Baker, and R. F. D'Amato. 1979. Rapid identification of *Prototheca* species by the API 20C system. *J. Clin. Microbiol.* **10:**579–582.

Pasarell, L., M. E. Kemna, M. R. McGinnis, and I. F. Salkin. 1993. Mycetoma caused by *Phialophora verrucosa,* abstr. F-31, p. 532. *Abstr. 93rd Annu. Meet. Am. Soc. Microbiol. 1993.* American Society for Microbiology, Washington, D.C.

Roberts, G. D. 1994. Laboratory methods in basic mycology, p. 689–775. *In* E. J. Baron, L. R. Peterson, and S. M. Finegold (ed.), *Bailey & Scott's Diagnostic Microbiology,* 9th ed. The C. V. Mosby Co., St. Louis, Mo.

Salfelder, K. 1990. *Atlas of Fungal Pathology.* Kluwer Academic Publishers, Dordrecht, The Netherlands.

Salkin, I. F., D. M. Dixon, M. E. Kemna, P. J. Danneman, and J. W. Griffith. 1990. Fatal encephalitis caused by *Dactylaria constrica* var. *gallopava* in a snowy owl chick *(Nyctea scandiaca). J. Clin. Microbiol.* **28:**2845–2847.

Scholer, H. J., E. Muller, and M. A. A. Schipper. 1983. Mucorales, p. 9–59. *In* D. H. Howard (ed.), *Fungi Pathogenic for Humans and Animals,* part A. Marcel Dekker, New York, N.Y.

Tintelnot, K., G. Haase, M. Seibold, F. Bergmann, M. Staemmler, T. Franz, and D. Naumann. 2000. Evaluation of phenotypic markers for selection and identification of *Candida dubliniensis. J. Clin. Microbiol.* **38:**1599–1608.

Walsh, T. J., G. P. Melcher, M. G. Rinaldi, J. Lecciones, D. A. McGough, P. Kelly, J. Lee, D. Callender, M. Rubin, and P. A. Pizzo. 1990. *Trichosporon beigelii,* an emerging pathogen resistant to amphotericin B. *J. Clin. Microbiol.* **28:**1616–1622.

Wang, C. J. K., and R. A. Zabel (ed.). 1990. *Identification Manual for Fungi from Utility Poles in the Eastern United States.* American Type Culture Collection, Rockville, Md.

Index

Note: Page number in **boldface type** indicates page of detailed description
          Italic type indicates color photograph
          t = tables for identification

A

Abscess, 13, 379
Absidia corymbifera, *364*
   characteristics and morphology, 35, 169
   differentiating from *Apophysomyces elegans*, 169, 170
Absidia spp.
   characteristics and morphology, 74
   differentiating from other zygomycetes, 165t
   differentiating from *Rhizopus* spp., 166
Acanthosis, 41
Acetate ascospore agar, 327
Acetate ascospore medium, 134
Achlorophyllous algae, 139
Acid-fast stain
   for ascospores, 316
   Coates-Fite, *355*
   modified Kinyoun, 22t, 34, 104, 300, 315-316
Acid mercuric chloride, 338
Acremonium spp., *377*
   characteristics and morphology, 72, 77, 88, 90, 186t, **279**
   hyalohyphomycoses, 38
   mycetoma, 32-33
Actinomadura madurae, differentiating from other actinomycetes, 103t
Actinomadura pelletieri, differentiating from other actinomycetes, 103t
Actinomadura spp.
   characteristics and morphology, 32, 68, 86, 89, **107**, 108
   mycetoma, 32-33, 107

Actinomyces bovis, 31
Actinomyces israelii, 31
Actinomyces spp., *355*
   stains for, 22t
Actinomycetes
   aerobic, **68**, 103t, 345, 347
   media for, 345, 347, 348
   Splendore-Hoeppli phenomenon, 3
   stains for, 22t
   tissue response to infection, 3
Actinomycosis, 24, **31**
Actinomycotic mycetoma, 24, **32-33**
Acute inflammation, 18
Adiaconidia, in *Emmonsia crescens*, 61
Adiaspiromycosis, 28, **61**, 264
Aerial hyphae, 379
Aerobic, definition, 379
Aerobic actinomycetes, **68**, 103t, 345, 347
Agar with indicator method, 330-331
AIDS patients
   cryptococcal meningitis in, 129
   Emmonsia spp. in, 264
Allergic aspergillosis, 36
Alternaria sp.
   characteristics and morphology, 83, 95, 221, *368*
   phaeohyphomycosis, 43
Angioinvasion, **19**, 36, *354*
Annellide, 379
Annelloconidia, yeasts and yeastlike organisms having, 70
Antibacterial agents, in culture media, 300, 301t

Sexual state, 385

Shimono-Hartman method, methenamine silver stain, 320

"Ship's wheel" appearance, 23, 173

Skin specimens
    collection and preparation, 296
    H&E stain, *355*

Slide culture, 7, 304-305

"Soap bubbles," 54

South American blastomycosis, 154

Spherule
    of *Coccidioides* spp., *353*
    defined, 385

Spiral hypha, 385

Splendore-Hoeppli phenomenon, 3, 15, **19**, 32, *355*

Spongiosis, 40

Sporangia
    defined, 386
    moulds having, 74, 83-84
    of *Prototheca wickerhamii*, 57
    of *Rhinosporidium seeberi*, 59

Sporangiola, moulds having, 74

Sporangiophores, 163
    of *Absidia corymbifera*, 169
    of *Apophysomyces elegans*, 170
    of *Cunninghamella bertholletiae*, 174
    defined, 386
    of *Rhinosporidium seeberi*, 59
    of *Rhizopus* spp., 166
    of *Saksenaea vasiformis*, 172
    of *Syncephalastrum racemosum*, 175

Spore, 386

Sporobolomyces salmonicolor, 131t, **133**, *361*

Sporobolomyces spp., 70

Sporothrix schenckii, *362*
    characteristics and morphology, **45**, 71, **148-149**, 182
    differentiating from *Histoplasma capsulatum*, 45, 46

Sporotrichosis, 26, **45**, 148

Sporotrichum pruinosum, **287**, *378*

Sporotrichum spp.
    differentiating from *Chrysosporium* spp., 286t
    morphology, 73, 80, 82, 87, 90

Sporulation
    of *Apophysomyces elegans* and *Saksenaea vasiformis*, induction, 310
    rapid sporulation medium (RSM), 343

Sputum specimens, collection and preparation, 297

Stachybotrys alternans, **214**

Stachybotrys atra, **214**

Stachybotrys chartarum, **214**

Stachybotrys spp., 73, 94

Staib agar, 332

Stains, 21-22, 298-300, 315-323; *see also under individual stains*

Starch hydrolysis agar, 345-346

Stemphylium sp., 83, 95, **223**

Sterigmata, 386

Stock fungal cultures, maintenance, 311-312

Stolon, 386

Stool specimens, collection and preparation, 297

Stratum corneum, 15

Streptomyces albus, 103t

Streptomyces anulatus, 106

Streptomyces griseus, 103t, 106

Streptomyces lavendulae, 103t

Streptomyces rimosus, 103t

Streptomyces somaliensis, 106

Streptomyces spp., *358*, *359*
    characteristics and morphology, 68, 72, 85, 89, **106**, 108
    differentiating from other actinomycetes, 103t
    direct microscopic examination of specimen, 32, *358*, *359*
    mycetoma, 32-33

"String of beads," 43

Subcutaneous, 386

Subcutaneous phaeohyphomycosis, 189

Subcutaneous tissue specimens, collection and preparation, 297

Subcutaneous zygomycosis, 35, 176

Sulfur granules, 24, 31

Suppurative inflammation, 15, 18, *352*, 386

Surface color
    beige, 76-81
    black, 92, 93-96
    brown, 82-85
    cream, 72-81
    dark gray, 92, 93-96
    green, 91
    greenish, 93-96
    light gray, 72-81
    orange, 86-88
    pink, 89-90
    tan, 82-85
    violet, 89-90
    white, 72-81
    yellow, 86-88

Sympodial growth, 216, 386

Syncephalastrum racemosum, **175**, *364*

Syncephalastrum spp., 92

T

Tan surface, moulds having, 82-85

Tease mount, 303

Terminal, 386

Thallus, 386

Truncate, 386

Trypanosoma cruzi, differentiating from *Histoplasma capsulatum*, 46

Tuberculate, 386

Tuberculoid granuloma, 18

Tween 80 agar, 104, 335

Tyrosine agar, 347

U

Ulocladium sp., 84, 95, **222**

Uniseriate, 387

Urea agar, 348

Urine specimens, collection and preparation, 297-298

U.S. Department of Transportation, packaging and shipping of fungi, 3-5

Ustilago sp., 70, 85, **138**

V

V-8 medium, 134, 327-328

Verticillium spp., 72, 82, 88, 90, 91, **278**, *377*

Vesicle, 387

Violet surface, moulds having, 89-90

W

Wangiella dermatitidis, 366, 367

characteristics and morphology, 93, 200t, **202**

differentiating from *Aureobasidium pullulans*, 207

phaeohyphomycosis, 43

Wangiella spp., media for, 347

Water agar, 348

Water culture technique, 312

White grain mycetoma, 279

White piedra, 140, 206

White surface, moulds having, 72-81

Whorl, 387

Wickerham broth method, 328-329

Wright's stain, 300

X

Xanthine agar, 347

Xanthine hydrolysis test, 347, *378*

Xylohypha bantiana, 7, **195**

Y

Yeast extract-phosphate agar with ammonia, 348-349

Yeastlike colony, 387

Yeasts and yeastlike organisms, **111-143**

characteristics, 114t, 116t-118t, 130t, 131t, 141t

fermentation broth for, 336-337

identification, techniques for, 305-306

media for, 301t, 328-331, 336-337, 348

mixed with bacteria, isolation, 307

morphology, 69-70

Yellow reverse, moulds having, 76-77

Yellow surface, moulds having, 86-88

Z

Zygomycetes, 163-177

as cycloheximide-sensitive fungus, 339

differentiating from hyphomycetes, 10, 35

differentiating from other zygomycetes, 165t

medium for, 339

stains for, 21-22, 22t, 35

tissue response to infection, 19, 35, *355*

Zygomycosis, 24, **35**, 163, 165t, 166-172

Zygospores, 173